The Treatment of Glomerulonephritis

DEVELOPMENTS IN NEPHROLOGY

Volume 40

The titles published in this series are listed at the end of this volume.

The Treatment of Glomerulonephritis

Edited by

C.D. Pusey

Imperial College School of Medicine,
Hammersmith Hospital, London, UK

KLUWER ACADEMIC PUBLISHERS
DORDRECHT / BOSTON / LONDON

Library of Congress Cataloging-in-Publication Data is available.

ISBN 0-7923-5332-3

Published by Kluwer Academic Publishers BV,
PO Box 17, 3300 AA Dordrecht, The Netherlands.

Sold and distributed in North, Central and South America
by Kluwer Academic Publishers, PO Box 358,
Accord Station, Hingham, MA 02018-0358, USA

In all other countries, sold and distributed
by Kluwer Academic Publishers, Distribution Center,
PO Box 322, 3300 AH Dordrecht, The Netherlands

Printed on acid-free paper

Printed and bound in Great Britain by MPG Books Limited, Bodmin, Cornwall

Contents

List of contributors

Shinichi Abe
Department of Internal Medicine, Keio University School of Medicine, Tokyo, Japan

Dwomoa Adu
Department of Nephrology, Queen Elizabeth Hospital, Birmingham, UK

Victoria Cattell
Department of Histopathology, Imperial College School of Medicine, St. Mary's Hospital, London, UK

Terry Cook
Department of Histopathology, Imperial College School of Medicine, Hammersmith Hospital, London, UK

Mark Denton
Laboratory of Transplantation and Immunogenetics, Brigham and Women's Hospital, Harvard Medical School, Boston, MA, USA

John Feehally
Department of Nephrology, Leicester General Hospital, Leicester, UK

Gill Gaskin
Renal Section, Division of Medicine, Imperial College School of Medicine, Hammersmith Hospital, London, UK

Marshall Lindheimer
Departments of Medicine and Obstetrics and Gynecology, University of Chicago Pritzker School of Medicine, Chicago, IL, USA

Peter Mathieson
Academic Renal Unit, University of Bristol, Southmead Hospital, Bristol, UK

Alain Meyrier
Service de Néphrologie et INSERM U 430, Hôpital Broussais, Paris, France

David Oliveira
Division of Renal Medicine, St George's Hospital Medical School, London, UK

Charles Pusey
Renal Section, Division of Medicine, Imperial College School of Medicine, Hammersmith Hospital, London, UK

Mohammed Sayegh
Laboratory of Transplantation and Immunogenetics, Brigham and Women's Hospital, Harvard Medical School, Boston, MA, USA

Colin Short
Department of Renal Medicine, Manchester Royal Infirmary, Manchester, UK

Wai Tse
Department of Nephrology, Queen Elizabeth Hospital, Birmingham, UK

Preface

Glomerulonephritis is one of the commonest causes of end-stage renal failure worldwide. Despite increasing knowledge of the underlying disease mechanisms, advances in treatment have been slow. However, in recent years it has become apparent that the prognosis in various forms of glomerulonephritis can be improved by appropriate immunosuppressive therapy. This book sets out to review current treatment options in the major types of glomerulonephritis. The focus is on specific treatment aimed at modulating the disease process, rather than on general aspects of management which are covered in the larger textbooks on renal disease. The introductory chapters review immune mechanisms and pathology in glomerulonephritis, since the understanding of these is necessary for consideration of treatment. The majority of chapters focus on specific histologically or immunologically defined types of glomerulonephritis. Brief consideration is given to pathogenesis where appropriate, but the main intention is to provide a balanced view of current approaches to treatment, including analysis of controlled clinical trials. All of the major types of glomerulonephritis are covered, as well as the more significant secondary causes such as systemic vasculitis and systemic lupus erythematosus. Finally, there are chapters on selected aspects of management, including recurrent glomerulonephritis following renal transplantation and glomerulonephritis in pregnancy. Although some of this information is also available in the larger textbooks, the aim of this volume is to provide a concise and accessible guide to treatment. This should be of interest to nephrologists and general physicians, including those in training, and to all concerned in the management of patients with glomerular disease. I hope that the contributions in this book will encourage an active and informed approach to the treatment of this important condition.

Charles Pusey
London
December 1998

C.D. Pusey (ed.), The Treatment of Glomerulonephritis, ix.

1. Immune mechanisms in glomerulonephritis

D.B.G. OLIVEIRA

Introduction

The immune mechanisms involved in glomerulonephritis can be considered at a number of different levels. First, there are mechanisms which involve specific recognition, that is binding of particular antigens or fragments of antigens by the recognition molecules of B cells (antibodies) or T cells (the T cell receptor). Second, there are a variety of non-specific mediator systems, often recruited by these specific elements, which are involved in the mediation of tissue damage. These include both cellular (e.g. neutrophils, monocytes) and non-cellular (e.g. complement) systems. Finally, a variety of mechanisms such as chemoattractant cytokines (chemokines) and adhesion molecules on endothelium are involved in recruiting cellular members of both the specific and non-specific systems into the site of inflammation in the glomerulus. As exemplified by this last level there is considerable overlap between these divisions. Thus deposition of immune complexes, although clearly involving specific antibody/antigen systems, can in some circumstances be non-specific in the sense that the resulting damage does not depend on the particular specificity of the antibody. Similarly, the damage caused by cytotoxic T cells is presumably mediated at the molecular level by non-specific molecules such as perforin, but this is so closely bound up with specific recognition that it is of little help to attempt to separate the two. However, these distinctions do have some force, both conceptually and with respect to the degree of therapeutic specificity which could ultimately be achieved by the blockade of the various mechanisms. The rest of this chapter will consider examples from both animal models and, where possible, human disease which will help illustrate these mechanisms.

Specific mechanisms

Historically, the involvement of the immune system in glomerulonephritis was first shown by the demonstration of deposits of antibody within the glomeruli. This influenced early ideas to such an extent that it was thought that all glomerulonephritis could be explained by antibody-mediated mechanisms, either a direct reaction with intrinsic glomerular antigens (as exemplified by anti-glomerular basement membrane (GBM) disease) or by the deposition of

C.D. Pusey (ed.), The Treatment of Glomerulonephritis, 1–13.

circulating immune complexes [1]. More recently, there has been a rapid development in our knowledge of the role of T cells in both experimental and human forms of glomerulonephritis. Indeed, it seems likely that T cells will prove to be the most important mediators of glomerulonephritis, either directly or indirectly via help for antibody production.

B cells

Formation of antibodies

Antibodies involved in the pathogenesis of glomerular disease may arise as a result of a number of processes. They may arise as a product (a paraprotein) of a monoclonal proliferation of B cells at varying stages of differentiation, or as a result of polyclonal B cell activation. Both of these processes may to a greater or lesser extent be T cell-independent, in contrast to a third mechanism, that of antigen-driven specific B cell proliferation, which is usually dependent upon help from T cells.

The deposition of paraproteins or fragments of such proteins is of course an important cause of glomerular disease but, as it does not usually involve inflammation, is outside the scope of this volume. A major exception is the mesangiocapillary glomerulonephritis seen typically in association with type II mixed essential cryoglobulinaemia [2]. In this particular condition, the monoclonal component, usually IgM, has rheumatoid factor activity and captures a polyclonal population of IgG antibodies. Deposition in the kidney produces an immune complex-mediated glomerulonephritis (considered further below in general terms). An interesting development in this condition over the past few years has been the realization that it is associated in many cases with underlying hepatitis C virus infection [3]. Though the details are obscure, the persistent virus infection, presumably via chronic immune stimulation, eventually triggers the formation of the monoclonal IgM rheumatoid factor.

Polyclonal activation has been well documented, both in animal models of lupus [4] and also in humans with lupus and primary Sjögren's syndrome [5]. Some animal models of membranous nephropathy are produced by the polyclonal activation of B cells with chemicals such as mercuric chloride [6] and gold salts [7]. The same agents may induce membranous nephropathy in humans and there has been speculation that a similar mechanism of polyclonal activation could underlie the pathogenesis here [8].

In contrast to polyclonal activation, antigen-driven responses are obviously of much more restricted specificity. In addition, they usually have the characteristics of a T cell-driven response in being of IgG class and high affinity. Molecular analysis of the genes encoding these antibodies shows that they have been subjected to somatic mutation (a T cell-dependent process), which alters the original germline-encoded antibody towards higher-affinity species. The formation of such antibodies may be to external antigens which become planted in the glomerulus, as seen for example in post-streptococcal glomerulonephritis. The formation of antibodies under these circumstances is easy to understand as it is part of the normal defence mechanisms to invading pathogens. More difficult to explain is the formation of antibodies to autoantigens, as this implies a breakdown in the normal mechanisms of tolerance which are still not well understood. Examples of human autoantibodies which are involved in glomerular disease, and which are not polyclonal but presumably antigen-driven, include anti-GBM antibodies [9] and at least some anti-DNA antibodies [10].

Mediation of damage

As mentioned above, the two traditional major mechanisms of antibody-mediated damage in the kidney are reactions with insoluble or tissue-fixed antigens on the one hand and reactions with soluble antigens with resulting immune complex deposition on the other [1]. The tissue-fixed antigens may either be intrinsic components of the kidney or extrinsic planted antigens. However, the distinction between these main mechanisms is not always clear-cut. Thus, many of the animal models which were originally thought to be due to the deposition of circulating immune complexes may in fact be due to an interaction with fixed antigens which are either intrinsic (Heymann nephritis, see below) or planted (e.g. cationic bovine serum albumin [11], DNA [12]). In addition, immune complexes in the kidney, even if formed *in situ*, are still exposed to circulating antigen and antibody. This may lead to further accumulation of material on the initial deposits [13] or, under suitable conditions, dissolution of the deposits [14]. Clearly the deposition of antigen/antibody in the kidney is a fluid process, with considerable scope for flexibility in the order in which components are laid down and potential for dynamic modification of components once formed.

Following reaction with either intrinsic or planted glomerular antigens, as seen in anti-GBM disease or post-streptococcal glomerulonephritis respectively, the antibodies fix complement and attract an inflammatory cell infiltrate. The importance of the cellular element, both specific (T cells) and non-specific (macrophages), is shown by experiments in which depletion of one or other of the cell populations markedly ameliorates glomerular injury without affecting antibody deposition [15]. By contrast, cellular elements appear to be less important in human membranous nephropathy and the relevant animal model, Heymann nephritis [16]. The pathogenesis of the latter model is well understood and involves reaction of an antibody with antigens on the glomerular epithelial cell. The resulting immune complexes are shed and aggregate on the epithelial surface of the glomerular basement membrane. They are, therefore, presumably inaccessible to cellular elements on the other side of the basement membrane. However, complement deposition certainly occurs and the subsequent formation of the membrane attack complex is involved in the pathogenesis of the proteinuria [17]. It is generally assumed that human membranous nephropathy has a similar pathogenesis, although the relevant intrinsic autoantigens have resisted identification.

Although the site of the reaction of antibodies with fixed glomerular antigens is clearly predetermined, the site of deposition of circulating immune complexes is both more variable and, as outlined above, dynamic. The important factors that determine the localization of circulating immune complexes seem to be charge, size of complex, and affinity of antibody involved; the latter two are probably closely related. The anionic charge of the glomerular basement membrane will favour the subepithelial and subendothelial localization of cationic complexes [18]. Smaller complexes, as formed with lower-affinity IgG antibodies, preferentially localize to the subepithelial area, whereas larger insoluble complexes formed from IgM or high-affinity IgG deposit in subendothelial and mesangial areas [19–21]. The load of immune complexes is also important; the initial site of mesangial deposition in chronic serum sickness is followed by glomerular capillary deposition if the quantity of the immune complexes increases [22]. Once deposited, immune complexes can recruit the same effector mechanisms as outlined previously.

Whether deposited in the kidney as a result of binding to fixed antigens or as a result of immune complex deposition, the subsequent mediation of damage by the deposited antibody is relatively easy to understand. All forms of aggregated antibody can activate the complement system, at least by the alternative pathway. Cells with receptors for the Fc portion of antibodies, such as neutrophils and monocytes, may also be recruited. These non-specific mediator systems are considered further below. In contrast, the mechanisms by which an important class of antibodies seen in association with renal disease, namely antineutrophil cytoplasm antibodies (ANCA), mediate disease, if indeed they are involved in pathogenesis, is much less clear. Perhaps the most powerful piece of evidence in favour of a role for ANCA in pathogenesis is a number of experiments showing that ANCA are able to activate neutrophils *in vitro* [23, 24], and that such activated neutrophils are able to damage endothelium [25, 26]. *In-vivo* activation of neutrophils could explain the exacerbating effect that ANCA have been shown to have on an animal model of anti-GBM disease [27]. Other possible pathogenic mechanisms include direct binding of ANCA to endothelial cells expressing the relevant autoantigen (although whether such expression actually occurs is controversial [28]), and stabilization of the proteases that are the targets of ANCA, with resulting prolonged proteolytic damage. There are, however, many unresolved issues. In contrast to the animal model mentioned above, human ANCA-associated glomerulonephritis is not associated with the consistent deposition of antibodies. Furthermore, there are many patients who have high titres of ANCA but are otherwise well. Even if ANCA are necessary for pathogenesis they are clearly not sufficient.

T cells

There is ample direct evidence for the involvement of T cells in a wide range of animal models of glomerulonephritis (reviewed in reference 29). In human disease the evidence is necessarily more indirect, but still persuasive. As mentioned in the previous section on B cells, several of the autoantibodies associated with human glomerulonephritis have the characteristics of a T cell-dependent response. Further indirect evidence is provided by the association between particular alleles of the major histocompatibility complex (MHC) and disease. This is perhaps best shown by the association between anti-GBM disease and DR2 [30]. Because it is T cells rather than B cells that recognize antigens in the context of products of the MHC, such associations clearly imply a role for T cells. It is important to note that absence of detectable MHC associations does not exclude the involvement of T cells. Thus, for example, ANCA-positive vasculitis is probably not positively associated with any particular MHC allele [31, 32], but the antibodies clearly have the characteristics of a T cell-dependent response.

Slightly more direct evidence is provided by the histological observation that T cells are actually present in the glomerulus in a variety of glomerulonephritides [33, 34]. The main problem in interpreting this observation is in determining whether such cells are playing a causal role in the inflammatory process or have simply been recruited in a relatively non-specific manner. Similarly the expansion in particular populations of T cells seen in the peripheral blood in some patients with vasculitis [35] is difficult to interpret.

Of potentially greater pathogenic significance would be the detection of specific T cell responses. These have been found in the peripheral blood in at least two circumstances: anti-GBM disease, with specificity for the α3 chain of type IV collagen [36], and ANCA-associated vasculitis, with specificity for neutrophil proteases [37]. Whether these relatively weak specific proliferative responses are a true reflection of a T cell-mediated attack in the glomerulus, or are simply a relatively non-specific response to autoantigens released as a result of glomerular damage or neutrophil turnover, is unclear [38].

Potentially the most direct piece of evidence for T cell involvement in humans would be amelioration of glomerulonephritis by therapy directed specifically at T cells. There have been anecdotal reports of intractable systemic vasculitis responding to treatment with a variety of monoclonal antibodies which have specificity for T cells [39]. There is likely to be further progress in this area with the development of strategies to target ever more restricted parts of the T cell repertoire. The ultimate development of such a strategy would be to tolerize just the putative autoreactive T cells and leave the rest of the T cell repertoire untouched. If such a strategy were to be successful it would also provide the best evidence in humans for T cell involvement in glomerulonephritis.

Mediation of damage

There are a number of mechanisms whereby T cells can potentially mediate glomerular damage. Indirectly they can do this by help for the production of pathogenic antibodies, such as anti-GBM antibodies. More directly, T cells can themselves be directly cytotoxic via mechanisms such as perforin release [40] and induction of apoptosis in the target cell via Fas/Fas ligand interactions [41]. Finally, T cells can release a variety of cytokines and chemokines which have the potential to recruit and activate non-specific mediators such as macrophages [15].

Non-specific mechanisms

Neutrophils

The importance of polymorphonuclear leukocytes (PMN) is suggested by their presence in several forms of glomerulonephritis in humans. A number of factors are involved in the recruitment of PMN into the glomerulus. These include chemotactic peptides produced as a result of activation of the complement system; the importance of this is demonstrated by the prevention of PMN accumulation in complement-depleted animals during the heterologous phase of nephrotoxic nephritis [42]. Other factors are also important, as shown by the fact that complement depletion does not affect PMN accumulation in the autologous phase of the same model [43]. These other factors will include neutrophil-specific chemokines, the relevant adhesion molecules involved in passage of cells from the circulation into the glomerulus (see below), and adherence via Fc receptors to immunoglobulin deposited in the glomerulus. Once within the glomerulus, PMN may mediate damage by the release of a variety of destructive enzymes [44] and will also be involved in the production, via the action of myeloperoxidase, of reactive oxygen species (see below). The importance of PMN in at least one experimental model is shown by the fact that beige mice, which have a congenital defect in PMN, are protected from the effects of nephrotoxic antiserum [45]. Following mediation of damage, neutrophils may be cleared from the glomerulus by a variety of mechanisms. These include direct emigration and also, at least in some experimental systems, apoptosis [46]. This last mechanism is of particular importance as it involves non-inflammatory disposal of the cell.

Macrophages

Macrophages may also be recruited into the inflamed glomerulus by a variety of mechanisms, including chemokines and Fc receptor-mediated mechanisms. They may also be recruited by both CD4+ and CD8+ T cells and, in at least one model of anti-GBM glomerulonephritis, the subsequent injury is mediated by such macrophages rather than by the T cells themselves [15]. As well as their contribution to endocapillary proliferation, macrophages also make a major contribution to crescent formation, particularly when this is associated with breaches in the glomerular basement membrane [47]. Macrophages have a variety of mediator systems that they can deploy to cause damage, including the production of procoagulant activity [48], the secretion of many potentially damaging enzymes [49] and the generation of reactive oxygen species [50]. They also produce a variety of cytokines which may play an important role in mediating renal injury [51]. A further theoretical property is that, in contrast to PMN, macrophages express class II MHC molecules. They therefore have the potential to act as antigen-presenting cells for T cells and, by virtue of this, could perpetuate autoimmune injury within the glomerulus.

Complement

The complement system plays a role in mediating damage in many forms of glomerulonephritis in which there is deposition of antibodies. Some antibodies (e.g. IgM and some subclasses of IgG) may activate complement via the classical pathway. Others (aggregated IgA or IgG4), although normally poor activators of the classical pathway, may activate the alternative pathway. In either event, chemotactic peptides will be produced, attracting inflammatory cells into the glomerulus, and ultimately the membrane attack complex, which appears to be involved in the genesis of proteinuria in both animal [17] and possibly human [52] membranous nephropathy, will be formed. In addition to this direct role, the complement system may also play a more indirect part in the pathogenesis of two forms of glomerulonephritis: lupus nephropathy and type II mesangiocapillary glomerulonephritis.

Lupus nephropathy

There is an extraordinarily high incidence of lupus-like immune complex diseases in patients with hereditary deficiencies of certain complement components [53]. This, together with the fact that an important role of the complement system in normal physiology is the solubilization and safe disposal of immune complexes, has led to the formulation of a general theory of the role of complement deficiency in the pathogenesis of lupus [54]. In normal individuals the bulk of immune complexes solubilized by the complement system are probably carried via the CR1 receptor (with specificity for C3b attached to the immune complex) on red blood cells to the liver for proteolytic disposal. In the presence of deficiencies of the complement system, either congenital or acquired, complexes are not cleared efficiently by this route, and can deposit in target organs such as the kidney. Here they start an inflammatory response which, by the release of cytokines and autoantigens may drive the production of autoantibodies. This leads to the formation of further immune complexes and the perpetuation of the cycle.

Type II mesangiocapillary glomerulonephritis

There is a strong association between type II mesangiocapillary glomerulonephritis and the presence of the autoantibody C3 nephritic factor, which binds to and stabilizes the alternative pathway C3 convertase [55], producing continuous complement activation. This autoantibody is also found in association with partial lipodystrophy, and in some individuals C3 nephritic factor, glomerulonephritis and lipodystrophy may all be present [56]. Other less well-defined autoantibodies which produce different patterns of complement activation may be associated with other forms of mesangiocapillary glomerulonephritis [57]. There has been some progress in understanding how activation of the complement system by C3 nephritic factor may be associated with partial lipodystrophy. It has become clear that the adipocyte is actually a synthetic source of a number of complement components, notably factor D [58], the key serine protease involved in the alternative pathway. This suggests that the balance between activation and control of the alternative pathway may be particularly delicate in the vicinity of the fat cell, and that the stabilizing influence of C3 nephritic factor may upset this balance. There is experimental evidence to support this, with damage of fat cells occurring in the presence of C3 nephritic factor as compared to control sera [59]. On the other hand the connection, if any, between C3 nephritic factor and type II mesangiocapillary glomerulonephritis remains obscure. Attempts to reproduce this pattern of glomerular injury by prolonged complement activation in animal models have not been successful [60, 61]. There are, however, technical problems in the interpretation of these experiments, not least the fact that there are important species differences in complement receptors and, uniquely, humans possess CR1 receptors on visceral epithelial cells in the glomerulus [62].

Chemokines

The chemokines are a group of chemoattractant cytokines which can be classified into a number of families depending upon the arrangements of cysteine residues in their structure [63]. Chemokines may be produced by a variety of cell types, including intrinsic renal cells [64]. The different species of chemokine have different cellular targets, with some, such as monocyte chemoattractant protein-1 (MCP-1), promoting the accumulation of monocytes/macrophages, whereas others attract neutrophils, T cells, or eosinophils. It would seem plausible that, whatever the initial cause of glomerular injury, the subsequent coordinated expression of chemokines by either intrinsic or extrinsic cells could play an important part in mediating the sequential changes in cellular infiltration seen in both experimental and human glomerulonephritis. There is indeed an accumulating body of evidence to support such a role for chemokines [65]. Increased expression of MCP-1 has been demonstrated both in animal models [66] and in human glomerulonephritis [67]. Direct evidence for a role in the pathogenesis of a mouse model of crescentic nephritis has been provided by blocking the function of either MCP-1 or another chemokine, RANTES, with antibodies, and demonstrating a significant decrease in both numbers of infiltrating leukocytes and proteinuria [68].

The frequent discovery of new chemokines, together with the obvious therapeutic potential of chemokine blockade, suggests that there should be further interesting developments in this field in the future.

Adhesion molecules

In order for cellular elements of either the specific (e.g. T cells) or non-specific (e.g. neutrophils, macrophages) immune systems to travel from within the circulation into the extravascular component of the glomerulus, a variety of steps are necessary. These various steps are mediated by a variety of adhesion molecules [69]. The initial rolling contact between cell and endothelium is mediated by molecules from the selectin family. The subsequent firm attachment is mediated by members of the β2 integrin family, such as intercellular adhesion molecule-1 (ICAM-1). Finally, diapedesis between endothelial cells, driven by a variety of chemotactic factors, is mediated largely by platelet–endothelial cell adhesion molecule (PECAM) [70]. Because these interactions occur at a very early stage, before the cells have a chance to carry out any of their effector functions, they represent attractive potential therapeutic targets. There are complications, in that there is considerable redundancy in the system. However, combinations of blocking antibodies to a number of these adhesion molecules and their counter-receptors have been shown to ameliorate experimental crescentic glomerulonephritis [71] and other animal models of inflammation [72].

Other non-specific mediator systems

A number of other effector systems may be involved in the mediation of immunological damage. These include the coagulation system, which is probably most efficiently activated by macrophages [48], although activated neutrophils via the production of reactive oxygen species may also be capable of initiating glomerular thrombosis [73]. The importance of the coagulation system is demonstrated by the amelioration of a number of forms of experimental glomerulonephritis by defibrination [74] or treatment with recombinant tissue plasminogen activator [75]. There is also anecdotal evidence for the effectiveness of a similar strategy in human lupus nephritis [76].

A number of products of arachidonic acid metabolism (prostaglandins, thromboxanes, leukotrienes) are important inflammatory and vasoactive mediators. Interference with such mediators may be one of the mechanisms whereby fish oil is able to ameliorate IgA nephropathy [77]. There has been considerable interest recently in the role of reactive oxygen species in the mediation of both glomerulonephritis and inflammation in general. Reactive oxygen species may be produced by a variety of cell types, but notably by PMN and macrophages, often triggered by immune complexes [78]. Myeloperoxidase, a product of PMN, is able to produce oxidant injury in the presence of hydrogen peroxide and halide ions [79]. This property has been used to create an animal model which has some similarities with human antimyeloperoxidase-associated autoimmune crescentic nephritis [80].

References

1. Wilson CB, Dixon FJ. The renal response to immunological injury. In: Brenner BM, Rector FC, editors. The Kidney, 3rd edn. Philadelphia, PA: W.B. Saunders; 1986:800–89.
2. D'Amico G, Colasanti G, Ferrario F, Sinico RA. Renal involvement in essential mixed cryoglobulinemia. Kidney Int 1989;35:1004–14.
3. Agnello V, Chung RT, Kaplan LM. A role for hepatitis C virus infection in type II cryoglobulinaemia. N Engl J Med 1992;327:1490–5.
4. Klinman DM. Polyclonal B cell activation in lupus-prone mice precedes and predicts the development of autoimmune disease. J Clin Invest 1990;86:1249–54.
5. Fauci AS, Moutsopoulos HM. Polyclonally triggered B cells in the peripheral blood and bone marrow of normal individuals and in patients with systemic lupus erythematosus and primary Sjögren's syndrome. Arthritis Rheum 1981;24:577–84.
6. Aten J, Veninga A, Bruijn JA, Prins FA, de Heer E, Weening JJ. Antigenic specificities of glomerular-bound autoantibodies in membranous glomerulopathy induced by mercuric chloride. Clin Immunol Immunopathol 1992;63:89–102.
7. Tournade H, Guery J, Pasquier R *et al.* Experimental gold-induced autoimmunity. Nephrol Dial Transplant 1991;6:621–30.
8. Oliveira DBG. Membranous nephropathy: an IgG4 mediated disease. Lancet 1997;351:670–1.
9. Pusey CD, Dash A, Kershaw MJ *et al.* A single autoantigen in Goodpasture's syndrome identified by a monoclonal antibody to human glomerular basement membrane. Lab Invest 1987;56:23–31.
10. Diamond B, Katz JB, Paul E, Aranow C, Lustgarten D, Scharff MD. The role of somatic mutation in the pathogenic anti-DNA response. Annu Rev Immunol 1992;10:731–57.
11. Border WA, Ward HJ, Kamis ES, Cohen AH. Induction of membranous nephropathy in rabbits by administration of an exogenous cationic antigen. Demonstration of a pathogenic role for electrical charge. J Clin Invest 1982;69:451–61.
12. Izui S, Lambert P, Miescher PA. *In-vitro* demonstration of a particular affinity of glomerular basement membrane and collagen for DNA. A possible basis for a local formation of DNA–anti-DNA complexes in systemic lupus erythematosus. J Exp Med 1976;144:428–43.
13. Ford PM, Kosatka I. A mechanism of enhancement of immune complex deposition following in situ immune complex formation in the mouse glomerulus. Immunology 1981;43:433–9.
14. Mannik M, Striker GE. Removal of glomerular deposits of immune complexes in mice by administration of excess antigen. Lab Invest 1980;42:483–9.
15. Huang XR, Tipping PG, Apostolopoulos J, Oettinger C, D'Souza M, Milton G. Mechanisms of T cell-induced glomerular injury in anti-glomerular basement membrane (GBM) glomerulonephritis in rats. Clin Exp Immunol 1997;109:134–42.
16. Farquhar MG, Saito A, Kerjaschki D, Orlando RA. The Heymann nephritis antigenic complex: Megalin (gp330) and RAP. J Am Soc Nephrol 1995;6:35–47.
17. de Heer E, Daha MR, Bhakdi S, Bazin H, Van Es LA. Possible involvement of terminal complement complex in active Heymann nephritis. Kidney Int 1985;27:388–93.
18. Gallo GR, Caulin-Glaser T, Lamm ME. Charge of circulating immune complexes as a factor in glomerular basement membrane localization in mice. J Clin Invest 1981;67:1305–13.
19. Cameron JS, Clark WF. A role for insoluble antibody–antigen complexes in glomerulonephritis? Clin Nephrol 1982;18:55–61.

20. Iskander SS, Jennette JC. Influence of antibody avidity on glomerular immune complex localization. Am J Pathol 1983;112:155–9.
21. Lew AM, Staines NA, Steward MW. Glomerulonephritis induced by pre-formed immune complexes containing monoclonal antibodies of defined affinity and isotype. Clin Exp Immunol 1984;57:413–22.
22. Wilson CB, Dixon FJ. Quantitation of acute and chronic serum sickness in the rabbit. J Exp Med 1971;134:7–18s.
23. Falk RJ, Terrell RS, Charles LA, Jennette JC. Anti-neutrophil cytoplasmic autoantibodies induce neutrophils to degranulate and produce oxygen radicals *in vitro*. Proc Natl Acad Sci USA 1990;87:4115–19.
24. Porges AJ, Redecha PB, Kimberley WT, Csernok E, Gross WL, Kimberley RP. Anti-neutrophil cytoplasmic antibodies engage and activate human neutrophils via Fc gamma R11a. J Immunol 1994;153:1271–80.
25. Ewert BH, Jennette JC, Falk RJ. Anti-myeloperoxidase antibodies stimulate neutrophils to damage human endothelial cells. Kidney Int 1992;41:375–83.
26. Savage COS, Pottinger BE, Gaskin G, Pusey CD, Pearson JD. Autoantibodies developing to myeloperoxidase and proteinase 3 in systemic vasculitis stimulate neutrophil cytotoxicity towards cultured endothelial cells. Am J Pathol 1992;141:335–42.
27. Heeringa P, Brouwer E, Klok PA *et al.* Autoantibodies to myeloperoxidase aggravate mild anti-glomerular-basement-membrane-mediated glomerular injury in the rat. Am J Pathol 1996;149: 1695–706.
28. King WJ, Adu D, Daha MR *et al.* Endothelial cells and renal epithelial cells do not express the Wegener's autoantigen, proteinase 3. Clin Exp Immunol 1995;102:98–105.
29. Tam FWK, Pusey CD. The role of T lymphocytes in extracapillary glomerulonephritis. J Nephrol 1995;8:305–16.
30. Rees AJ, Peters DK, Compston DAS, Batchelor JR. Strong association between HLA DRw2 and antibody mediated Goodpasture's syndrome. Lancet 1978;i:966–8.
31. Zhang L, Jayne DRW, Zhao MH, Lockwood CM, Oliveira DBG. Distribution of MHC class II alleles in primary systemic vasculitis. Kidney Int 1995;47:294–8.
32. Hagen EC, Stegeman CA, D'Amaro J *et al.* Decreased frequency of HLA-DR13DR6 in Wegener's granulomatosis. Kidney Int 1995;48:801–5.
33. Nolasco FEB, Cameron JS, Hartley B, Coelho A, Hildreth G, Reuben R. Intraglomerular T cells and monocytes in nephritis: study with monoclonal antibodies. Kidney Int 1987;31:1160–6.
34. Neale TJ, Tipping PG, Carson SD, Holdsworth SR. Participation of cell-mediated immunity in deposition of fibrin in glomerulonephritis. Lancet 1988;ii:421–4.
35. Simpson IJ, Skinner MA, Geursen A *et al.* Peripheral blood T lymphocytes in systemic vasculitis: increased T cell receptor Vβ2 gene usage in microscopic polyarteritis. Clin Exp Immunol 1995;101:220–6.
36. Derry CJ, Ross CN, Lombardi G *et al.* Analysis of T cell responses to the autoantigen in Goodpasture's disease. Clin Exp Immunol 1995;100:262–8.
37. Griffith ME, Coulthart A, Pusey CD. T cell responses to myeloperoxidase (MPO) and proteinase 3 (PR3) in patients with systemic vasculitis. Clin Exp Immunol 1996;103:253–8.
38. Mathieson PW, Oliveira DBG. The role of cellular immunity in systemic vasculitis. Clin Exp Immunol 1995;100:183–5.
39. Lockwood CM, Thiru S, Isaacs J, Hale G, Waldmann H. Long-term remission of intractable systemic vasculitis with monoclonal antibody therapy. Lancet 1993;341:1620–2.
40. Griffiths GM, Mueller C. Expression of perforin and granzymes *in vivo*: potential diagnostic markers for activated cytotoxic cells. Immunol Today 1991;12:415–19.
41. Nagata S, Suda T. Fas and Fas ligand: lpr and gld mutations. Immunol Today 1995;16:39–43.
42. Cochrane CG, Unanue ER, Dixon FJ. A role of polymorphonuclear leukocytes and complement in nephrotoxic nephritis. J Exp Med 1965;122:99–116.
43. Thomson NM, Naish PF, Simpson IJ, Peters DK. The role of C3 in the autologous phase of nephrotoxic nephritis. Clin Exp Immunol 1976;24:464–73.

44. Janoff A. Neutrophil proteases in inflammation. Annu Rev Med 1972;23:177–90.
45. Schrijver G, Schalkwijk J, Robben JCM, Assman KJM, Koene RAP. Antiglomerular basement membrane nephritis in beige mice. Deficiency of leukocytic neutral proteinases prevents the induction of albuminuria in the heterologous phase. J Exp Med 1989;169:1435–48.
46. Hughes J, Johnson RJ, Mooney A, Hugo C, Gordon K, Savill J. Neutrophil fate in experimental glomerular capillary injury in the rat. Emigration exceeds in situ clearance by apoptosis. Am J Pathol 1997;150:223–34.
47. Boucher A, Droz D, Adafer E, Noel LH. Relationship between the integrity of Bowman's capsule and the composition of cellular crescents in human crescentic glomerulonephritis. Lab Invest 1987;56:526–33.
48. Brentjens JR. Glomerular procoagulant activity and glomerulonephritis. Lab Invest 1987;57: 107–11.
49. Werb Z, Bainton DF, Jones PA. Degradation of connective tissue matrices by macrophages. III. Morphological and biochemical studies on extracellular, pericellular, and intracellular events in matrix proteolysis by macrophages in culture. J Exp Med 1980;152:1537–53.
50. Boyce NW, Tipping PG, Holdsworth SR. Glomerular macrophages produce reactive oxygen species in experimental glomerulonephritis. Kidney Int 1989;35:778–82.
51. Tomosugi NI, Cashman SJ, Hay H *et al.* Modulation of antibody-mediated glomerular injury *in vivo* by bacterial lipopolysaccharide, tumour necrosis factor, and IL-1. J Immunol 1989;142: 3083–90.
52. Coupes BM, Kon SP, Brenchley PEC, Short CD, Mallick NP. The temporal relationship between urinary C5b-9 and C3dg and clinical parameters in human membranous nephropathy. Nephrol Dial Transplant 1993;8:397–401.
53. Rynes RI. Inherited complement deficiency states and SLE. Clin Rheum Dis 1982;8:29–47.
54. Lachmann PJ. Complement – friend or foe? Br J Rheumatol 1987;26:409–15.
55. Daha MR, Fearon DT, Austen KF. C3 nephritic factor (C3Nef): stabilization of fluid phase and cell-bound alternative pathway convertase. J Immunol 1976;116:1–7.
56. Sissons JGP, West RJ, Fallows J *et al.* The complement abnormalities of lipodystrophy. N Engl J Med 1976;294:461–5.
57. Varade WS, Forristal J, West CD. Patterns of complement activation in idiopathic membranoproliferative glomerulonephritis, types I, II, III. Am J Kidney Dis 1990;16:196–206.
58. Rosen BS, Cook KS, Yaglom J *et al.* Adipsin and complement factor D activity: an immune-related defect in obesity. Science 1989;244:1483–7.
59. Mathieson PW, Würzner R, Oliveira DBG, Lachmann PJ, Peters DK. Complement-mediated adipocyte lysis by nephritic factor sera. J Exp Med 1993;177:1827–31.
60. Verroust PJ, Wilson CB, Dixon FJ. Lack of nephritogenicity of systemic activation of the alternative complement pathway. Kidney Int 1974;6:157–69.
61. Simpson IJ, Moran J, Evans DJ, Peters DK. Prolonged complement activation in mice. Kidney Int 1978;13:467–71.
62. Moran JE, Peters DK. Studies on the glomerular C3b receptor. In: Kincaid-Smith P, d'Apice AJF, Atkins RC, editors. Progress in Glomerulonephritis. New York: John Wiley & Sons; 1979:109–17.
63. Adams DH, Lloyd AR. Chemokines: leucocyte recruitment and activation cytokines. Lancet 1997;349:490–5.
64. Wolf G, Aberle S, Thaiss F *et al.* TNF-alpha induces expression of the chemoattractant cytokine RANTES in cultured mouse mesangial cells. Kidney Int 1993;44:795–804.
65. Wu X, Dolecki GJ, Sherry B, Zagorski J, Lefkowith JB. Chemokines are expressed in a myeloid cell-dependent fashion and mediate distinct functions in immune complex glomerulonephritis in rat. J Immunol 1997;158:3917–24.
66. Stahl RAK, Thaiss F, Disser M, Helmchen U, Hora K, Schlondorff D. Increased expression of monocyte chemoattractant protein-1 in anti-thymocyte antibody-induced glomerulonephritis. Kidney Int 1993;44:1036–47.
67. Rovin BH, Rumancik M, Tan L, Dickerson J. Glomerular expression of monocyte chemoattractant protein-1 in experimental and human glomerulonephritis. Lab Invest 1994;71:536–42.

68. Lloyd CM, Minto AW, Dorf ME *et al.* RANTES and monocyte chemoattractant protein-1 (MCP-1) play an important role in the inflammatory phase of crescentic nephritis, but only MCP-1 is involved in crescent formation and interstitial fibrosis. J Exp Med 1997;185:1371–80.
69. Springer TA. Traffic signals for lymphocyte recirculation and leucocyte emigration: the multi-step paradigm. Cell 1994;76:301–14.
70. Liao F, Ali J, Greene T, Muller WA. Soluble domain 1 of platelet-endothelial adhesion molecule (PECAM) is sufficient to block transendothelial migration *in vitro* and *in vivo*. J Exp Med 1997; 185:1349–57.
71. Nishikawa K, Guo Y, Miyasaka M *et al.* Antibodies to intercellular adhesion molecule 1/ lymphocyte function-associated antigen 1 prevent crescent formation in rat autoimmune glomerulonephritis. J Exp Med 1993;177:667–77.
72. Issekutz AC, Issekutz TB. Monocyte migration to arthritis in the rat utilizes both CD11/CD18 and very late activation antigen 4 integrin mechanisms. J Exp Med 1995;181:1197–203.
73. Poelstra K, Hardonk MJ, Koudstaal J, Bakker WW. Intraglomerular platelet aggregation and experimental glomerulonephritis. Kidney Int 1990;37:1500–8.
74. Holdsworth SR, Thomson NM, Glasgow EF, Atkins RC. The effect of defibrination on macrophage participation in rabbit nephrotoxic nephritis. Clin Exp Immunol 1979;37:38–43.
75. Mathieson PW, Thiru S, Peters DK, Oliveira DBG. Effects of Ancrod and rTPA on fibrin accumulation, glomerular inflammation and renal function in nephrotoxic nephritis. Int J Exp Pathol 1991;72:679–93.
76. Hariharan S, Pollak VE, Kant KS, Weiss MA, Wadhwa NK. Diffuse proliferative lupus nephritis: long-term observations in patients treated with ancrod. Clin Nephrol 1990;34:61–9.
77. Cheng IK, Chan PC, Chan MK. The effect of fish-oil dietary supplement on the progression of mesangial IgA glomerulonephritis. Nephrol Dial Transplant 1990;5:241–6.
78. Ward PA, Duque RE, Sulavik MC, Johnson KJ. *In vitro* and *in vivo* stimulation of rat neutrophils and alveolar macrophages by immune complexes. Am J Pathol 1983;110:297–309.
79. Johnson RJ, Guggenheim SJ, Klebanoff SJ *et al.* Morphologic correlates of glomerular oxidant injury induced by the myeloperoxidase-hydrogen peroxide-halide system of the neutrophil. Lab Invest 1988;58:294–301.
80. Brouwer E, Huitema MG, Klok PA *et al.* Antimyeloperoxidase-associated proliferative glomerulonephritis: an animal model. J Exp Med 1993;177:905–14.

2. Pathology of glomerulonephritis

V. CATTELL and H.T. COOK

Introduction

Classification of glomerulonephritis depends on examination of the kidney by light and electron microscopy and immunohistochemical assessment of the glomerular localization of immunoglobulins and complement. In this chapter we discuss the appearances found in glomerular diseases under these three headings.

Primary glomerulonephritis

Minimal change disease

Light microscopy
One of the defining features of the disease is that the glomeruli show no changes by light microscopy. However, a small proportion of cases, which appear to behave clinically in a typical fashion, may have a slight increase in mesangial cells with three or four nuclei in some mesangial areas. Eosinophilic droplets of reabsorbed protein are often seen in tubular epithelial cells and, as with other causes of the nephrotic syndrome, foam cells may be seen in the interstitium.

Immunohistology
Classically, no immunoglobulins or complement components are seen in the glomeruli but in a few cases there may be small amounts of mesangial IgM. Segmental IgM should raise the suspicion of focal and segmental glomerulo-sclerosis.

Electron microscopy
The foot processes of the visceral epithelial cells are extensively obliterated (Figure 2.1), and the cells may have microvilli over their surface away from the basement membrane, increased cellular organelles, and vacuoles or cysts.

C.D. Pusey (ed.), The Treatment of Glomerulonephritis, 15–37.

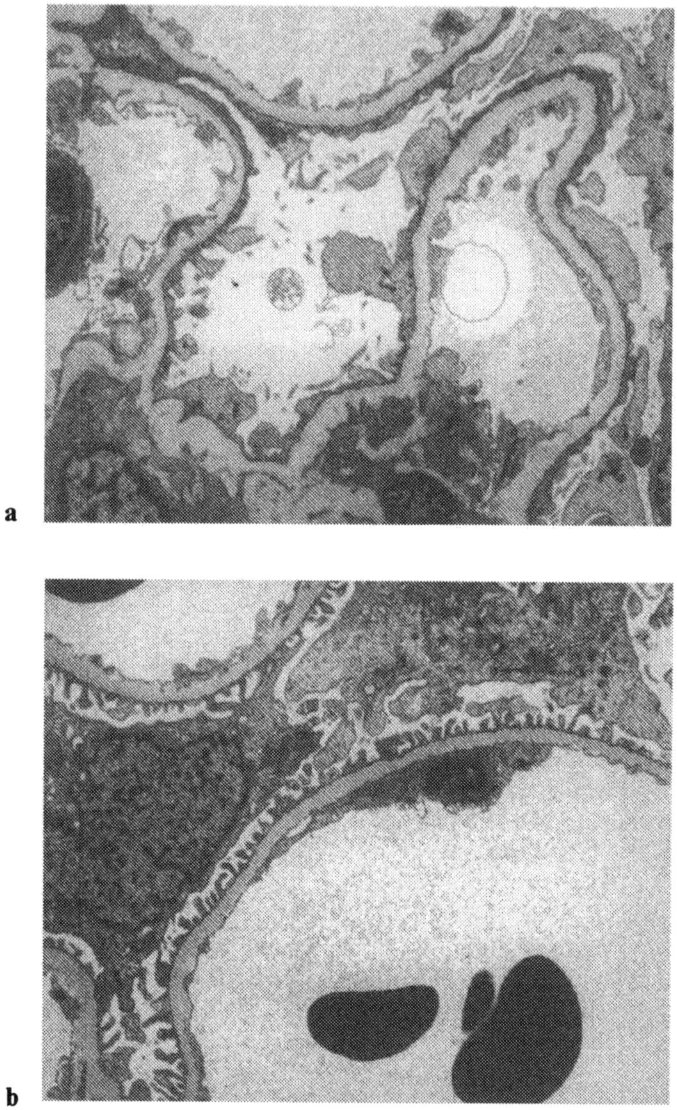

Figure 2.1 Minimal change disease. (**a**) Electron micrograph of minimal change disease showing extensive loss of epithelial cell foot processes (original magnification ×7280). (**b**) Normal glomerulus for comparison (original magnification ×7280)

Focal and segmental glomerulosclerosis (FSGS)

This morphological pattern of glomerular disease may represent a primary glomerular disease associated with the nephrotic syndrome (idiopathic) or may be a secondary glomerular response to a variety of other renal diseases, particularly those in which there is loss of functioning nephrons. Distinguishing these two possibilities is often difficult and sometimes impossible; a full clinical history is essential.

Light microscopy
The characteristic lesion is an area of solidification involving one segment of the glomerular tuft (Figure 2.2). A variable number of glomeruli may show such lesions and early in the course of the disease the lesions are more commonly seen in juxtamedullary glomeruli. The sclerotic lesion shows collapse and wrinkling of the capillary walls and obliteration of the capillary lumens. There may also be an area of adhesion to Bowman's capsule. Adjacent visceral epithelial cells often appear prominent and may contain eosinophilic protein droplets. In some sclerotic areas there is eosinophilic material within capillary loops, known as a hyalinosis lesion. Foam cells are commonly seen in the area of sclerosis. In the classical form of the disease any segment of the glomerulus may be involved although the lesions are slightly more common near the hilum. Uninvolved glomerular segments appear normal or show mild mesangial hypercellularity. Eventually the segmental sclerosis may progress to global obsolescence.

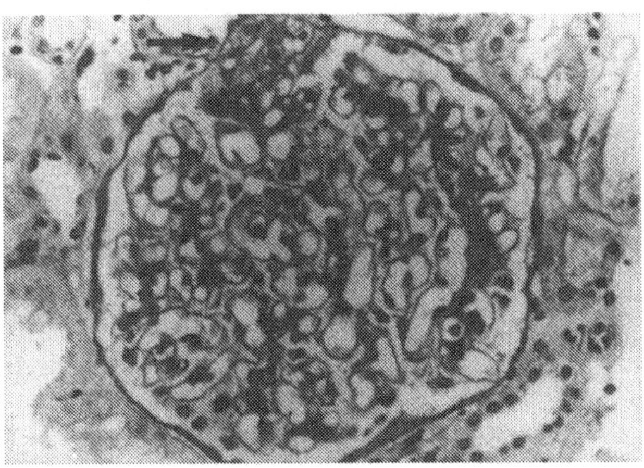

Figure 2.2 Focal and segmental glomerulosclerosis . At the tubular pole of the glomerulus there is an area of adhesion to Bowman's capsule and occlusion of the capillary lumen by cells with foamy cytoplasm (arrow). (Haematoxylin and eosin, original magnification ×250)

There are variations on this typical appearance. In the *cellular variant* the sclerotic area appears hypercellular and may contain nuclear fragments leading to possible confusion with a scarring focal and segmental glomerulonephritis. The *collapsing variant* is particularly associated with HIV infection but may be seen in the absence of identifiable infection (Figure 2.3). It is characterized by marked wrinkling and collapse of glomerular capillaries which, in some glomeruli, may be global rather than segmental; visceral epithelial cell swelling is often very marked. In some cases of FSGS the segmental lesions occur exclusively at the tubular pole of the glomerulus (*tip lesion*); it has been suggested that this may be a group with a better response to steroids and a more favourable prognosis.

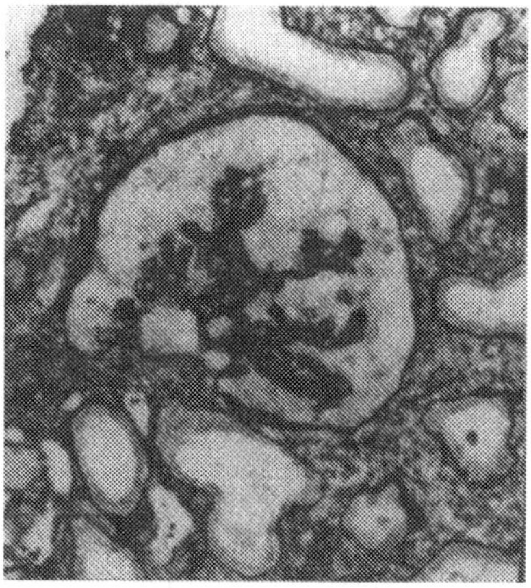

Figure 2.3 Collapsing glomerulopathy. There is collapse of the glomerular tuft, without increase in mesangial matrix, and hyperplasia of the visceral epithelial cells. (Jones methenamine silver, original magnification × 150)

The tubules show focal atrophy associated with interstitial fibrosis in proportion to the severity of the glomerulosclerosis. The presence of such scarring in a biopsy from a patient with the nephrotic syndrome and apparently normal glomeruli should prompt a careful search for segmental sclerosis. Collections of foam cells may be present in the interstitium. In the collapsing variant, particularly when associated with HIV infection, there may be marked tubular damage with cystic dilatation, and tubulointerstitial inflammation.

Immunohistochemistry

The sclerotic areas stain for IgM and C3 but the uninvolved glomerular segments are negative. Focal and segmental staining for IgM and C3 may precede recognizable changes by light microscopy.

Electron microscopy

The most significant feature in idiopathic FSGS is extensive loss of the foot processes of the visceral epithelial cells, which is diffuse and not just confined to the sclerotic areas. These cells may also show vacuolation and protein resorption droplets as well as focal detachment from the basement membrane. In the secondary form of the disease foot process loss may be much less widespread and confined mainly to areas of sclerosis. The sclerotic areas show collapse of basement membranes with matrix increase and there may be granular electron-dense material corresponding to the hyalinosis lesions seen by light microscopy. In HIV infection a characteristic finding is the presence of cytoplasmic tubuloreticular structures (Figure 2.4).

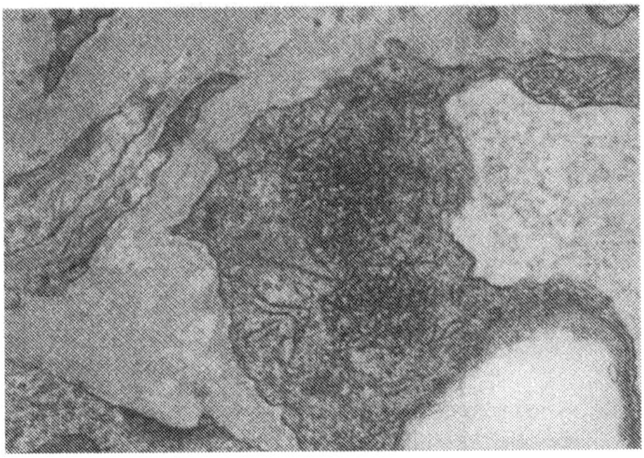

Figure 2.4 HIV nephropathy. Two clusters of tubuloreticular structures in the cytoplasm of a glomerular endothelial cell. (original magnification × 30 000)

Membranous glomerulonephritis

This disease is characterized by the deposition of immune complexes on the outside of the glomerular basement membrane followed by a thickening of the membrane.

Light microscopy

There is thickening of glomerular capillary walls affecting all glomeruli in a uniform fashion. In the earliest stage, when deposits are present but there is no basement membrane thickening, it may be impossible to recognize the changes by light microscopy. As the thickening of the membrane progresses silver stains show the characteristic spikes of new membrane forming next to deposits and later, when the deposits become incorporated, the basement membrane shows a lattice-like appearance in PAS or silver stains. The mesangial matrix may show a slight increase but there is no mesangial hypercellularity. Segmental scars appear to be associated with a worse prognosis. Marginating neutrophils in glomerular capillaries are suggestive of secondary renal vein thrombosis as a result of the nephrotic syndrome.

Immunohistochemistry
There is a granular capillary wall IgG and C3. The presence of additional immunoglobulins or complement components raises the possibility of systemic lupus erythematosus (SLE).

Electron microscopy
The appearances can be used to classify the stage of the disease. In *stage I* there are multiple discrete electron-dense deposits on the outside of the glomerular basement membrane beneath the visceral epithelial cells which show obliteration of their foot processes over the deposits. In *stage II* the basement membrane is thickened by projections (spikes) adjacent to the deposits (Figure 2.5), while in *stage III* the deposits are encircled by newly formed basement membrane. During the late stage of the disease (*stage IV*) the deposits may gradually lose their electron-density and the basement membrane becomes vacuolated and thickened.

Diffuse endocapillary proliferative glomerulonephritis

This usually follows an infection, typically with a beta-haemolytic *Streptococcus.*

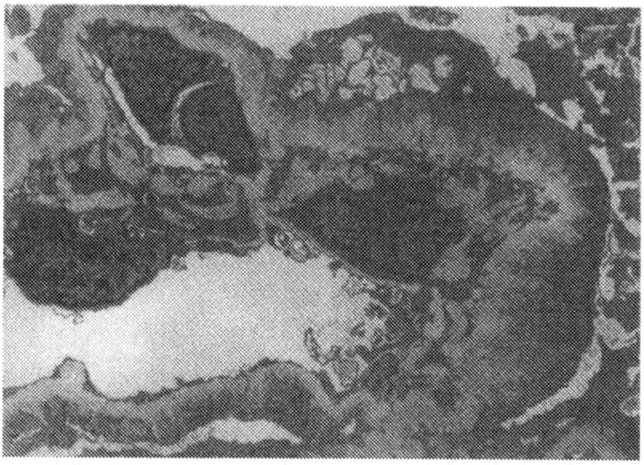

Figure 2.5 Membranous glomerulonephritis, stage II. There is thickening of the basement membrane with multiple subepithelial electron-dense deposits and projections of basement membrane between the deposits. (original magnification ×4000)

Light microscopy

The glomeruli are enlarged and globally hypercellular with increased cells in the mesangium, and neutrophils and monocytes in capillary lumens (Figure 2.6). The number of neutrophils is very variable, with more early in the course of the disease. Crescents may be present. Oedema and focal chronic inflammation are usually seen in the interstitium. Rarely there is a necrotizing arteritis.

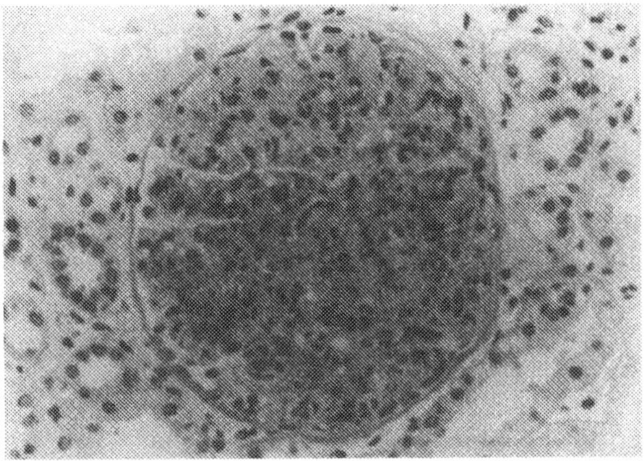

Figure 2.6 Diffuse endocapillary proliferative glomerulonephritis. The glomerular tuft is markedly hypercellular due to infiltration by monocytes and occasional neutrophils and increased mesangial cells. (Haematoxylin and eosin, original magnification ×250)

Immunohistology

There is granular IgG and C3 on capillary walls and sometimes in the mesangium.

Electron microscopy

There are large, dome-shaped, electron-dense deposits ('humps') on the subepithelial aspect of the basement membrane, often accompanied by smaller subendothelial and mesangial deposits. Leukocytes infiltrating capillary loops may be in contact with the basement membrane.

Mesangiocapillary glomerulonephritis type I

Light microscopy

Glomeruli show a combination of mesangial hypercellularity and capillary wall thickening which involves all the glomeruli fairly uniformly. The glomeruli are enlarged and may show accentuated lobulation. The capillary walls show a characteristic double contour, or 'tram-track', appearance which results from the interposition of mesangial cells between the original basement membrane on the outside and newly formed membrane on the inside, with immune deposits lying between. In addition to the increase in mesangial cells there may also be an increase in inflammatory cells within capillary lumens.

Immunohistochemistry
There is granular IgG and C3 along the capillary walls and in the mesangium, and this may be accompanied by IgM, C1q and C4.

Electron microscopy
Electron-dense immune deposits are seen in the mesangial areas and on the inner (subendothelial) aspect of the basement membrane. On the endothelial side of the deposits there are extensions of mesangial cell cytoplasm (mesangial cell interposition). In some cases there may also be small subepithelial deposits. In patients with proteinuria there may be loss of the epithelial cell foot processes.

Dense deposit disease (mesangiocapillary glomerulonephritis type II)

In this disease there is deposition in basement membranes of very electron-dense material.

Light microscopy
The glomerular capillary walls show a prominent eosinophilic, refractile, ribbon-like thickening. Early in the disease this change may be present only in a few segments. There is an increase in mesangial matrix and mesangial cells although the amount of cellular proliferation is variable. Eosinophilic deposits may also be present in the mesangium, in Bowman's capsule, along tubular basement membranes and in arteriolar walls. Neutrophils may be seen in capillary lumens and crescent formation is relatively common.

Immunohistology
There is staining for C3 along capillary walls and granular staining for C3 in the mesangium. Examination at high power shows that the C3 staining is around the dense deposits but the deposits themselves do not stain. In a minority of patients there is no staining for immunoglobulins or complement.

Electron microscopy
The lamina densa of the glomerular basement membranes is replaced by very electron-dense material which appears almost black (Figure 2.7). There is moderate thickening of the membrane in areas where the deposit is present. The changes may be segmental. Similar electron-dense material may also be seen in the mesangium, in Bowman's capsule, in tubular basement membranes and in arterioles.

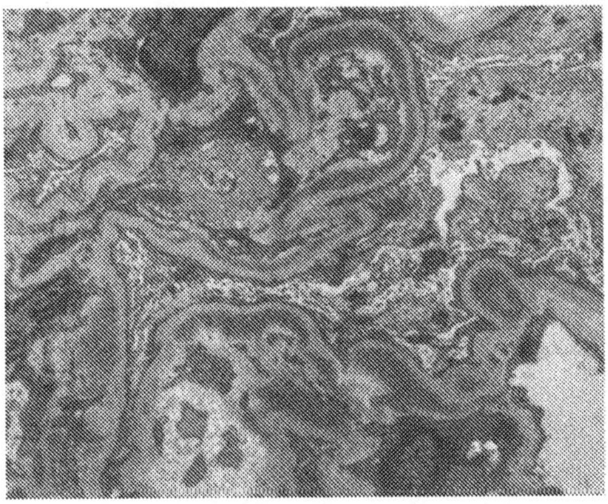

Figure 2.7 Dense deposit disease. There is a ribbon-like deposit within the basement membrane and mesangial cell interposition. (original magnification ×7280)

IgA nephropathy

Light microscopy

There is usually a mild increase in the number of glomerular mesangial cells with a slight expansion of mesangial matrix (Figure 2.8); this may affect all the glomeruli or only some. Immune deposits in the mesangium may be recognized as densely PAS-positive nodules which are more clearly seen with a Masson's trichrome stain. In some cases there may be more prominent segmental proliferative lesions with intraluminal inflammatory cells, segmental fibrinoid necrosis and, sometimes, crescent formation. There may also be segmental scars with adhesions to Bowman's capsule identical to those seen in focal and segmental glomerulosclerosis. Red cell casts may be seen in the tubules, particularly in patients biopsied during episodes of macroscopic haematuria, and there is often focal tubulointerstitial scarring in proportion to the degree of glomerular damage.

Immunohistology

The defining feature of the disease is the presence of predominant deposits of IgA in the mesangium usually accompanied by C3 (Figure 2.9). It is sometimes present on the adjacent capillary wall and there may be smaller amounts of mesangial IgM, IgG and C1q. In most cases the IgA is mainly of the IgA_1 subclass.

Electron microscopy

The mesangium contains large electron-dense deposits. In a significant number of cases there are also deposits at subendothelial, subepithelial and intramembranous sites. Segments of mesangial cell interposition may occasionally be present.

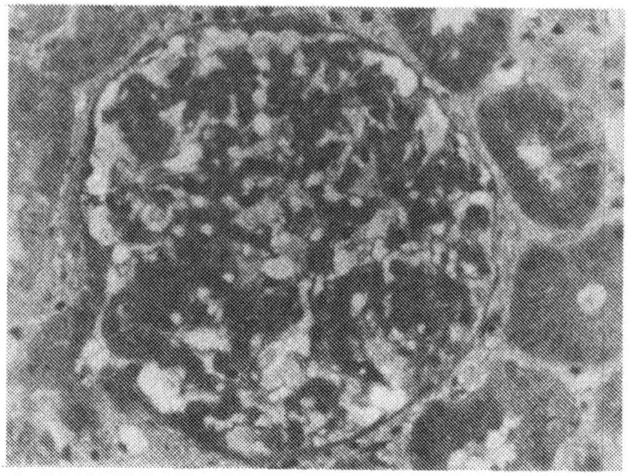

Figure 2.8 IgA nephropathy. The glomerulus shows increased mesangial matrix and segmental increase in mesangial cells (Periodic acid-Schiff, original magnification ×250)

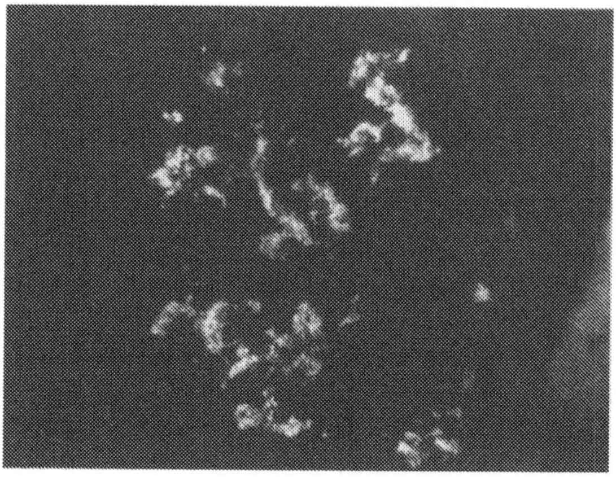

Figure 2.9 IgA nephropathy. Immunofluorescence demonstrating deposition of IgA in the mesangium. (Direct immunofluorescence, original magnification ×250)

Other diseases with mesangial IgA

Henoch–Schönlein purpura shows mesangial proliferation together with segmental proliferative or necrotizing lesions and crescent formation. In comparison with typical IgA nephropathy, focal necrosis and crescents are more prominent, and IgA is more commonly found on capillary walls as well as in the mesangium. The deposits, when examined by electron microscopy, are rarely as large or nodular as those in IgA nephropathy.

Deposition of mesangial IgA with similar appearances to idiopathic IgA nephropathy may also be seen in patients with chronic liver disease and intestinal disease, including ulcerative colitis and Crohn's disease.

Recurrence of glomerulonephritis in renal allografts

Recurrence of glomerulonephritis in grafts is reported to occur in up to 30%, although exact figures for the rate of recurrence may be unreliable due to failure to document the original disease in native kidneys by renal biopsy. There can be difficulties in the histological distinction of recurrent glomerulonephritis from chronic allograft glomerulopathy. All types of glomerulonephritis have recurred after transplantation but some are much more likely to do so than others. The most common forms of recurrent glomerulonephritis are dense deposit disease (90%), IgA nephropathy (50%), mesangiocapillary glomerulonephritis type I (40%), focal and segmental glomerulosclerosis (30%) and membranous glomerulonephritis (10%). In most cases recurrent disease shows only slow progression. A major exception is focal and segmental glomerulosclerosis where there may be very rapid onset of recurrent disease after transplantation with heavy proteinuria and early graft loss. Once transmission of FSGS has occurred in the first graft there is an increased chance of recurrence in subsequent grafts.

The criteria for the histological diagnosis of glomerulonephritis in renal allografts are the same as for native kidneys.

Glomerulonephritis in systemic diseases

It is beyond the scope of this chapter to deal with all the diseases which may be associated with glomerulonephritis or glomerulopathy, particularly as in some the association is tenuous. Here the systemic diseases which are most commonly seen in clinical practice and biopsied for diagnostic and prognostic purposes are described.

Systemic lupus erythematosus (SLE)

The glomerular appearances in SLE are variable, depending on severity of renal involvement, and these have been classified into five separate groups.

Light microscopy
In summary:

Class I	Normal light microscopy, with or without immune deposits by immunohistochemistry or electron microscopy.
Class II	Mesangial proliferative glomerulonephritis.
Class III	Focal proliferative glomerulonephritis.
Class IV	Diffuse proliferative glomerulonephritis.
Class V	Membranous glomerulonephritis.

The highly characteristic lesions of lupus nephritis are seen in Class III and IV disease: focal and segmental in Class III, and diffuse and global in Class IV. The proliferation is a combination of mesangial cell increase and leukocyte infiltration. In Class IV this may take the form of a mesangiocapillary glomerulonephritis (Figure 2.10). The capillary walls are irregularly thickened, mainly due to large subendothelial deposits, which have a refractile appearance ('wire loops'). There may also be mesangial matrix expansion with refractile deposits in the mesangium. The capillary lumens are narrowed or obliterated by the cellular increase, and may contain hyaline thrombi. The pathognomonic *haematoxylin bodies* are seen in only about 3% of biopsies. Signs of activity are areas of fibrinoid necrosis, crescents, neutrophil infiltration, and nuclear fragments. Chronic changes (sclerosis, adhesions, fibrous crescents) are often present together with active lesions. Whether formal scoring of activity and chronicity can be used prognostically is still uncertain.

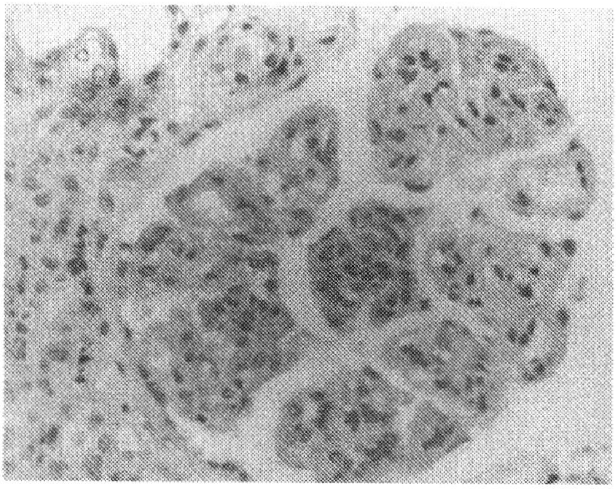

Figure 2.10 Systemic lupus erythematosus. Glomerulus showing mesangiocapillary glomerulonephritis with increased mesangial cells and capillary wall thickening. (Haematoxylin and eosin, original magnification ×250)

There may be tubular atrophy and fibrosis, and focal dense mononuclear cell infiltrates are often prominent, a feature not seen in primary forms of proliferative glomerulonephritis. In some cases there is an active vasculitis.

In patients with circulating 'lupus anticoagulant', glomerular thrombi and changes resembling haemolytic uraemic syndrome kidneys may be present.

Immunohistology

A 'full house' of immunoglobulins and complement components (IgG, IgM, IgG, C1q, C3, C4) is almost diagnostic of SLE. These may occur at all sites, depending on the class of nephritis.

Electron microscopy

This is most useful for defining the sites of immune deposits (Figure 2.11). It may allow the differentiation of primary from lupus-associated membranous glomerulonephritis. In the latter, deposits are not only epimembranous, but are also present in smaller amounts subendothelially and in the mesangium. One fascinating feature of lupus is the presence of tubuloreticular strictures in glomerular and peritubular capillary endothelium (similar to those in HIV nephropathy) (Figure 2.4).

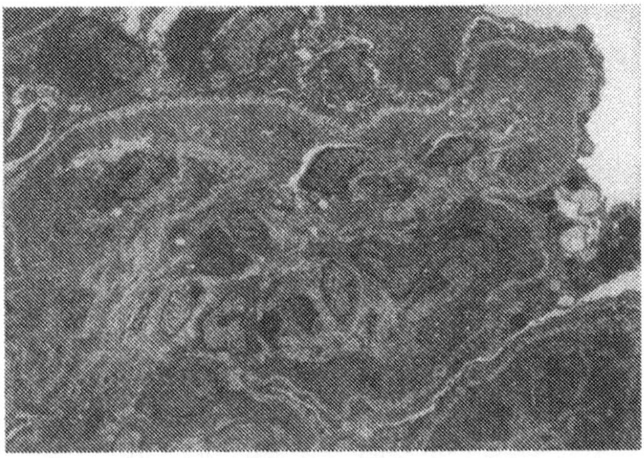

Figure 2.11 Systemic lupus erythematosus. Electron micrograph of diffuse proliferative (WHO Class IV) lupus nephritis. There is hypercellularity and subepithelial, subendothelial and mesangial electron-dense deposits are present. (original magnification ×2000)

Diabetes mellitus

A variety of pathological changes can be found in the kidneys of diabetics, including non-specific ischaemic changes and pyelonephritis. The specific glomerular lesion is diabetic glomerulosclerosis. It is important to recognize that diabetics can also have other important forms of glomerulonephritis, alone and/or combined with diabetic glomerulosclerosis, and the incidence of primary glomerulonephritis in biopsied diabetics can be as high at 50%. The diagnosis of a superimposed form of primary glomerulonephritis can rarely be made without electron microscopy.

Diabetic glomerulosclerosis

Light microscopy

The glomeruli are often enlarged. In the *diffuse* form there is a global increase in mesangial matrix and capillary wall thickness. The mesangial changes are more obvious than the capillary wall thickening, which may only be detectable by electron microscopy. In some cases the number of mesangial cells is also increased, and this may simulate a mild mesangial proliferative glomerulonephritis. In the *nodular* form the excessive accumulation of matrix forms irregular nodules (*Kimmelstiel–Wilson nodules*) which have narrowed capillary lumens around their margins (Figure 2.12). These have to be distinguished from nodules of amyloid or light chain deposits. There may be other non-specific changes as glomeruli become obsolete. One lesion which is thought to be specific for diabetes is the *capsular drop*.

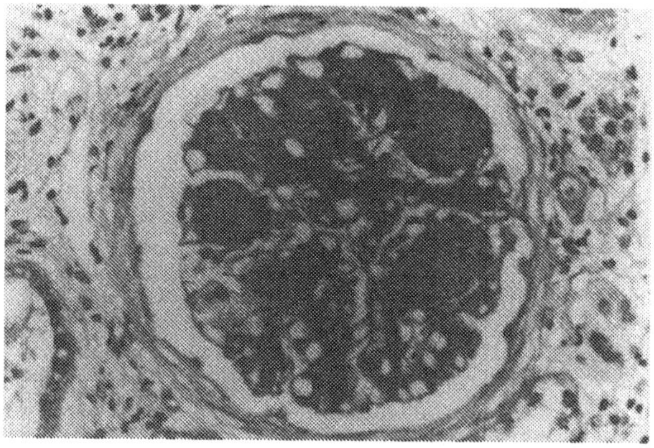

Figure 2.12 Diabetes mellitus. Nodular diabetic glomerulosclerosis. There are rounded homogeneous nodules in several lobules of the glomerulus. (Periodic acid-Schiff, original magnification ×250)

The arterioles have large hyaline deposits, which affect both afferent and efferent vessels (and are usually more extensive than in hypertension). The arteries often are narrowed by non-specific arteriosclerosis.

Immunohistology

There is no immune complex deposition. In some biopsies there is faint linear staining for immunoglobulins on glomerular capillary walls.

Electron microscopy

The lamina densa of the glomerular basement membranes is thicker than normal. There are no discrete deposits unless a primary form of glomerulonephritis is superimposed. The mesangial nodules have a homogeneous bland appearance with no deposits or fibril deposition. The degree of epithelial foot process loss depends on the level of proteinuria.

Amyloidosis

Classical amyloidosis involving the kidneys has been known for many years. More recently rare types of fibrillary glomerulopathies, where the deposits do not have the tinctorial properties defining amyloid, have been described. The description here is confined to classical amyloid.

Light microscopy

In the majority of cases most of the amyloid is in glomeruli, with smaller amounts in arterioles and, in advanced disease, in the interstitium and tubular basement membranes. On haematoxylin and eosin staining, amyloid is an amorphous pale pink material first detectable in the mesangium, and gradually encroaching on the capillary walls. There is no cellular reaction. When stained with Congo red , amyloid shows apple green birefringence with polarized light. AA amyloid congophilia is sensitive to potassium permanganate treatment; AL and most other forms of amyloid are resistant. Amyloid can also be detected at a light microscopic level by staining with methyl violet.

Immunohistochemistry

Amyloid deposits may have a weak smeary positive reaction with immunoglobulin and complement antibodies. Specific antibodies are very useful for confirming AA amyloid and may be of help in determining the type of non-AA amyloid.

Electron microscopy

Electron microscopy confirms the 8–10 nm diameter fibrillar structure of amyloid (Figure 2.13). Fibrils may be present in the mesangium, in the capillary walls, and in some cases at epimembranous sites simulating spike formation, which could be confused with a focal stage II membranous glomerulonephritis.

There are no ultrastructural differences between the different amyloid subtypes. The special value of electron microscopy is in detecting early disease.

Subacute bacterial endocarditis (SBE)

The commonest lesion is a focal proliferative glomerulonephritis. There are no diagnostic features by light microscopy.

Immunohistochemistry

This is the most useful investigation for differentiating SBE from the other causes of a focal proliferative glomerulonephritis. C3 is usually the predominant immunodeposit. There may be IgG and IgM, but no IgA, and this distinguishes the condition from IgA nephropathy or Henoch–Schönlein purpura-associated glomerulonephritis. The deposits are granular, contrasting

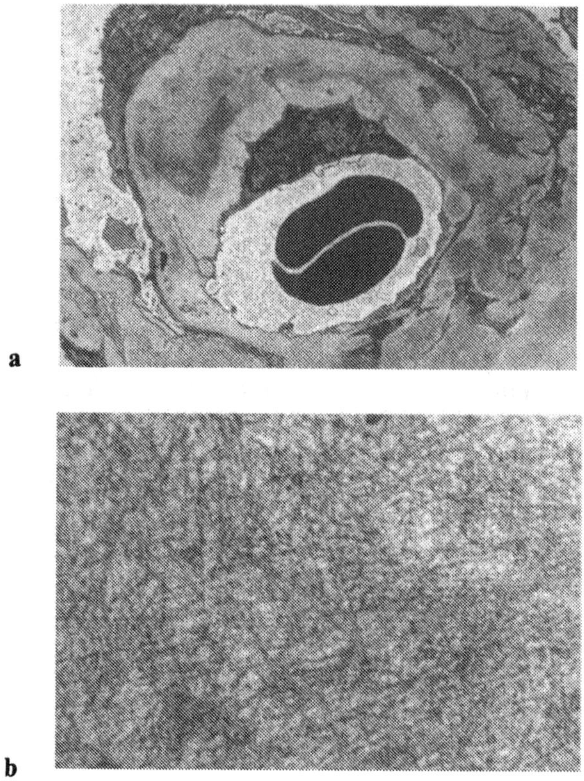

Figure 2.13 Amyloid. (**a**) Thickening of the glomerular capillary wall with loss of the lamina densa, and mesangial matrix expansion (original magnification ×6500). (**b**) High-power electron micrograph showing the fibrillar structure (original magnification ×78 000)

with the linear staining found in anti-GBM glomerulonephritis. Deposits are not a feature of systemic vasculitis (see below).

Electron microscopy

Immune deposits should always be present, and it is hazardous to diagnose SBE in their absence. They are usually scanty, but can be present at all sites.

Light chain nephropathy

Light chain nephropathy is characterized by the deposition of monoclonal light chains in the glomerular and tubular basement membranes and in the mesangium. Approximately two-thirds of patients have multiple myeloma or some other lymphoplasmacytic disease such as Waldenstrom's macroglobulinaemia or lymphoma. Only certain light chains (usually of kappa type) appear to cause this lesion; light chains which cause light chain nephropathy do not cause amyloid deposition, and vice-versa.

Light microscopy
Light chains deposit predominantly in the mesangium. The appearances can therefore resemble amyloid. The material, however, does not have the tinctorial properties of amyloid. Where deposits are large they form well-defined nodules which can be very like nodular diabetic glomerulosclerosis.

There is often extensive tubular atrophy with a characteristic refractile thickening and wrinkling of tubular basement membranes due to light chain deposits.

Immunohistology
Glomerular nodules and tubular basement membranes may stain with antibodies against IgG. Staining for specific kappa or lambda light chains is diagnostic, but these antibodies are notoriously fickle, particularly in paraffin-embedded material.

Electron microscopy
This is diagnostic. The ultrastructural appearances of amyloid and light chain disease paraproteins are different. Amyloid has a fibrillar structure, while in light chain disease the deposits have a granular or amorphous and very electron-dense appearance (Figure 2.14). They are present in mesangial nodules and the subepithelial aspect of the capillary walls.

Cryoglobulinaemia

Several forms of glomerulonephritis are associated with 'essential' cryoglobulinaemia; in addition cryoglobulin deposits may be a component of post-infectious glomerulonephritis and SLE. The increasing frequency of cryoglobulinaemic glomerulonephritis is now ascribed to hepatitis C infection.

Light microscopy
The commonest appearance is of a mesangiocapillary glomerulonephritis, although diffuse proliferative glomerulonephritis, and crescentic glomerulonephritis, can occur. The additional features which are characteristic of cryoglobulinaemia are prominent neutrophil and macrophage infiltration and eosinophilic thrombi in capillary lumens. There may be a necrotizing vasculitis in arterioles and small arteries.

Immunohistology
This will depend on the composition of the deposited cryoglobulins. These are most frequently type II, mixed monoclonal IgM and polyclonal IgG. C3 is usually present.

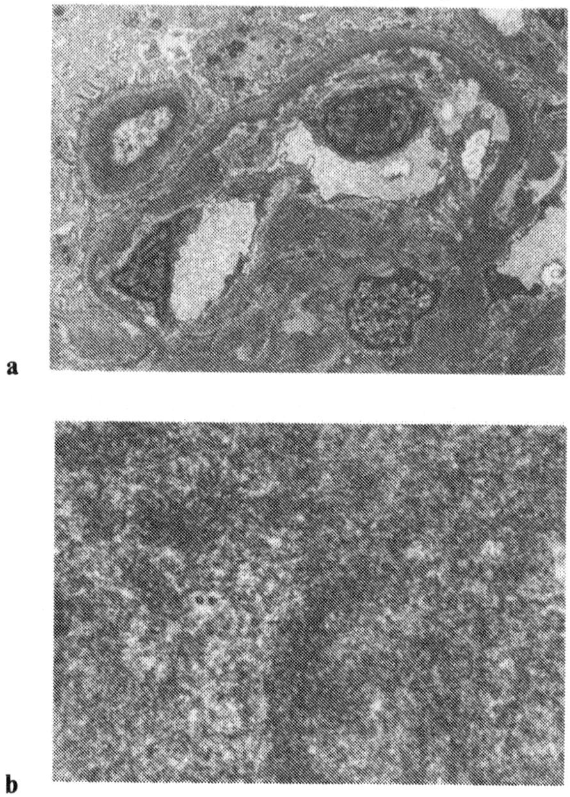

Figure 2.14 Light chain nephropathy. (**a**) There is thickening of the capillary wall by subendothelial granular electron-dense material and similar material is present in the expanded mesangium (original magnification × 5400). (**b**) High-power electron micrograph showing the granular structure of light chain deposits. Compare with Figure 2.13b (original magnification × 78 000)

Electron microscopy

The characteristic deposits are predominantly subendothelial and structured. A typical appearance is of curved cylinders (Figure 2.15). There may also be rhomboid crystalline structures in the cytoplasm of glomerular cells.

Haemolytic uraemic syndromes (HUS)

The glomerular changes in the various coagulopathies that affect the kidneys are exemplified by the changes in HUS. These changes can therefore be seen in HUS, thrombotic thrombocytopenic purpura, scleroderma, severe malignant hypertension, severe pre-eclampsia, and post-partum renal failure.

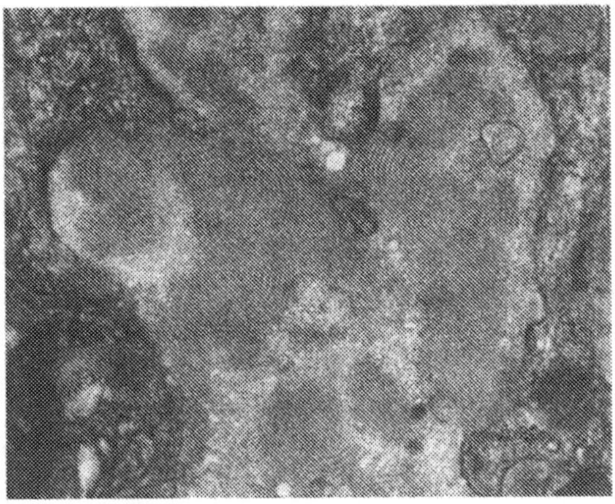

Figure 2.15 Cryoglobulinaemia. The deposits are composed of curved cylinders giving a fingerprint appearance. (original magnification ×48 000)

Light microscopy
The glomeruli show thickening and splitting of the capillary walls best seen with methenamine silver staining. The loops may appear bloodless, or have segmental necrosis or thrombosis.

The arterioles are often abnormal with thrombi, fibrinoid necrosis or endothelial swelling initially and later pale intimal thickening. Where there is arterial involvement this affects interlobular more often than larger vessels, and causes a concentric cellular intimal thickening indistinguishable from malignant hypertension or scleroderma.

Immunohistology
Negative, or scanty, scattered granular deposits of immunoglobulin and complement.

Electron microscopy
This shows that the capillary wall thickening is due to the formation of a characteristic lucent subendothelial widening. The split appearance is due to new layers of lamina densa being laid down inside the lucent area. There may be dense material (most probably non-polymerized fibrinogen) in the subendothelia and capillary lumens; there are no discrete electron-dense deposits of the type found in immune complex glomerulonephritis.

Pre-eclampsia/eclampsia

The clinical criteria for this condition are somewhat confusing, and the pathogenesis is still unclear. From a pathological viewpoint there are characteristic glomerular changes on renal biopsy, the most important task being to differentiate them from a primary or secondary form of glomerulonephritis.

Light microscopy
The glomeruli are enlarged and have a solid, bloodless appearance, due to endothelial swelling. There may be mild proliferation, but this is not usually a prominent feature and when present raises the possibility of an underlying proliferative glomerulonephritis. There may be splitting of the basement membranes. The lesions are global, and the presence of a focal and segmental distribution suggests a glomerulonephritis rather than pre-eclampsia. In severe cases the appearances are indistinguishable from HUS (see above).

The blood vessels may have no changes, show endothelial swelling, or in severe cases have HUS-type lesions. Hyaline deposits may be present. The tubulo-interstitium is usually normal.

Immunohistology
There may be small amounts of granular or smeary capillary wall IgM, IgG and C3, and this is not indicative of an underlying glomerulonephritis.

Electron microscopy
The glomerular endothelium is swollen with loss of fenestrations. There is granular subendothelial material, and there may be segmental mesangial cell interposition. In most cases the ultrastructure is the most helpful technique for distinguishing pre-eclampsia from a proliferative form of glomerulonephritis (Figure 2.16).

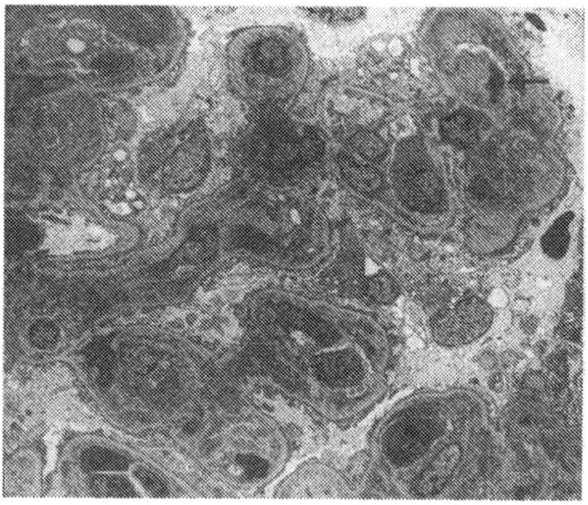

Figure 2.16 Pre-eclampsia. Electron micrograph of a glomerulus showing a reduction in capillary lumens due to endothelial swelling, and increase in subendothelium with scattered subendothelial deposits. Visceral epithelial cells show focal foot process loss and cystic change. A mitosis is present in an endothelial cell (arrow). (original magnification ×2000)

The natural history is for resolution, in most cases by 3–6 months, although in a few patients the lesions may persist for up to 2 years. Further persistence of lesions indicates a diagnosis other than pre-eclampsia.

Liver disease

The association between liver diseases and glomerulonephritis is complex. Mesangial IgA deposits can be found in a variety of diseases with liver involvement, including those without a recognizable immune complex aetiology. More specific is the association between hepatitis viruses and glomerulonephritis. Hepatitis B has been associated with several forms of glomerulonephritis, most commonly with membranous glomerulonephritis. Recently, the strong association between hepatitis C virus and cryoglobulinaemic glomerulonephritis (see above) has become apparent.

Crescentic glomerulonephritis and vasculitis

Crescents may be present in many forms of proliferative glomerulonephritis. When 50% or more glomeruli are affected the disease is classified as a crescentic glomerulonephritis, although this definition is somewhat arbitrary. There are three principal pathogenic groups: (a) anti-GBM disease, (b) vasculitic renal disease – by some designated pauci-immune crescentic glomerulonephritis, and (c) immune complex disease. Renal biopsy is the most important investigation for distinguishing between these.

(a) Anti-GBM disease (Goodpasture's syndrome).

Light microscopy
The number and size of crescents varies with severity of disease, and the cellularity depends on their age. With severe acute disease, large cellular crescents may occupy nearly the whole capsular circumference (circumferential crescents) and fill Bowman's space. Fibrin is also present in Bowman's space. Experimental studies show that a mixture of epithelial cells and macrophages form the crescent, but their identity is not apparent by light microscopy. The underlying glomeruli may show a variety of changes, including foci of fibrinoid necrosis, proliferation, and apparent collapse and compression of glomerular capillaries. There is often quite extensive acute tubular injury, with numerous red cell casts, or tubules filled with fresh red cells, and interstitial oedema. Focal interstitial mononuclear infiltrates can be prominent. Classically the blood vessels are normal, and this is helpful in distinguishing it from a vasculitic crescentic nephritis, but in some cases there is a vasculitis with fibrinoid necrosis in arterioles and distal interlobular arteries.

Immunohistology
The diagnostic feature is linear deposition of IgG and C3 diffusely on the capillary walls of all glomeruli, irrespective of whether they have crescents or not. In a few cases IgM or IgA is present. It is important to note that not all cases of anti-GBM disease have crescents. In some mild cases there is only a focal proliferative glomerulonephritis.

Electron microscopy
The main features are the lack of discrete electron-dense deposits, and breaks in the basement membranes in relation to the crescents. Elsewhere the basement membranes look surprisingly normal. It is therefore possible to differentiate this from immune complex disease.

(b) Vasculitic crescentic glomerulonephritis

This is now the most frequent form of crescentic glomerulonephritis, and is usually associated with circulating antineutrophil cytoplasmic antibodies (ANCA).

Light microscopy
The appearances can be identical to anti-GBM disease. Helpful distinguishing features are the lack of glomerular hypercellularity, often much more prominent fibrinoid necrosis in the underlying tufts (Figure 2.17), and the presence of vasculitis in arterioles and arteries, sometimes with eosinophils in interstitial infiltrates.

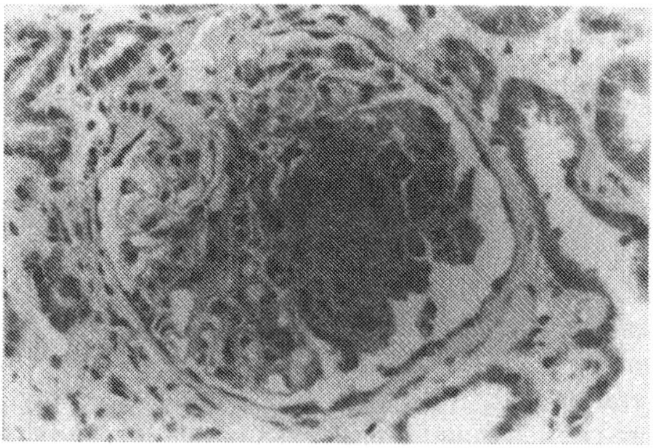

Figure 2.17 Vasculitic (pauci-immune) glomerulonephritis. The glomerulus shows a segmental area of fibrinoid necrosis without hypercellularity in the rest of the tuft. Other glomeruli contained crescents. (Haematoxylin and eosin, original magnification ×250)

Immunohistology
Negative.

Electron microscopy
As anti-GBM glomerulonephritis.

(c) Immune complex crescentic glomerulonephritis.

The morphological appearances depend on the underlying disease and crescents can occur in most types of immune complex disease, including diffuse endocapillary proliferative glomerulonephritis, IgA nephropathy, mesangiocapillary glomerulonephritis and SLE.

Acknowledgement

Ms Jill Collar is thanked for expert electron microscopy.

Suggested further reading

1. Jennette JC, Olson JL, Schwartz MM, Sieva FG, editors. Heptinstall's Pathology of the Kidney, 5th edn. Philadelphia, PA: Lippincott-Raven; 1998.
2. Tisher CC, Brenner BM. Renal Pathology, 2nd edn. Philadelphia, PA: JB Lippincott; 1994.
3. Churg J, Bernstein J, Glassock RJ. Renal Disease: Classification and Atlas of Glomerular Diseases, 2nd edn. New York: Igaku-Shoin; 1995.

3. Minimal change disease and focal segmental glomerulosclerosis

A. MEYRIER

Introduction

The denomination 'idiopathic nephrotic syndrome' (INS) is progressively replacing the time-honoured term 'nephrosis' to define a disease comprising: (a) nephrotic syndrome; (b) on renal biopsy, absence of any lesions by light microscopy and immunofluorescence (minimal change disease, MCD), or with lesions of focal and segmental glomerulosclerosis (FSG); and (c) absence of concomitant identified disease. Of note, this last element can be assessed only after sufficient follow-up, as some rare cases of MCD may herald lymphoma [1] or discovery of a solid tumour [2]. Similarly, FSG cannot be considered 'idiopathic' before a host of conditions have been ruled out [3]. That MCD and FSG represent the same entity has never been definitely proven [4]. FSG can be overlooked on renal biopsy [5, 6], and a transition from MCD to FSG is common in corticosteroid-resistant forms [7]. This is why paediatricians, who rarely carry out renal biopsy at first contact with a nephrotic child, consider that the sole point of interest in INS (or nephrosis – I shall use both terms) is its mode of response to corticosteroid treatment. In fact, FSG differs from MCD in many ways. Even when the glomerular tuft appears normal by standard microscopy, the glomerular size is larger in FSG than in cases which remain MCD over time [8]. Proteinuria selectivity index [9] is poor in FSG and to some extent helps predict a poor response to therapy. Finally, FSG usually develops along with tubulointerstitial damage, interstitial fibrosis and vascular lesions, in which the part played by massive proteinuria [10, 11] and by the offending substance responsible for the podocyte changes of FSG [12], remains an open question. The response of FSG to corticosteroids, alkylating agents and cyclosporin A (CsA) is disappointing. Its development is usually progression of the glomerular lesions, leading to end-stage renal disease, especially in case of steroid resistance [13–15]. In such cases, the nephrotic syndrome and the glomerular lesions often relapse after renal transplantation, but this is not the rule, which might conceivably indicate an heterogeneity in the pathophysiology of the disease.

C.D. Pusey (ed.), The Treatment of Glomerulonephritis, 39–53.

Pathophysiological mechanisms relevant to treatment

INS is characterized by an abnormal permeability of the glomerular basement membrane (GBM) to serum albumin. This is obviously the consequence of an abnormal environment on primarily normal kidneys [16, 17]. A yet-unidentified substance induces loss of the GBM polyanion which normally repulses negatively charged serum albumin [18]. At least in FSG this is deleterious to the glomerular visceral epithelial cell, and may also induce defects in the GBM which might be pathways allowing passage of the serum albumin molecules [19].

In 1974 Shalhoub postulated that a lymphokine might be responsible for increased permeability of the GBM [20]. In fact, many observations point to a T-cell-driven substance interfering with glomerular permselectivity. It is beyond the scope of this review to analyse them in detail. Overall, the basis of these experiments was to provoke proteinuria in laboratory animals by injection of a supernatant of lymphocytes cultured from patients with nephrotic syndrome, leading to the concept of a glomerular permeability factor (GPF) [21–23]. Other tests, which consisted of injecting the T-cell product subcutaneously, disclosed increased capillary permeability, leading to the notion of 'vascular permeability factor' (VPF) [24, 25]. The most convincing argument for immune production of GPF/VPF stems from clinical observations [16, 17], and especially relapse of nephrosis and FSG after transplantation [26–30].

These data indicate that therapy should be geared to controlling a disorder of cellular immunity, and also the consequences of impaired glomerular permselectivity.

Natural history of nephrosis

It is worth recalling that, prior to the advent of mechlorethamine and corticosteroid treatment of nephrosis, the main causes of death in children with nephrosis were infection, thromboembolism and, to a much lesser extent, renal insufficiency. The reports of Barness *et al.* in the US [31] and of Arneil in the UK [32], including respectively 161 and 164 untreated cases, showed that survivors (respectively 41% and 56%) were symptom-free after 2 years and that spontaneous remission was a common feature of childhood nephrosis. These historical data are important, as they indicate that remission obtained with corticosteroids or CsA may buy time to reach a phase of spontaneous extinction of the ill-understood process causing proteinuria.

Drug treatment

Corticosteroids

Children

Glucocorticoids are the mainstay of treatment [33]. However, given that about 5% of cases undergo spontaneous remission, treatment is not an emergency, except in cases of acute onset with vascular collapse and hypotension, which is a possible, although rare, mode of presentation in childhood. The corticosteroid most commonly used is prednisone, at a dosage of 60 mg/m^2 per day. In case of a response, proteinuria disappears between the 7th and the 14th day. Once proteinuria is nil, treatment is pursued for 4 weeks and, after switching to an alternate-day schedule with the same dosage, prednisone is tapered to a stop over the following 12 weeks, decreasing by one-fourth of the dosage every other week. Thus, treatment of a first episode of nephrotic syndrome is in the order of 4.5 months. Shorter treatment schedules entail the risk of early relapse. The overall pattern of response to corticosteroids in children with MCD in the ISKDC 1977 report [34] is the following. Of 100 children with MCD, 94 were responders and six early non-responders. Responders developed into non-relapsers in 36%, infrequent relapsers in 18% and frequent relapsers in 46%. Two-thirds of early nonresponders ended up as responders and one-third remained non-responders.

When remission is not obtained after 1 month of full-dose treatment, paediatricians usually administer three pulses of methylprednisolone, 1 g/ 1.73 m^2, over 3 days [35]. Persistence of proteinuria despite this treatment defines corticosteroid resistance. In such cases, paediatricians usually consider renal biopsy, as corticosteroid resistance may indicate that the glomerular lesions might be other than MCD.

The course after remission is unpredictable. Persistent remission 2 years after stopping steroid treatment usually means cure. However, INS of childhood is a multi-relapsing disease in more than two-thirds of cases. Early relapses require a new course of corticosteroids, continued for more than a year on an alternate day basis, with the maintenance dosage being 15–30 mg/ m^2 every other day. Corticosteroid dependency is characterized by relapse of nephrotic syndrome when dosage is reduced below a threshold or by multiple relapses despite complete efficacy of each course. In both instances the child is exposed to the multiple consequences of steroid toxicity, and an alternative regimen must be envisaged.

Adults

The results of corticosteroid treatment of adult INS were reviewed in 1988 [14]. In 302 patients with MCD, corticosteroids obtained complete remission in 74.8% of cases, partial remission in 7% and were a failure in 18.2%. The response of nephrotic FSG to corticosteroids was 15.6% complete remission, 20.2% partial remission and 64.2% failure. However, since this publication, better knowledge of the response rate to corticosteroids in adults has been acquired [15], although treatment of a first attack of nephrosis in the adult is less well defined than in children. The initial dosage is identical, comprising 1 mg/kg per day of prednisone, or, for better tolerance, a double dose on an alternate-day schedule [36–38]. An important point is that the response of adult nephrosis to corticosteroids is much slower than that in children [15, 39–41]. Fujimoto *et al.* studied 33 patients with adult-onset MCD [42]. The longest time to remission was 4 months. In some patients it occurred when tapering of corticosteroid dosage had begun. In the series of Mak *et al.* [43], of 37 patients given full-dose oral prednisolone, 30% had not achieved remission by the 8th week and 11% by the 16th week. Contrary to the situation in children, corticosteroid resistance in adults should not be pronounced before a 4-month course of full-dosage prednisone has been completed [15]. In too many publications adult nephrotics are considered corticosteroid-resistant after a 6-week course of corticosteroids and are embarked on more aggressive treatment, whereas remission might have been obtained with a longer course of steroids. Such additional immunosuppressive agents are often prescribed along with steroids and it is conceivable that the apparent favourable effect of the new treatment is in fact explained by the continuing course of steroids.

Another difference between adult-onset and childhood MCD is the trend towards a reduced incidence of relapses after a first successful course of treatment [41, 43]. With increasing age, and especially after 30, corticosteroid-sensitive nephrotics usually experience a single attack of nephrotic syndrome. However, although its incidence is not easily found in the literature, corticosteroid dependency remains common and entails the risks of steroid toxicity, including the worrisome prospect of hip osteonecrosis. In such cases a course of alkylating agents may be beneficial [43], but cytotoxicity and the oncogenic potential of these drugs remain a problem. CsA is an alternative non-cytotoxic treatment of steroid-dependent nephrosis [44].

A suggested schedule for treating an adult with nephrotic syndrome and MCD is the following [45]: prednisone 1 mg/kg per day (up to 80 mg/day) for 8–12 weeks, followed by 0.5 mg/kg per day (or 60 mg every other day) for 6–8 weeks, then tapering to a stop over 8 weeks. In fact, as specified above, the initial full-dose treatment can be prolonged to 16 weeks if remission is not obtained earlier.

Cytotoxic agents

Three cytotoxic agents have been used in the treatment of INS: mechlorethamine, chlorambucil and cyclophosphamide. Let us recall that mechlorethamine, a nitrogen mustard derived from mustard gas used in chemical warfare in 1917, and which had been known since 1921 to inhibit antibody formation [46], was the first agent tried in the treatment of childhood nephrosis [47], before corticosteroids became available. Nitrogen mustard, which had been abandoned for newer drugs, was again proposed for this indication in the 1980s [48, 49]. However, its poor venous tolerance and its borderline efficacy do not make its indication convincing.

Cyclophosphamide

Cyclophosphamide (CYC) is the alkylating agent most commonly used in nephrosis. Apart from a single publication [50], it is not considered a first-line treatment. Its best indication is the steroid-dependent or multi-relapsing case with steroid toxicity. It is also used in steroid-resistant cases, but the results in this indication are poor. In corticosteroid-responsive children the Arbeitsgemeinschaft für pädiatrische Nephrologie determined that a 12-week course using 2 mg/kg per day was superior to an 8-week course, as the relapse rate after 12 weeks was 33% whereas it was 78% for the shorter course [51]. Duration of treatment longer than 12 weeks, or cyclophosphamide dosage greater than 3 mg/kg per day, are not superior in terms of efficacy but entail greater risk of side-effects. The same group also showed that the incidence of prolonged remission was greater in multi-relapsers than in steroid-dependent children [52]. In adults CYC has been used in steroid-responsive as well as in steroid-resistant INS, but the published results are less readily interpretable than those presented by the more rigorous paediatric nephrologists.

The side-effects of CYC are many. In the short term they include loss of hair, bladder irritation and the risk of leukopenia with the attending hazards of opportunistic infection. In the long run the drug compromises male fertility. The risk of azoospermia is great when cumulative dosage exceeds 150 mg/kg [53], and in our opinion this should always be clearly explained to the patient or the parents before embarking on this treatment. There is also a risk of leukaemia, mucous membrane cancer and bladder malignancy [54].

Chlorambucil

Chlorambucil (CHL) has also been used in steroid-dependent and steroid-resistant nephrosis. Several studies [55–59], including controlled trials, showed that at a dosage of 0.2–0.4 mg/kg per day for 6–12 weeks this agent induced prolonged remission in steroid-dependent or multi-relapsing children. The short-term side-effects of CHL are somewhat less than those of CYC, especially in terms of bladder irritation. However, the risk of leukopenia is the same. Male gonadal toxicity appears at a cumulative dosage over 8 mg/kg. The risk of leukaemia [60] must be seriously considered. The response to CHL compares with that to CYC, with a high yield of complete stable remissions in steroid-responsive cases and rather disappointing results in steroid-resistant nephrosis. In the experience of Broyer *et al.* [58], of 74 steroid-resistant children only 14 (19%) went into full or partial remission during or shortly after treatment.

Owing to the lack of large-scale studies like those conducted in children, the results of CYC or CHL treatment in adults can be deduced only from retrospective analysis of publications which often include both adults and children. In 1988 we analysed nine papers published between 1966 and 1986, totalling 94 patients who were considered to have an indication for treatment with cyclophosphamide [14]. The results were 66% complete remission, 10.6% partial remission and 23.4% failure.

Overall, the foregoing data show that the best indication for alkylating agents is the patient (child or adult) with steroid-dependency or multiple relapses. A majority of steroid-resistant cases are also failures with cytotoxic agents. In such failures, an aggressive rescue protocol comprising repeated high-dose intravenous pulses of methylprednisolone and alkylating agents was proposed recently [61, 62], with an increased success rate but obviously entailing more risk of side-effects.

Azathioprine

The results of azathioprine (AZA) treatment in INS are controversial. In 1970 Abramowicz *et al.* [63] conducted a controlled study which demonstrated the inefficacy of this antimetabolite in the child, a conclusion ratified by Linshaw and Gruskin on behalf of the International Study Group of Kidney Disease in Children [64]. Conversely, occasional publications presented several cases in which AZA induced complete remission in children [65] and in adults [14, 66]. Cade *et al.* [66] treated 13 adults in whom INS had appeared in childhood in two and after age 14 in 11. Eight had MCD and five FSG. Six had been steroid-resistant from the outset. Seven others were multi-relapsers, of whom four evolved to steroid-resistance. AZA was given at a dosage of 2–2.5 mg/kg per day. At 3 months all patients showed clinical improvement. At 18 months the six patients with selective proteinuria were in remission. At 24 months 12 out of 13 of the patients who were still followed up were in complete remission. Since that time AZA has occasionally been cited in papers dealing with treatment of INS, but there are no hard data on the place of this drug in the limited therapeutic panoply for steroid-resistant or steroid-dependent INS. Obviously, we lack a wide-scale, multicentre trial to settle the issue.

Levamisole

Levamisole (L) was originally developed for the treatment of parasitic infections by worms. It was shown that this drug was also an immunostimulant when the immune system was depressed, which is the case in nephrotic syndrome. L restores *in vitro* and *in vivo* most functions of T cells. Occasional non-randomized studies of L therapy have been published since 1980. The British Association for Paediatric Nephrology (BAPN) [67] randomized a group of 61 children with steroid-dependent or multi-relapsing nephrosis. Thirty-one received 2.5 mg/kg of L every other day over a maximum period of 112 days. After inclusion, the dosage of prednisolone was tailed off to a stop at day 56. At day 112 there was persistent remission in 14 patients treated with L, and in only four patients receiving the placebo. L can induce neutropenia or, more rarely, agranulocytosis. A screening of 140 published cases found that neutropenia occurred in 3/140 patients and was rapidly reversible after stopping the drug. The BAPN concluded that alternate-day treatment with L for 6–12 months might be justified in patients suffering from steroid toxicity and might be an alternative to more aggressive forms of therapy such as CsA or alkylating agents.

Cyclosporin A

Cyclosporin A (CsA) impairs IL-2 gene transcription in T cells. However, despite the fact that IL-2 or IL-2 R plasma levels are elevated in some cases of INS [68], there is no evidence that IL-2 is responsible for the increased glomerular permeability to albumin which characterizes this condition. In fact, the mode of action of CsA in INS appears to be both immunological and pharmacological.

Tomizawa *et al.* [25] studied the effect of CsA on the production of VPF/GPF isolated from T lymphocyte cultures from children with MCD. They found a dose-dependent inhibition of VPF production. However, CsA significantly reduces proteinuria in a wide variety of non-immunological glomerular diseases [69]. Diminution of proteinuria simply by the renal vasoconstrictive action of CsA is not a fully satisfactory explanation. *In-vitro* study of glomerular permeability to albumin [70], animal experiments [71, 72] and sieving curves of dextran infusion in humans [73] demonstrated that CsA exerts an antiproteinuric effect by reducing glomerular membrane permeability to albumin through increased charge selectivity. This notion must be kept in mind when interpreting cases of partial remission induced by CsA.

Efficacy and tolerability

The first trials of CsA treatment of nephrosis, reported between 1986 and 1988 [74], were followed by numerous contributions which confirmed that the response of nephrosis to CsA is essentially predicted by previous response to corticosteroid treatment, and that CsA nephrotoxicity is reasonably low when dosage does not exceed 5.5 mg/kg per day.

Children. Corticosteroid-sensitive INS. The best indication for CsA is the patient with steroid-responsive nephrosis in whom steroid dependency or a multi-relapsing course induces steroid toxicity.

Niaudet and Habib [75] reviewed the results of CsA treatment in 129 children with steroid-sensitive or steroid-dependent INS. CsA produced complete remission in 109 (84.5%). Tejani *et al.* [76], using CsA as first-line treatment, obtained remission in 13/14 children, compared with 8/14 children receiving prednisone alone. In most studies, dosage in children was in the order of 6 mg/kg per day. However, Ingulli and Tejani [77], analysing the results of a 2-month CsA treatment in 47 children, identified 13 non-responders whose serum cholesterol levels were significantly greater than in responders. Increasing dosage to 10–14 mg/kg body weight, they obtained remission without evidence of nephrotoxicity. Lieberman and Tejani [78] in a randomized, double blind placebo-controlled trial, included 25 patients with a mean age just over 11 years, who were treated for 6 months. All of the 12 patients who received CsA experienced a significant reduction in proteinuria, as opposed to only 2/12 in the placebo subset. A significant correlation was found between the percentage of change in proteinuria and the pre-study serum cholesterol levels. Ten patients were continued on CsA in doses ranging from 6 to 12 mg/kg per day, and maintained normal renal function.

CsA induces remission of nephrotic syndrome in about 80% of steroid-sensitive cases. It allows suppression or drastic reduction in corticosteroid needs, with regression of steroid toxicity, but contrary to alkylating agents [79] most children relapse when dosage is tailed off to a stop, which means that CsA exerts a suppressive not a curative effect on the process responsible for INS. This raises the question of CsA nephrotoxicity following prolonged exposure. Niaudet *et al.* [80] and Melocoton *et al.* [81] studied long-term tolerance in CsA-dependent children. Serial renal biopsies disclosed increasing interstitial fibrosis despite apparently stable renal function. Such findings raise the question whether it is preferable to trade off the cytotoxicity of alkylating agents for the nephrotoxicity of CsA in steroid-dependent cases.

Corticosteroid-resistant INS. The results of CsA treatment in steroid-resistant forms are disappointing. Niaudet and Habib [75] reviewed eight uncontrolled studies involving 60 steroid-resistant patients. Complete remission was attained in only 12 (20%). In the US, Melocoton *et al.* [81] treated 18 patients with steroid-resistant nephrotic syndrome and steroid-dependent nephrotic syndrome for 2–29 months. CsA therapy did not achieve remission in 10 patients with steroid-resistant INS, regardless of the presence of FSG or MCD on renal biopsy. Following 11–29 months of CsA, seven patients underwent renal biopsy, which showed nephrotoxicity in all seven and led to stopping CsA in four. The authors expressed reservations concerning efficacy and safety of CsA in steroid-resistant INS.

The association of CsA and low-dose prednisone slightly improves results. Niaudet *et al.* [82] prospectively studied 65 children treated with a combination of CsA and prednisone for 5 months: 42% went into complete remission, 6% into partial remission and 52% failed to respond. The longest time to remission was 6 months. Eight patients who relapsed after CsA treatment responded further to prednisone alone, and nine patients had not relapsed more than 1 year after CsA withdrawal.

Adults. The results in adult INS are comparable to the foregoing data in children (for review, see reference 83). This is reflected by the study of the

French Collaborative Group of the Société de Néphrologie [39, 84]. It enrolled 112 patients, among whom 98 were considered valid for evaluating efficacy. There were 52 cases with MCD and 46 with FSG; 37/98 (38%) were steroid-dependent and 61/98 (62%) were steroid-resistant. Of 52 patients with MCD, 36 (69.23%) went into remission and 16 (30.76%) were failures. Of 46 patients with FSG, 11 (24%) underwent remission and 35 (76%) failed to respond. The rate of remission was highest in steroid-dependent MCD (71%) and lowest in steroid-resistant FSG (20%). Ponticelli *et al.* [85] confirmed the poor results of CsA treatment of steroid-resistant adult INS. In 12 adults, including 10 with FSG and two with MCD, they obtained partial remission in seven and five were failures.

Tolerance was analysed by Meyrier *et al.* [39]. Minor side-effects were common but led to withdrawal in less than 10% of cases. Renal tolerance was evaluated on the basis of renal function tests and in 36 cases on repeat renal biopsies. Renal function and histology were remarkably stable in patients with MCD. Conversely, when renal biopsy disclosed FSG, tubulointerstitial lesions which were already present on pre-CsA biopsies increased with time, along with declining renal function. This was interpreted as a combination of drug toxicity and the natural history of the primary renal disease. Multivariate analysis identified three predictive factors of CsA toxicity: FSG with accompanying tubulointerstitial injury, incipient renal insufficiency with serum creatinine levels >180 mmol/L, and CsA dosage >5.5 mg/kg per day. Aggravation of interstitial fibrosis and of FSG was observed in some cases in which CsA had obtained partial or even complete remission, indicating the necessity of repeat renal biopsies in patients so treated. An encouraging finding was that in 14/36 adults who had been treated with CsA for steroid-dependent or steroid-resistant INS during 26 ± 14.5 months, tailing off CsA to a stop was followed by stable remission, indicating that CsA dependency is not the rule. The same had been noted in children by Yoshikawa *et al.* [86].

Time to remisssion

The time to remission in CsA-responsive INS was analysed [87] by pooling data from seven studies including 104 steroid-dependent and 226 steroid-resistant patients, both children and adults. The cumulative rate of complete remission in steroid-dependent cases was in the order of 60% at 2 months, 75% at 3 months, reached 80% at 6 months, and thereafter increased very little. The same type of progression was observed in steroid-resistant cases, where the maximum cumulative rate of remission (20%) was achieved at 6 months. These figures indicate that failure of CsA can be declared at 6 months of treatment, provided dosage has been adequate, that is not less than 5 mg/kg per day.

FK 506

McCauley and co-authors published a report on their experience of FK 506 in the management of steroid-resistant nephrotic syndrome [88]. To the best of our knowledge, this is the only pilot trial of *Tacrolimus* in this condition. There were seven cases, including three with various glomerulopathies and four children with FSG. Prior therapy consisted of prednisone in all four with FSG, associated with CYC in one, CYC and CsA in two, and CsA in one. The initial response was no improvement in the case on prednisone and CYC, and a partial response in the three others on CsA. FK 506 induced complete remission in one case and a significant decline in proteinuria with a rise in serum albumin levels in the three others. Creatinine clearance decreased in all patients and renal function returned towards pretreatment values when the dosage was reduced or the drug was stopped. However, follow-up in this pilot trial was too short to appreciate long-term nephrotoxicity. The first case was followed up for 14 months and two attempts to stop FK 506 induced a flare-up in proteinuria, which resolved within days of reinstituting the drug. The overall impression left by this publication is that, similarly to CsA, FK 506 is variably effective in controlling proteinuria. It may induce complete remission in some cases and fail in others. McCauley *et al.* [88] speculated that differing responses to T-cell-directed therapy might indicate that nephrosis with lesions of FSG might be the consequence of various pathogenetic mechanisms.

Pefloxacin

Pefloxacin (P) is a fluoroquinolone. Its possible activity on nephrotic proteinuria due to MCD or FSG was serendipitously discovered in 1992 [89]. The present experience amounts to 32 cases enrolled in a French multicenter study [90]. Owing to cartilage toxicity of fluoroquinolones in children, only adults with MCD were included. Dosage was 400 mg b.i.d. for 1 month. In seven cases, P was first-line treatment of a first episode of nephrotic syndrome. The six other patients had previously experienced 2.7 ± 0.9 episodes; five had responded at least once to steroids and three had required an immunosuppressive regimen. Thirteen out of 32 patients (40.6%) went into remission. Complete (nine cases) or partial (four cases) remission was obtained within 2 months, that is during or after the end of P treatment. Three patients relapsed 3 months after obtaining complete remission. Two responded to a new course of P, and a third to glucocorticoids alone. The investigators were unable to identify predictive elements of success or failure. The mode of action of P in MCD is unknown. However, it is worth noting that another fluoroquinolone, ciprofloxacin, has been considered to have immunomodulating properties [91].

Other treatments

Other treatments have been proposed. Angiotensin-converting enzyme inhibitors reduce proteinuria in nephrotic patients, but their efficacy in INS stubbornly resistant to conventional therapy is distinctly less than in diabetic nephropathy [92]. Non-steroidal anti-inflammatory drugs, which in the past were also used for lowering nephrotic proteinuria, are now considered extremely hazardous in this situation. Finally, there are anecdotal reports of plasmapheresis [28], and plasma protein [27] or lipoprotein [93] adsorption, especially in cases of relapse of nephrotic FSG after renal transplantation, leading to transitory improvement in proteinuria. These manoeuvres await further assessment.

Conclusion

Nephrosis must still be considered a whimsical disease of unknown aetiology. That INS proceeds from an immunological derangement is more than probable. That MCD and FSG represent but two facets of the same condition remains to be indisputably established. The same applies to steroid-sensitive versus steroid-resistant forms, and to CsA-responsive versus CsA-resistant patients. Such uncertainties leave the prescribing nephrologist with the prospect of treating a disease of unknown pathophysiology with drugs whose mode of action is poorly understood. Such empiricism leads but to one practical recommendation: when every treatment has failed it is preferable to accept failure with humility rather than pursue therapeutic escalation with drugs which, in the long run, may prove to be more harmful than the disease itself.

Acknowledgements

Doreen Broneer typed this manuscript and prepared the bibliography with her usual care.

References

1. Fouque D, Laville M, Colon S *et al.* Cyclosporine A-sensitive nephrotic syndrome preceding Hodgkin's disease by 32 months. Clin Nephrol 1990;34:1–4.
2. Meyrier A, Delahousse M, Callard P, Rainfray M. Minimal change nephrotic syndrome revealing solid tumors. Nephron 1992;61:220–23.
3. D'Agati V. The many masks of focal segmental glomerulosclerosis. Kidney Int 1994;46:1223–41.
4. Habib R, Churg J, Bernstein J *et al.* Minimal change disease, mesangial proliferative glomerulonephritis and focal sclerosis: individual entities or a spectrum of disease? In: Robinson RR, Dennis VW, Ferris TF, Glassock RJ, Kokko JP, Tisher CC, editors. Nephrology. Proceedings of the IXth International Congress of Nephrology. New York: Springer-Verlag; 1984:634–44.
5. Fogo A, Glick AD, Horn SL, Horn RG. Is focal segmental glomerulosclerosis really focal? Distribution of lesions in adults and children. Kidney Int 1995;47:1690–6.

6. Fuiano G, Comi N, Magri P *et al.* Serial morphometric analysis of sclerotic lesions in primary 'focal' segmental glomerulosclerosis. J Am Soc Nephrol 1996;7:49–55.
7. Tejani A. Morphological transition in minimal change nephrotic syndrome. Nephron 1985;39: 157–9.
8. Fogo A, Hawkins EP, Berry PL *et al.* Glomerular hypertrophy in minimal change disease predicts subsequent progression to focal glomerular sclerosis. Kidney Int 1990;38:115–23.
9. Ramjee G, Coovadia HM, Adhikari M. Comparison of noninvasive methods for distinguishing steroid-sensitive nephrotic syndrome from focal glomerulosclerosis. J Lab Clin Med 1997;129: 47–52.
10. Burton C, Harris KPG. The role of proteinuria in the progression of chronic renal failure. Am J Kidney Dis 1996;27:765–75.
11. Benigni A, Zoja C, Remuzzi G. The renal toxicity of sustained glomerular protein traffic. Lab Invest 1995;73:461–8.
12. Schwartz MM, Lewis EJ. Focal segmental glomerular sclerosis: the cellular lesion. Kidney Int 1985;28:968–74.
13. Pei Y, Cattran D, Delmore T, Katz A, Lang A, Rance P. Evidence suggesting under-treatment in adults with idiopathic focal segmental glomerulosclerosis. Am J Med 1987;82:938–44.
14. Meyrier A, Simon P. Treatment of corticoresistant idiopathic nephrotic syndrome in the adult: minimal change disease and focal segmental glomerulosclerosis. Adv Nephrol 1988;17:127–50.
15. Korbet SM. Management of idiopathic nephrosis in adults, including steroid-resistant nephrosis. Curr Opin Nephrol Hypertens 1995;4:169–76.
16. Lagrue G, Branellec A, Niaudet P, Heslan JM, Guillot F, Lang P. Transmission d'un syndrome néphrotique à deux nouveau-nés. Régression spontanée. Presse Méd 1991;20:255–7.
17. Ali AA, Wilson E, Moorhead JF *et al.* Minimal-change glomerular nephritis. Normal kidneys in an abnormal environment? Transplantation 1994;58:849–51.
18. Guasch A, Deen WM, Myers BD. Charge selectivity of the glomerular filtration barrier in healthy and nephrotic humans. J Clin Invest 1993;92:2274–82.
19. Ota Z, Shikata K, Ota K. Nephrotic tunnels in glomerular basement membrane as revealed by a new electron microscopic method. J Am Soc Nephrol 1994;4:1965–73.
20. Shalhoub RJ. Pathogenesis of lipoid nephrosis: a disorder of T cell function. Lancet 1974;ii: 556–9.
21. Wilkinson AH, Gillespie C, Hartley B, Williams DG. Increase in proteinuria and reduction in number of anionic sites on the glomerular basement membrane in rabbits by infusion of human nephrotic plasma *in vivo*. Clin Sci 1989;88:43–8.
22. Tanaka R, Yoshikawa N, Nakamura H, Ito H. Infusion of peripheral blood mononuclear cell products from nephrotic children increases albuminuria in rats. Nephron 1992;60:35–41.
23. Koyama A, Fujisaki M, Kobayashi M, Igarashi M, Narita M. A glomerular permeability factor produced by human T cell hybridomas. Kidney Int 1991;40:453–60.
24. Heslan JM, Branellec AI, Laurent J, Lagrue G. The vascular permeability factor is a T lymphocyte product. Nephron 1986;42:187–8.
25. Tomizawa S, Nagasawa N, Maruyama K, Shimabukuro N, Arai H, Kuroume T. Release of the vascular permeability factor in minimal change nephrotic syndrome is related to CD4+ lymphocytes. Nephron 1990;56:341–2.
26. Zimmerman SW. Increased urinary protein excretion in the rat produced by serum from a patient with recurrent focal glomerular sclerosis after renal transplantation. Clin Nephrol 1984; 22:32–8.
27. Dantal J, Bigot E, Bogers W *et al.* Effect of plasma protein adsorption on protein excretion in kidney-transplant recipients with recurrent nephrotic syndrome. N Engl J Med 1994;330:7–14.
28. Artero M, Biava C, Amend W, Tomlanovich S, Vincenti F. Recurrent focal glomerulosclerosis: Natural history and response to therapy. Am J Med 1992;92:375–83.
29. Li PKT, MacMoune Lai F, Leung DB, Lui SF, Wang A, Lai KN. Plasma exchange in the treatment of early recurrent focal glomerulosclerosis after renal transplantation. Am J Nephrol 1993;13:289–92.

30. Savin VA, Sharma R, Sharma M *et al.* Circulating factor associated with increased glomerular permeability to albumin in recurrent focal segmental glomerulosclerosis. N Engl J Med 1996; 334:878–83.
31. Barness LA, Moll GH, Janeway CA. Nephrotic syndrome. Pediatrics 1950;5:486–503.
32. Arneil GC. 164 children with nephrosis. Lancet 1961;ii:1103–10.
33. Melvin T, Bennett W. Management of nephrotic syndrome in childhood. Drugs 1991;42:30–51.
34. ISKDC (International Study of Kidney Disease in Children) Ten years of activity: a report for the International Study of Kidney Disease in Children. In: Batsford SR *et al.*, editors. Glomerulonephritis. New York: John Wiley & Sons; 1977:201–9.
35. Murnaghan K, Vasmant D, Bensman A. Pulse methylprednisolone therapy in severe idiopathic childhood nephrotic syndrome. Acta Paediatr Scand 1984;73:733–9.
36. Bolton WK, Atuk NO, Sturgill BC, Westervelt FBJ. Therapy of the idiopathic nephrotic syndrome with alternate day steroids. Am J Med 1977;62:61–70.
37. Wang F, Looi LM, Chua CT. Minimal change glomerular disease in Malaysian adults and use of alternate day steroid therapy. Q J Med 1982;203:312–28.
38. Nair RB, Date A, Kirubakaran MG, Shastry JCM. Minimal-change nephrotic syndrome in adults treated with alternate day steroids. Nephron 1987;47:209–10.
39. Meyrier A, Noël LH, Auriche P, Callard P. Long-term renal tolerance of cyclosporin A treatment in adult idiopathic nephrotic syndrome. Kidney Int 1994;45:1446–56.
40. Nolasco F, Cameron JS, Heywood EF, Hicks J, Ogg C, Williams DJ. Adult-onset minimal change nephrotic syndrome: a long-term follow-up. Kidney Int 1986;29:1215–23.
41. Korbet SM, Schwartz MM, Lewis EJ. Minimal change glomerulopathy of adulthood. Am J Nephrol 1988;8:291–7.
42. Fujimoto S, Yamamoto Y, Hisanaga S, Morita S, Eto T, Tanaka K. Minimal change nephrotic syndrome in adults: response to corticosteroid therapy and frequency of relapse. Am J Kidney Dis 1991;17:687–92.
43. Mak SK, Short CD, Mallick NP. Long-term outcome of adult-onset minimal-change nephropathy. Nephrol Dial Transplant 1996;11:2192–201.
44. Meyrier, A. Treatment of idiopathic nephrotic syndrome with cyclosporine Am J Nephrol 1997; 10:14–24.
45. Glassock RJ. Therapy of idiopathic nephrotic syndrome in adults. Am J Nephrol 1993;13:422–8.
46. Balow JE. Cytotoxic drugs: rationale for management of glomerulonephritis. In: d'Amico G, Colasanti G, editors. Eclampsia, Glomerulonephritis, Uremia. Milano: Wichtig Editore; 1991: 106–10.
47. Chasis H, Goldring W, Baldwin DS. Effect of febrile plasma, typhoid vaccine and nitrogen mustard on renal manifestations of human glomerulonephritis. Proc Soc Exp Biol Med 1949; 71:565.
48. Schoeneman MJ, Spitzer A, Greifer, I. Nitrogen mustard therapy in children with frequent-relapsing nephrotic syndrome and steroid toxicity. Am J Kidney Dis 1983;2:526–9.
49. Broyer M, Meziane A, Kleinknecht D, Niaudet P. Nitrogen mustard therapy in idiopathic nephrotic syndrome of childhood. Int J Pediatr Nephrol 1985;6:29–34.
50. Al-Khader AA, Lien JW, Aber GM. Cyclophosphamide alone in the treatment of adult patients with minimal change glomerulonephritis. Clin Nephrol 1979;11:26–30.
51. Arbeitsgemeinschaft für Pädiatrische Nephrologie. Short versus standard prednisone therapy for initial treatment of idiopathic nephrotic syndrome in children. Lancet 1988;i:380–3.
52. Arbeitsgemeinschaft für Pädiatrische Nephrologie, Oemar BS, Brodehl J. Cyclophosphamide treatment of steroid dependent nephrotic syndrome: comparison of eight week with 12 week course. Arch Dis Child 1987;62:1102–6.
53. Bogdanovic R, Banicevic M, Cvoric A. Testicular function following cyclophosphamide treatment for childhood nephrotic syndrome: long-term follow-up study. Pediatr Nephrol 1990;4:451–4.
54. Talar-Williams C, Hijazi YM, Walther MM *et al.* Cyclophosphamide-induced cystitis and bladder cancer in patients with Wegener granulomatosis. Ann Intern Med 1996;124:477–84.

55. Arbeitsgemeinschaft für Pädiatrische Nephrologie. Effect of cytotroxic drugs in frequently relapsing nephrotic syndrome with or without steroid dependency. N Engl J Med 1982;306: 451–4.
56. Grupe WE. Cytotoxic drugs for nephrotic syndrome. N Engl J Med 1982;307:313.
57. Grupe WE, Makker SP, Ingelfinger JR. Chlorambucil treatment of frequently relapsing nephrotic syndrome. N Engl J Med 1976;295:746–9.
58. Broyer M, Meyrier A, Niaudet P, Habib R. Minimal changes and focal segmental glomerulosclerosis. In: Cameron S, Davison AM, Grünfeld JP, Kerr D, Ritz E, editors. Oxford Textbook of Clinical Nephrology. Oxford: Oxford University Press; 1992:298–339.
59. Elzouki AY, Jaiswal OP. Evaluation of chlorambucil therapy in steroid-dependent and cyclophosphamide-resistant children with nephrosis. Pediatr Nephrol 1990;4:459–62.
60. Kleinknecht C, Guesry P, Lenoir G, Broyer M. High-cost benefit of chlorambucil in frequently relapsing nephrosis. N Engl J Med 1977;296:48.
61. Mendoza SA, Tune BM. Treatment of childhood nephrotic syndrome. J Am Soc Nephrol 1992; 3:889–94.
62. Tune BM, Kirpekar R, Sibley RK, Reznik VM, Griswold WR, Mendoza SA. Intravenous methylprednisolone and oral alkylating agent therapy of prednisone-resistant pediatric focal segmental glomerulosclerosis: a long-term follow-up. Clin Nephrol 1995;43:84–8.
63. Abramovicz M, Barnett HI, Edelmann CMJ *et al.* Controlled trial of azathioprine in children with nephrotic syndrome. Lancet 1970;ii:959–61.
64. Linshaw MA, Gruskin AB. Management of the nephrotic syndrome. A summary of progress in the use of immunosuppressive therapy. Clin Pediatr 1974;13:45–51.
65. Lagrue G, Bariéty J, de Boisdeffre B, Milliez P. L'azathioprine dans les glomérulopathies primitives. Résultats préliminaires dans 24 cas. J Urol Néphrol 1968;74:327–33.
66. Cade R, Mars D, Privette M *et al.* Effect of long-term azathioprine administration in adults with minimal-change glomerulonephritis and nephrotic syndrome resistant to corticosteroids. Arch Intern Med 1986;146:737–41.
67. British Association for Paediatric Nephrology. Levamisole for corticosteroid-dependent nephrotic syndrome in childhood. Lancet 1991;337:1555–7.
68. Tejani A, Ingulli E. Current concepts of pathogenesis of nephrotic syndrome. In: Tejani A, editor. Cyclosporin in the Therapy of Renal Disease. Basel: Karger; 1995:1–5.
69. Meyrier A. Antiproteinuric and immunologic effects of cyclosporin A in the treatment of glomerular diseases. Nephrol Dial Transplant 1992;7:80–4.
70. Jameson MD, Savin VJ, Sharma R, Lovell HB, Diederich DA. Cyclosporine treatment decreases glomerular ultrafiltration coefficient. National Kidney Foundation 19th Scientific Meeting. Abstract A12; 1989.
71. Berden JHM, Schrijver G, Assmann KJM, Koene RAP. Antiproteinuric effect of cyclosporin (CsA) in anti-GBM nephritis in the mouse. Proceedings of the 2nd Congress on Immunointervention in Autoimmune Diseases, Paris: 185, 1991.
72. Desassis JF, Raats CJI, Bakker MAH, van den Born J, Berden JHM. Antiproteinuric effect of ciclosporin A in adriamycin nephropathy in rats. Nephron 1997;75:336–41.
73. Zietse R, Derkx FHM, Schalekamp MADH, Weimar W. Cyclosporin and the glomerular filtration barrier in minimal change disease and membranous glomerulopathy. In: Tejani A, editor. Cyclosporin in the Therapy of Renal Disease. Basel: Karger; 1995:6–18.
74. Meyrier A. Treatment of glomerular disease with cyclosporine A. Nephrol Dial Transpl 1989;4: 923–31.
75. Niaudet P, Habib R. Cyclosporine in the treatment of idiopathic nephrosis. J Am Soc Nephrol 1994;5:1049–56.
76. Tejani A, Suthanthiran M, Pomerantz A. A randomized controlled trial of low-dose prednisone and ciclosporine versus high-dose prednisone in nephrotic syndrome of children. Nephron 1991;59:96–9.
77. Ingulli E, Tejani A. Severe hypercholesterolemia inhibits cyclosporin A efficacy in a dose-dependent manner in children with nephrotic syndrome. J Am Soc Nephrol 1992;3:254–59.

78. Lieberman KV, Tejani A. A randomized double-blind placebo-controlled trial of cyclosporine in steroid-resistant idiopathic focal segmental glomerulosclerosis in children. J Am Soc Nephrol 1996;7:56–63.
79. Niaudet P, and French Society of Pediatric Nephrology. Comparison of cyclosporine and chlorambucil in the treatment of steroid-dependent idiopathic nephrotic syndrome: a multicenter randomized controlled trial. Pediatr Nephrol 1992;6:1–3.
80. Niaudet P, Broyer M, Habib R. Serial renal biopsies in children with idiopathic nephrosis receiving cyclosporin. In: Tejani A, editor. Cyclosporin in the Therapy of Renal Disease. Basel: Karger; 1995:78–83.
81. Melocoton TL, Kamil ES, Cohen AH, Fine RN. Long-term cyclosporine A treatment of steroid-resistant and steroid-dependent nephrotic syndrome. Am J Kidney Dis 1991;18:583–8.
82. Niaudet P, and French Society of Pedicatric Nephrology. Treatment of childhood steroid-resistant idiopathic nephrosis with a combination of cyclosporine and prednisone. J Pediatr 1994;125:981–6.
83. Meyrier A. Use of cyclosporin in the treatment of idiopathic nephrotic syndrome in adults. In: Tejani A, editor. Cyclosporin in the Therapy of Renal Disease. Basel: Karger; 1995:28–48.
84. Meyrier A, Niaudet P, Brodehl J. Optimal use of Sandimmun in nephrotic syndrome (monograph). Berlin: Springer-Verlag; 1992:1–34 .
85. Ponticelli C, Rizzoni G, Edefonti A *et al.* A randomized trial of cyclosporine in steroid-resistant idiopathic nephrotic syndrome. Kidney Int 1993;43:1377–84.
86. Yoshikawa N, Tanaka R, Kitano Y, Nakamura H, Ito H. Long-term cyclosporin in steroid-dependent nephrotic syndrome. In: Tejani A, editor. Cyclosporin in the Therapy of Renal Disease. Basel: Karger; 1995:19–27.
87. Collaborative Study Group of Sandimmun in Nephrotic Syndrome. Safety and tolerability of cyclosporin A (Sandimmun) in idiopathic nephrotic syndrome. Clin Nephrol 1991;35(Suppl.1): S48–60.
88. McCauley J, Shapiro R, Ellis D, Igdal H, Tzakis A, Starzl TE. Pilot trial of FK 506 in the management of steroid-resistant nephrotic syndrome. Nephrol Dial Transplant 1993;8:1286–90.
89. Pruna A, Metivier F, Akposso K *et al.* Pefloxacin as first-line treatment in nephrotic syndrome [letter]. Lancet 1992;340:728–9.
90. Pruna A, Barka A, Nochy D, Hauet T, Boulanger H, Landais P. Pefloxacine comme traitement de première intention du syndrome néphrotique à lésions glomérulaires minimes de l'adulte. Etude multicentrique de 32 malades. Néphrologie 1997;18:95–101.
91. Riesbeck K, Gullberg M, Forsgren A. Evidence that the antibiotic ciprofloxacin counteracts cyclosporine-dependent suppression of cytokine production. Transplantation 1994;57:267–72.
92. Korbet S, Schwartz M, Lewis E. Primary focal segmental glomerulosclerosis: clinical course and response to therapy. Am J Kidney Dis 1994;23:773–83.
93. Faucher C, Albert C, Beaufils H, Jouanneau C, Dupouet L. Remission of a refractory nephrotic syndrome after low-density lipoprotein apheresis based on dextran sulphate adsorption. Nephrol Dial Transplant 1997;12:1037–9.

4. Membranous glomerulopathy

C.D. SHORT

Introduction

Membranous nephropathy (MN) defines a state of variable and evolving histopathological change within the glomeruli of the renal cortex [1]. It is referred to as idiopathic disease when it occurs for reasons that are as yet uncertain. Less commonly it can be found in association with other clinical disorders or, rarely, it may become manifest after exposure to certain drugs or toxins; in these situations it is termed secondary MN [2]. While perhaps somewhat artificial, because the term 'idiopathic' merely emphasizes our current ignorance of the aetiology and pathogenesis of the condition, this division is probably vital to the development of further understanding of MN, and certainly has particular relevance when considering the therapeutic options that are available.

Interestingly, a histological picture which is virtually identical to human membranous nephropathy (HMN) may be found in a number of other animals, occurring either spontaneously, for example in cats and dogs [3], or induced deliberately in experimental animals, usually rats [4] or rabbits [5]. Laboratory studies performed under the controlled conditions of experimentation have clearly contributed to unravelling what may eventually prove to be the pathogenetic mechanisms responsible for the development of idiopathic HMN (IHMN) in some patients [6]. However, this approach has made little or no progress towards determining the aetiological agent(s) responsible for the majority of cases of HMN, and neither has it yet led directly to any significant improvement in the design of treatment regimens.

There are no pathognomonic clinical, serological or radiographic features associated with membranous nephropathy, and thus a definitive diagnosis is dependent upon an adequate renal biopsy thoroughly examined by the appropriate techniques of immunofluorescence, light and electron microscopy.

Clinical features

In 70% of cases, IHMN presents to the clinician as a typical nephrotic syndrome (NS) when the patient has noticed the development of progressive, dependent oedema [7]. Perhaps the most commonly associated clinical feature,

C.D. Pusey (ed.), The Treatment of Glomerulonephritis, 55–79.

yet one that is frequently overlooked, is the non-specific complaint of generalized lethargy. This symptom is extremely common and undoubtedly genuine. Initially, the oedema may be intermittent; often it is accompanied by excessive frothing of the urine, although patients frequently forget to mention this phenomenon until asked directly. Less than 10% of patients give a history of antecedent infection [8] and only very occasionally, in less than 5% of adults, is macroscopic haematuria reported [9]. Presentation with uraemia is particularly rare. It is important to recognize that the time of clinical manifestation of the disorder does not necessarily equate with onset of the disease. Indeed, analysis of (a) long-term follow-up studies of patients who went into remission and subsequently suffered relapse, (b) observations on the development of HMN following drug exposure, and (c) serial investigations when there has been recurrence of the disease in a renal allograft, suggests that proteinuria may gradually increase over several months before the condition becomes symptomatic [10, 11].

Virtually all patients with idiopathic disease who do not present with oedema will have come to clinical attention because of asymptomatic proteinuria, that is with dipstick-positive proteinuria or a formally quantified abnormal amount of protein in the urine. This is most commonly detected at a medical examination for insurance or employment purposes; occasionally it follows routine urinalysis during investigation of an unrelated condition. Approximately 50% of patients whose initial manifestation of IHMN is with asymptomatic proteinuria alone eventually become frankly oedematous [10]; the rest almost invariably go into biochemical remission without progression of the disease, either in terms of increased proteinuria or impairment of renal function. This implies that there is an untold number of individuals in the community who develop IHMN, remain symptom-free, never have their urine tested at the appropriate time, and thus are never investigated or documented. Presumably, the condition heals spontaneously in these circumstances. It should be remembered that these observations are based on the available published reports, the vast majority of which emanate from the industrialized societies of Europe, North America, Australasia and Japan [12–20] and may not be representative of other parts of the world from where, for the most part, detailed information is still lacking. Patients with secondary MN may or may not exhibit symptoms referable to the underlying disease. Furthermore, such symptoms may not always be present at the time the nephropathy becomes obvious, although they may appear later.

Epidemiology

While the nephrotic syndrome may be associated with a variety of underlying glomerular lesions, in most reported series from westernized societies IHMN remains the commonest cause, usually accounting for 20–25% of the total nephrotic presentations [2]. An analysis of the Glomerular Disease Registry in the North West of England of nearly 1000 first native kidney biopsies performed during the years 1990–94 inclusive has confirmed that this percentage currently remains unchanged. It is virtually identical both to the figure derived from a similar population undergoing renal biopsy between the years 1960 and 1980 [21] and to the data published by the UK Medical Research Council for the years 1978–1985 [22]. It has been claimed, though, that the proportion of patients with NS due to IHMN increases with age, possibly reaching 35% in patients over 60 years [23]. The true incidence of IHMN cannot be known for the reasons discussed in consideration of patients with asymptomatic proteinuria.

Most series of IHMN report that males are twice as frequently affected as females in adult-onset disease [12–20, 24–26]. In children, though, the two sexes are probably affected in equal proportion, although in absolute numbers children are affected only rarely [27, 28]. While the diagnosis of IHMN is made most commonly during the fourth and fifth decades of life [14, 29, 30], it has been reported at both extremes of age [31, 32]. In children, secondary HMN is more likely to be found in association with SLE or infection [2], especially with hepatitis B, and in the elderly the commoner association is with an underlying malignancy, usually a carcinoma [33].

Aetiology

For the majority of patients with IHMN, no aetiological agent has yet been documented. Furthermore, it remains possible that, given the wide variety of agents incriminated in secondary disease, more than one factor will eventually prove responsible. Despite this deficit in current knowledge, and the fact that the pathological features clearly implicate, but do not conclusively prove, an immunological pathogenesis, it has become clear from many studies that IHMN appears to develop in immunologically predisposed individuals [34]. A number of reports from across the world have confirmed, in Caucasian [35, 36] and Chinese [37] populations, that IHMN will develop preferentially in individuals who are HLA DR3 positive. Interestingly, IHMN in Japan is associated with HLA DR2 [38]. A number of other immunogenetic markers in different communities have been reported to be associated with IHMN, including: (a) deletion of the C4A gene [39]; (b) a specific C7 phenotype [40]; (c) the presence of the HLA genotypes DQA1 and DQw1 [41]; and (d) homozygosity for HLA DRB1 [42]. Other immunological aberrations reported, including Gm allotypes [43], CD4/8 T cell ratios in peripheral blood [44], Fc receptor function [45], and TNF-α production from peripheral blood mononuclear cells, have proved to be more contentious [46]. However, the concept of the immunologically predisposed individual would seem to hold true, although it should be remembered that only a proportion of patients with HMN exhibit the genetic markers mentioned.

Consideration of secondary HMN is of particular importance in discussion of the management of membranous nephropathy. Appropriate treatment of any associated or underlying condition may alleviate or even cure the nephropathy and therefore assiduous assessment of the patient is warranted. Around 20% of patients from most unselected series have secondary disease [2]. The main conditions associated with HMN can be grouped conveniently into: (a) rheumatological diseases; (b) infectious diseases; (c) malignancies; (d) drug or toxin related; and (e) miscellaneous disorders. A detailed discussion and comprehensive list of secondary HMN is outside the scope of this chapter, but can be found in more exhaustive texts [7]. Moreover, some of the reputed associations are dependent on isolated case reports and may, therefore, have occurred solely by chance. Other associations, though, are undoubtedly authentic and probably even causally related. Even when the coexistence of two disorders is uncommon, antigen and/or antibody from the putative primary condition has occasionally been demonstrated in, or eluted from, the glomeruli [47–50]; these observations would suggest a genuine aetiological relationship. A list of the more common or important associated or underlying conditions is given in Table 4.1. I have omitted the oft-quoted and, world-wide, probably the commonest causes of secondary MN: malaria, filaria and schistosomiasis. Although these conditions have a high prevalence in the populations at risk, the finding of antigen or antibody in the glomeruli of patients with coexistent HMN is reported rarely.

Table 4.1 Conditions associated with membranous nephropathy

Rheumatological
Systemic lupus erythematosus
Rheumatoid arthritis
Infectious
Hepatitis B
Hepatitis C
Syphilis
Malignancies
Carcinomata: lung, gastrointestinal tract, breast, cervix
Lymphoma
Leukaemia
Drugs and toxins
Gold
Penicillamine
Mercury compounds
NSAID
Miscellaneous
Sarcoidosis
Thyroid disease
Diabetes mellitus

Glomerular involvement is common in systemic lupus erythematosus (SLE), with a membranous lesion accounting for perhaps 25% of patients with lupus nephropathy [51]. Overt nephropathy may predate clinical features of SLE, or vice-versa, or both may be manifest coincidentally [52]. Careful histological appraisal of the light microscopy changes, immunofluorescence pattern, or the electron micrographs may reveal changes that suggest SLE is the underlying disorder even in the absence of typical clinical findings [53]. The development of HMN in conjunction with rheumatoid arthritis (RA) is most frequently associated with exposure to gold [54], penicillamine [55] or non-steroidal anti-inflammatory agents (NSAID) [56], but it can undoubtedly occur in the absence of such treatment [57]. Like SLE, however, a number of other glomerular lesions may be responsible for the finding of proteinuria or haematuria in a patient with RA.

Hepatitis B, with the 'e' antigen now implicated as the specific aetiological agent [58], is one of many reported infectious agents capable of eliciting the characteristic histological change of HMN. This has been a particular feature of the disorder in the Far East and in children. Although the 'e' antigen is probably causal, 'e' and core antigen may not be detected in the serum which usually tests positive for the 's' antigen. More recently, the association of HMN with hepatitis C has received increasing attention and remains to be defined more fully [59]. The association with syphilis [60], despite being reported rarely, deserves mention because: (a) it is documented in both congenital and acquired disease; (b) it is one of the few conditions where implicated antigen and antibody (treponemal) have been demonstrated in the glomeruli; and (c) it responds to anti-treponemal antibiotic treatment, stressing the importance of considering secondary HMN before embarking on relatively non-specific forms of therapy.

The association of malignancy and nephropathy is well known [33]. When present, the associated tumour in HMN is nearly always derived from an epithelial cell lineage, i.e. it will be a carcinoma. It most frequently originates in lung or gastrointestinal tract but many other sites are reported [61]. Experience over the past three decades suggests that the overall incidence of carcinoma with HMN is approximately 5%, or less, and not 10% as was originally suggested [62]. However, the incidence may be as high as 20% in patients initially presenting over the age of 60 years [2]. Very occasionally, successful treatment of the malignancy has been followed by resolution of the nephropathy [63]. This is highly suggestive of a causal role for the tumour, rather than this being a coincidental finding, or both malignancy and nephropathy arising in response to a common predisposing factor.

Therapeutic agents are implicated in the genesis of HMN in perhaps 10% of patients. Those affected may be of any age, unlike infection-associated HMN which is usually found in children or malignancy-associated HMN which is almost exclusively restricted to the older patient. The clinical manifestation, usually proteinuria, most often occurs soon after initial exposure. The vast majority of such patients have RA and have received the drugs mentioned earlier. Resolution is virtually assured with withdrawal of the offending agent [64]. With gold and penicillamine treatment, patients are usually monitored for the development of such side-effects and either are not biopsied or are investigated soon after urinary abnormalities have become apparent. In these circumstances, the light microscopic changes may not have become obvious and immunofluorescence and electron microscopy techniques will be essential to confirm the clinical diagnosis. It has become clear in recent years that exposure to a number of NSAID can be temporally related to the onset of nephrotic syndrome, which on biopsy is shown to be due to HMN [65]. Despite the widespread use of these drugs the number of reports is relatively small. Finally, and perhaps more of historical interest, the occasional report still documents contact with mercury as a precipitant in the development of HMN, no longer after treatment with mercury-containing diuretics or industrial exposure, but following the use of mercury-based skin-lightening creams [66].

A number of distinct medical conditions have been observed to occur disproportionately in patients with HMN. In some, such as Graves' disease [67], insulin-dependent diabetes mellitus [68] and Sjögren's syndrome [69], the increased incidence may be because they are also HLA DR3-associated disorders. In others, such as sickle-cell disease [70], sarcoidosis [71] and primary biliary cirrhosis [72], the association remains unexplained.

HMN may also be found in up to 3% of renal allografts [73]. In a minority of patients it occurs as proven recurrent disease but it is a *de-novo* occurrence in probably twice as many [74]. Renal transplant recipients are the subject of close medical supervision and thus allograft HMN is most frequently discovered by routine dipstick urinalysis. In recurrent disease there is usually evidence of rejection in the biopsy [75]; *de-novo* HMN has been documented as being associated with episodes of post-transplantation obstruction [76]. The explanation for these phenomena is unclear.

Investigation

Urinary analysis reveals that, at some time during the course of the illness, 80% of adult patients will exhibit proteinuria in excess of 3.5 g/24 h and in 30% it will exceed 10 g/24 h; in the occasional patient, values of more than 20 g/24 h have been recorded [77]. As previously mentioned, macroscopic haematuria is particularly rare, but up to 50% of patients will have demonstrable microscopic haematuria – the frequency is reported as being even higher in children [14]. Glycosuria in the presence of a normal blood sugar is not uncommon. The terminal complex of the complement activation pathway, C5b-9, is frequently detectable in urine and probably indicates on-going immunological insult [78].

Renal function at presentation, as judged by serum creatinine, is normal in more than 90% of patients [14, 15]. Other biochemical investigations reveal a variably decreased plasma albumin, usually accompanied by low or low-normal levels of circulating IgG but frequently with a raised serum IgM [79].

Plasma fibrinogen is also present in increased amounts, as may be other components of the coagulation cascade [80]. Raised low-density lipoprotein (LDL) and very-low-density lipoprotein (VLDL) concentrations are responsible for high total cholesterol and triglyceride values, respectively [81]. These are well-known characteristics of the nephrotic syndrome in general. In membranous nephropathy in particular, a normal total high-density lipoprotein (HDL) concentration has been reported, but with raised and lowered levels, respectively, of the HDL3 and HDL2 components [82]. Furthermore, the serum concentration of lipoprotein (a) is raised in patients with proteinuria >3.5 g/24 h but within the normal range in IHMN patients in remission [83]. Unless the underlying condition is SLE, C3 and C4 levels are usually normal [84]. Other evidence of an associated condition may, of course, be detected, e.g. anti-DNA antibodies or hepatitis markers.

Most of the pertinent investigations have been mentioned in the preceding paragraphs and, along with additional investigative procedures, they are listed in Table 4.2. In the case of a patient presenting with a history, symptoms and signs of underlying glomerular disease, a renal biopsy is usually indicated. The purpose of investigation is to: (a) further specify the diagnosis; (b) determine if there is an underlying or associated condition; (c) detect non-renal morbidity; (d) assess prognosis; and (e) quantify the degree of end-organ damage. Progress or resolution, either with or without active therapeutic intervention, can then be accurately documented and assessed. Certain investigations will only be indicated in some patients, such as a search for gastrointestinal malignancy in an elderly patient with positive faecal occult blood tests or an iron-deficiency anaemia.

Table 4.2 Investigations for membranous nephropathy

24-hour urinary protein	Lipoprotein profile
Urine microscopy	Complement profile
Serum creatinine	Antinuclear factor
Creatinine clearance	Anti-DNA antibodies
Plasma albumin	Hepatitis serology
Serum immunoglobulin profile	Cryoglobulins
Serum (immuno)electrophoresis	Chest X-ray
Urine (immuno)electrophoresis	Renal biopsy

Pathology

The histological characteristics of HMN are: (a) diffuse, global and uniform thickening of the peripheral capillary loops, in the absence of a significant increase in cellular components of the glomerular tuft, as seen on light microscopy with PAS or H and E staining; (b) thickening and 'spiking' of the basement membranes outwards from the subepithelial aspect, best demonstrated with the silver methanamine stain which is preferentially taken up by the matrix of the glomerular basement membrane (GBM); (c) the demonstration, by an immunofluorescence method using FITC-labelled antibodies, of IgG and C3 along the GBM in a discrete and beaded fashion; and (d) the visualization on electron micrographs of distinct collections of electron-dense material along the subepithelial aspect of the GBM between, and even around, which the thickened GBM may extend [9].

The histology of HMN is best interpreted as representing an evolutional process, starting (probably) with the formation in the subepithelial space of immune deposits, which may be followed by a glomerular reaction to this phenomenon and, sometimes, its subsequent resolution [1]. The timing of the biopsy and extent of progression of any of these phases, together with whether or not any underlying condition is present, appears to dictate the findings in any given biopsy. Thickening of the GBM may not be apparent on light microscopy early in the course of the disease or if the insult is mild. Similarly, the extension of the GBM between the deposits may not have occurred; at the other extreme it may have surrounded the deposits giving the appearance of chain links. Careful examination may reveal a slight increase in mesangial cellularity, more particularly if there is an underlying rheumatological condition. Crescentic lesions have also been described, previously in association with circulating anti-GBM antibodies in the context of super-added anti-GBM disease [85], but most recently in association with circulating antineutrophil cytoplasmic antibodies (ANCA) with coincident evidence of either renally restricted or systemic vasculitis [86]. There may be a degree of coexistent interstitial damage which has been shown to be a sensitive indicator of a poor prognosis [87]. The immunofluorescence staining may sometimes reveal IgA or IgM in place of, or in addition to, IgG, most often if SLE is present. Occasionally neither C3 nor even IgG may be demonstrated.

It is the electron microscopic appearance, though, that is the defining hallmark of HMN [9]. The deposits may: (a) be very small and lie along the lamina rara externa, apparently having elicited no histopathological reaction; (b) appear somewhat larger with interposing projections of GBM-like matrix; (c) be surrounded by the GBM; or (d) have even disappeared from the middle of the grossly thickened, enlarged and distorted GBM, leaving it full of holes and looking like a 'Swiss cheese'. These varying appearances have been described as 'stages' by some authors, but unfortunately without much consistency, such that it is necessary to know which author's classification is being used for any given appearance [88–91]. There is limited evidence, after biochemical remission has occurred, that the histology resolves and the GBM remodels with time, although it is stated that there is a greater possibility of resolution if the lesion is less advanced.

The pathogenesis of HMN remains an enigma, despite the advances made in unravelling the processes involved in experimental animal models [92]. The available evidence would suggest that HMN is an immunologically mediated disorder. First, the known immunogenetic associations of IHMN, and some groups of secondary HMN, indicate that a perturbation in the immunological response may be involved. Secondly, characteristic immunoglobulin and complement deposition along the GBM is strong evidence that the pathogenesis is immunologically driven. Thirdly, evidence accrued from animal models, such as Heymann nephritis, which produce a virtually identical histological picture although with a different clinical course, provides strong evidence for the hypothesis [6]. There is no single explanation in IHMN, however, as to how and why the immunoglobulin is deposited along the subepithelial border of the GBM.

For many years it was believed that appropriately sized immune complexes circulating in the blood traversed the GBM intact and lodged there, in a more or less 'innocent bystander' scenario [93]. It took little imagination to suggest the possibility that these complexes dissociated before crossing the GBM and re-formed on the urinary aspect of the membrane. A great deal of work with the Heymann model has shown that, in this experimental model, newly formed or preformed antibodies directed against an intrinsic epitope(s) on the basal surface of the glomerular epithelial cell (GEC) will induce the membranous lesion. In the 'active' variant of this animal model, following immunization with a crude tubular brush-border extract, the injected animals produce antibody against the Heymann nephritis antigenic complex (HNAC), which is a structural component of the GEC composed of a glycoprotein, GP330, and a receptor-associated protein (RAP) [94]. Unfortunately, this antigen complex is not present in human GEC. In other animal models it has been demonstrated that endogenous or exogenous antigen may become lodged ('planted') in the subepithelial space and that appropriate specific antibody binds to it subsequently [95]. The precise process in IHMN is unknown and may even be due to more than one of the mechanisms described, the antigenic component being either an intrinsic part of the GBM or GEC, or a 'planted' endogenous or exogenous molecule. In some cases of secondary HMN, associated with hepatitis B or malignancy, there is good reason to believe that an antigenic component has become lodged in the capillary wall, and then attracts the relevant antibody.

Recently, the claim for the formation of circulating complexes followed by dissociation and reformation in the subepithelial space, has been restated [96]. The hypothesis suggests that the pathogenetic mechanism involves the production of low-affinity IgG4 antibodies against diverse antigenic stimuli. The IgG4/antigen complexes then formed would not be cleared in the usual way via complement-mediated pathways and the liver, since IgG4 does not bind to C1q. However, IgG4 does activate the complement cascade via the alternative pathway, which would explain why C3 deposition along the GBM takes place and how C5b-9 may be found in the urine in human IMN as well as in experimental animals. It should be remembered, however, that although IgG4 is usually found along the GBM when specific subclasses are looked for, most studies report finding the other IgG subclasses in addition [97].

Natural history

The prognosis of patients with secondary MN may be dependent upon the progress of the underlying disease rather than that of the nephropathy. The outcome for a patient with a malignancy may be poor whatever treatment is offered, drug-induced HMN usually responds to withdrawal of the offending agent, and effective treatment of underlying infection is followed by resolution of the nephropathy.

The clinical course of patients with IHMN, however, is extremely variable. If all patients are considered together, that is those with asymptomatic proteinuria and those with a nephrotic syndrome, then remission, usually with a normal glomerular filtration rate, is the most frequent outcome although this may take many years. Following remission, up to 30% of patients will subsequently relapse; however, the outlook for these patients is still good with further remission likely [11, 14, 98]. The most recently reported series and analyses suggest that by 20 years between 25% and 30% of patients will have developed end-stage renal failure [17, 30, 99–101]. The data are difficult to find, but in patients who are not exposed to immunosuppressive therapies it appears that, once started, the decline in renal function is relentlessly progressive [102]. The remainder of the patients will have persisting proteinuria, generally with stable normal renal function, over many years. By implication, patients who undergo remission and those with persisting proteinuria and stable, albeit occasionally mildly impaired, renal function do not die from renal failure, but the complications associated with IHMN, such as hypertension and ischaemic heart disease, may be contributory.

A number of factors have been documented, but not always confirmed in other reports or upon rigorous analysis, to have prognostic significance in IHMN. Undoubtedly, patients who never develop an overt nephrotic syndrome are less likely to develop end-stage renal failure. Furthermore, women and children are relatively infrequently reported as becoming dialysis-dependent [103]. Conversely, heavy proteinuria, hypertension and impaired renal function when first assessed, indicate a worse prognosis. The staging of the glomerular lesion may have some bearing on outcome, particularly if advanced, but the extent of tubulo-interstitial damage has long been known to correlate more accurately with subsequent impairment of renal function.

For reasons that are not entirely clear, there is significant variability in the capacity of otherwise similar patients, with similar amounts of proteinuria, to maintain a given level of plasma albumin. Nevertheless, patients with membranous nephropathy, particularly those with heavy proteinuria, are at risk of developing a number of clinical sequelae, which are directly or indirectly related to urinary protein loss. Certainly, hypoalbuminaemia will contribute to the development of dependent oedema, although this is probably also a function of intrarenal perturbation of salt and water retention in association with circulating or locally produced vascular permeability factor(s). Minimal ankle oedema is probably of little clinical consequence; however, larger amounts are not only cosmetically undesirable but may predispose to infection if the local area is traumatized, particularly as serum IgG is almost invariably diminished and especially if the patient is receiving immunosuppressive drugs.

The nephrotic state in general, and probably HMN in particular, is regarded as a hypercoagulable state. Typically, raised plasma levels of fibrinogen and the coagulation cascade factors V and VIII, in association with low levels of the anticoagulant factor antithrombin III, are found [104]. The increased concentration of apolipoprotein (a), the protein moiety of Lp(a), which has sequence homology with plasminogen but lacks the active protease domain and thus may act to inhibit thrombolysis, could indirectly promote thrombosis. In conjunction with the clotting factor abnormalities already described, this combination may be responsible for the observed increased incidence of venous thrombosis. The renal vein in particular may be affected; the event may be symptomatic, with flank pain and haematuria, or clinically silent leading to an abrupt yet unexpected decline in renal function. A sudden decline in renal function should also prompt the search for other rare but recognized complications of IHMN such as uncontrolled hypertension, superimposed anti-GBM disease, or ANCA-positive glomerulonephritis, in addition to treatment-related problems such as diuretic-induced interstitial nephritis [105] or hypovolaemia [106].

The raised Lp(a) level may also be a factor in the development of ischaemic heart disease, which has now been clearly documented in a series of patients with NS, in which the commonest underlying glomerulopathy was HMN [107]. Hypertension, hypercholesterolaemia and hypertriglyceridaemia are almost certainly additional contributory factors.

Treatment

The various aspects of HMN have been dealt with at length quite intentionally. In the absence of specific therapies aimed at known aetiological agents or well-defined pathogenetic processes, it remains probable that no single, empirically derived therapeutic regimen will be ideal treatment for all patients with HMN. It is clear that HMN is unlikely to be a homogeneous condition – much variability exists in the clinical features, pathology, course, complications and prognosis – and there is no universal consensus on the best treatment options, even for the secondary effects of this condition, such as hypoalbuminaemia, hypertension, hypercholesterolaemia or hypercoagulability, let alone the presumed immunologically mediated process. The therapeutic approach to each individual, therefore, may need a significant amount of consideration based upon the features outlined previously.

Undoubtedly of paramount importance is the need to exclude secondary causes of HMN. Appropriate treatment of an incriminated malignancy or infection, withdrawal of an implicated drug, or cessation of exposure to a suspected toxin may be all that is needed to effect complete and lasting cure.

Furthermore, steroids, which may be considered in the treatment of a patient with IHMN, may have a disastrous effect on a patient who has hepatitis B [108]. Conversely, while there are few available data on the specific treatment of allograft membranous nephropathy, high-dose steroid treatment has been reported as effective [109].

Further consideration of the treatment of patients with IHMN then falls into a number of areas, which can be regarded as supportive, prophylactic or therapeutic. The measures employed are directed predominantly at the metabolic consequences of proteinuria, or are used in an endeavour to change the immunopathogenetic processes of the nephropathy.

General measures

Initially, and where appropriate, an attempt should be made to alter certain facets of the patients' lifestyle. They should be strongly advised to stop smoking, not only as a general health education measure, but more specifically in the context of the increased risk of cardiovascular disease. Similarly, a relevant exercise programme should be encouraged.

Following professional assessment, suitable modifications to the diet may need to be suggested. These would include salt restriction where hypertension or marked oedema is present. Protein and calorie intake may also require adjustment. Very high protein diets are no longer recommended. However, hypoalbuminaemia can be minimized by a daily protein intake of 1 g per kg body weight plus 1 g per gram of urinary protein. It is important to provide sufficient non-protein calories in addition, and 200 kcal/g of nitrogen intake is recommended. In severely nephrotic patients a vicious cycle of nausea, anorexia and progressive hypoalbuminaemia may ensue, such that a period of overnight supplemental nasogastric feeding may be indicated.

From the patients' perspective, the most important symptom to be dealt with is usually the oedema. Careful titration of drug dose with effect, initially with a loop diuretic such as frusemide or bumetanide (the latter is better absorbed in nephrotic states), and subsequently with the addition of spironolactone, is usually sufficient to minimize the peripheral swelling. On occasions the potent additive effect of the thiazide diuretic metolazone will be required. Weight loss of around 1 kg per day should be attempted; if it exceeds this for more than a couple of days there is a risk of circulatory collapse, precipitation of acute renal failure, and theoretically exacerbation of the risk of thromboembolic phenomena. It frequently becomes clear with the disappearance of the excess fluid that a significant amount of body weight has been lost during the course of the illness. Current evidence suggests that there is no indication for the use of intravenous albumin since it is rapidly lost in the urine [110] and while bed rest is known to promote diuresis, the risk of venous thrombosis must be considered.

Some authorities advise the use of full prophylactic anticoagulation in all patients with membranous nephropathy and the nephrotic syndrome [111]. Experience suggests that a generally successful approach is to institute treatment with subcutaneous heparin twice daily for as long as the plasma albumin level remains below 20 g/L, but to anticoagulate fully with warfarin for a period of 3 months if venous thrombosis or thromboembolism develops, whatever the level of plasma albumin [112]. If a period of immobilization is considered, or enforced for clinical reasons, then the anticoagulant policy would need to be reviewed.

The lipoprotein profile of many nephrotic patients with IHMN is clearly one that in the general population would be regarded as atherogenic. However, until relatively recently, nephrologists appear to have been somewhat reticent about using hypolipidaemic agents, presumably due to the perceived lack of safe and effective hypocholesterolaemic drugs, combined with the paucity of evidence for an increase in incidence of ischaemic heart disease (IHD) in the proteinuric population. There have been three significant events which have altered this perspective. First was the development of the HMG Co-A reductase class of drugs which appear to be safe and can reliably lower the serum cholesterol concentration in patients with the nephrotic syndrome, usually by around 30% [113, 114]. Some agents may also possess significant triglyceride lowering potential. Second was the outcome of a prospective study which demonstrated clearly the increased risk of coronary artery disease developing in nephrotic individuals [107]. Third was the suggestion that hyperlipidaemia may be involved in the progressive deterioration in renal function that is observed not only in glomerular disease but also in many conditions where impaired renal function and associated perturbations of lipoprotein metabolism are present [115]. It is essential to point out that the rationale for treating hypercholesterolaemic IHMN patients in respect of IHD is based on extrapolation from the non-nephrotic population. In the absence of indications aimed specifically at patients with renal disease, it seems reasonable to adopt the published criteria regarding the level of cholesterol at which treatment should be instituted, taking into account other factors such as previous IHD, hypertension, diabetes and age [116]. No data yet exist as to the clinical (as opposed to biochemical) effectiveness of hypolipidaemic treatment on reduction in morbidity or mortality from IHD, or on progression of renal disease, in this population. Since remission may take place either spontaneously or in association with the use of immunosuppressive drugs, it is generally proposed that treatment with HMG Co-A reductase inhibitors should be withheld for the first 6 months after diagnosis. It is important to remember that if remission occurs subsequently, then serum cholesterol levels may return to normal [83] and the hypolipidaemic agent may no longer be required.

Hypertension is relatively uncommon at presentation but develops with time in a number of patients. Treatment with an ACE inhibitor would be appropriate, since it has been shown that, if salt intake is kept below 100 mmol/day, use of this class of drugs may have an antiproteinuric effect [117]. Indeed, some authors have used ACE inhibitors in the absence of hypertension for just that reason, with the rationale that reducing urinary protein loss may have a beneficial effect not only on the nephrotic state itself, i.e. raising the plasma albumin, but also on prognosis, because a better outcome is noted with smaller amounts of proteinuria. If ACE inhibitors are not effective or not tolerated then other hypotensive agents should be employed to keep blood pressure within the acceptable range. A recent controlled trial of diet alone, or diet plus simvastatin, in 17 patients with IHMN has shown, after a mean follow-up in excess of 1 year, no difference in glomerular filtration rate (GFR) but a significant decrease in LDL cholesterol and proteinuria in the treated group [118]. Proteinuria may also be diminished by the use of NSAID [119], but this is not promoted because of the concomitant deleterious effect on GFR. As end-stage renal failure (ESRF) approaches, as it does inevitably in some patients, the standard measures for treating this should be instituted.

Immunosuppressive therapy

Most of the therapeutic decisions discussed so far in this section are either self-evident, only mildly contentious, relatively well supported by extensive clinical experience or formal trials, can be readily extrapolated from the normal population, or at least are not likely to cause serious side-effects. The same cannot be said about the immunomodulating drug regimens proposed by a number of authors and used in IHMN. Quite clearly they are toxic in varying degrees, and injudicious and indiscriminate use of these agents without a clear understanding of their desirable and undesirable effects, and of the natural history of IHMN and its complications, is to be deprecated. The use of immunosuppressive drugs in the treatment of IHMN continues to engender heated debate [20, 101, 120–126]. It remains far from clear what drugs should be used, in what dosage and in what combination, which patients they should be given to, how and when they are best administered, and for how long treatment should be continued. A number of reports incorporating mathematical modelling, decision analysis, and meta-analyses of controlled trials have failed to provide totally convincing guidelines for therapeutic intervention [127–132].

The primary aim of treatment with these agents, if they are prescribed, should be to prevent the development of ESRF with minimal risk to the patient. They may also be considered if the manoeuvres described earlier fail to control a severe nephrotic syndrome, with its attendant complications, irrespective of attempts to prevent the development of renal failure. These objectives are, of course, not unconnected, since patients with heavy proteinuria are just those at risk of progressing to ESRF. The questions regarding the use of the immunosuppressive agents should be: first, can the primary aim be achieved and with what drug regimen; and second, when should treatment be instituted given that most patients with normal renal function will not progress to dialysis dependency? Assuming that answers to the first question can be found, the second question raises further problems. Should all patients be treated, even when GFR is normal, or should treatment be restricted to subsets of patients with poor prognostic features, such as males with heavy proteinuria? Should treatment be reserved until renal function is already declining, in which case progression may be irreversible and the 'window of opportunity' already lost? Certainly, few authorities would consider offering cytotoxic treatment to a woman with reproductive potential, asymptomatic proteinuria, and normal GFR who is not hypertensive. These considerations notwithstanding, there is an extensive literature regarding the use of immunosuppressive agents in patients with IHMN with relatively normal GFR, although there are fewer data concerning patients with declining renal function. Relatively few controlled studies have been reported for either group of patients.

Corticosteroids, cyclophosphamide, chlorambucil, cyclosporin and intravenous immunoglobulin have all been employed in uncontrolled trials [25, 26, 133–142]. These trials have usually been reported in the context of treating patients with well-maintained renal function on entry. The data on gammaglobulin treatment in humans remain sparse [143, 144] and will not be considered further in this chapter, although recent results from animal experiments look promising [145]. The clinical heterogeneity of the patients assessed, and variability of the clinical course followed, makes meaningful assessment of the numerous regimens employed difficult. Furthermore, the absence of a universally accepted independent marker of on-going injury has meant that, while we continue to rely on the measurement of proteinuria and serum creatinine to evaluate efficacy, they are probably relatively insensitive indicators of immunological activity within the kidney. Recently, the assessment of C5b-9 in the urine has suggested that immunological activity may be more accurately determined in future, which will allow more specific assessment of therapeutic effect [78]. Furthermore, studies of urinary β_2-microglobulin [146], urinary IgG excretion [147], and the pattern of low molecular weight urinary proteins [148] suggest that these markers may have prognostic value and be of potential use in indicating which patients should be treated aggressively.

Data from a number of uncontrolled trials, which have included patients who have or have not received immunosuppressive drugs, have been reevaluated by various authors [9, 149, 150]. The consensus of opinion from these analyses of many hundreds of patients is that the use of immunosuppressive therapy appears to have a real effect on proteinuria, and thus promotes complete or partial biochemical remission, but is of no significant consequence in the long-term prevention of the development of renal failure; this occurs in approximately 30% of patients whether or not they have been treated. One recently reported uncontrolled study on the use of cyclosporin deserves further consideration [151]; 15 patients with poor prognostic features were treated with 4–5 mg/kg per day of the drug for between 12 and 30 months. There was no response in four patients, partial remission in seven and complete remission in four. Only three of nine patients relapsed when cyclosporin was withdrawn. Unfortunately no randomized, controlled trial of cyclosporin in patients with IHMN and well-maintained renal function has yet appeared in the literature.

The conclusions from controlled studies on the effect of corticosteroid therapy used alone in the treatment of IHMN are at variance with each other. The original trial [152], on less than 20 patients and reported nearly three decades ago, suggested a beneficial effect on both proteinuria and serum creatinine, but for neither variable did the differences between the treated and untreated groups reach statistical significance. The two major prospective, randomized, double-blind, placebo-controlled trials, i.e. the US Collaborative Study [24] of 72 patients reported in 1979, and the UK Medical Research Council (MRC) study [153] of over 100 patients published in 1990, both used virtually identical regimens of high-dose alternate-day oral steroids (or placebo) for 8 weeks followed by a short tapering course, in patients who had proteinuria in excess of 3.5 g/24 h and well-maintained renal function at entry. The UK study found no effect of this regimen on renal function or proteinuria after 4 years follow-up, while the US trial reported a significant effect on serum creatinine at 6 months. Both series, however, showed a significant effect on proteinuria in the short term, which was not maintained once the drug was stopped. This observation has led some authorities to use longer courses of relatively high doses of corticosteroids, with a starting dose of up to 100 mg of prednisolone on alternate days and tapering to zero over a 6-month period, in order to effect an improvement in an unremitting and severe nephrotic state. The only report of a large controlled study using this approach, however, suggests that no significant benefit can be detected after a mean follow-up of 4 years [154].

Controlled studies of other immunosuppressive agents used in the treatment of IHMN are similarly limited in number. The MRC study [155] of prednisolone and azathioprine, reported in 1971, involved only 14 patients and showed no effect after a short course of treatment. Further studies involving cyclophosphamide [156], azathioprine alone [157], and cyclophosphamide in association with anticoagulant agents [158] all documented that no significant benefit could be found. One small study carried out in France and reported in 1975, which was only partially controlled and generally overlooked, is of some historical interest in that it claimed a remission rate of over 80% in patients receiving chlorambucil while the comparable figure for patients treated with azathioprine, or with supportive therapy only, was only 25% [159]. A recent meta-analysis of the five controlled trials on the treatment of IHMN, which used the cytotoxic agents chlorambucil or cyclophosphamide versus supportive therapy or prednisolone alone, came to the conclusion that these agents only had the effect of diminishing proteinuria but did not have any sustained effect on renal function [132].

The most widely recognized, and best validated regimen of combination therapy with corticosteroids and a cytotoxic agent is that developed and promoted by a group of nephrologists in Italy [160]. Eighty-one patients were enrolled in a randomized fashion to receive supportive therapy only, or 6 months immunosuppressive treatment, with alternating monthly courses of intravenous methylprednisolone daily for 3 days and then oral corticosteroid (prednisolone 0.5 mg/kg or methylprednisolone 0.4 mg/kg) for the remainder of the month, combined with chlorambucil at a dose of 0.2 mg/kg per day for the second, fourth and sixth months. After a minimum follow-up period of 5 years, 14 of 30 patients in the treated group were in remission and four had serum creatinine values more than double their baseline, of whom one had reached ESRF. The 25 patients in the control arm fared significantly worse, with only four in remission (16% vs. 47%), while 19 had doubled their baseline serum creatinine (76% vs. 13%), four of whom had reached ESRF (16% vs. 3%) [161]. After 10 years the probability of dialysis-free survival was 92% in the treated group but only 60% in the control group [162]. A recent study from the same group has shown that cyclophosphamide substituted for chlorambucil may give even better results, at least in the short term [163].

There are far fewer published reports which have addressed the problem of patients with already declining renal function. In uncontrolled studies, investigators have used various regimens which have included steroids alone [164], or in combination with azathioprine [25, 165, 166] or chlorambucil [167–169] or cyclophosphamide [170–173]; the reports have usually suggested some useful response, although this may not have been dramatic or long-lasting. Only two randomized, controlled studies have been reported concerning IHMN and declining renal function. Falk *et al.* in 1992, in a study involving 26 patients, compared the effect of oral steroid therapy versus oral steroid plus intravenous cyclophosphamide; at the end of the study they found no differences in the measured variables between the two groups [174]. However, Cattran and colleagues reported in 1995 on the effect of a 1-year course of oral cyclosporin treatment in nine patients with declining function and a comparable, randomized control group of eight patients receiving placebo [175]. They showed that the rate of decline of GFR in the treated group was less at 1 year; they also documented that this reduced rate of functional decline was maintained in some patients evaluated nearly 2 years after therapy was initiated. This is an interesting finding, but as it is based on small numbers of patients it can only be regarded as a preliminary result.

Some of the outstanding questions regarding immunosuppressive treatment and IHMN with declining function will hopefully be answered by a new, prospective, randomized trial to be carried out in the near future under the auspices of the UK Renal Association. Patients will have already have demonstrated a 20% fall in GFR before randomization into one of three arms and will then receive: (a) a modified Ponticelli regimen, consisting of 0.5 mg/kg per day of prednisolone alternating on a monthly basis with 0.1 mg/kg per day of chlorambucil for a total of 6 months; or (b) a 12-month course of cyclosporin at 5 mg/kg per day, adjusted to maintain whole blood trough levels of between 100 and 200 ng/ml; or (c) supportive therapy only. The observation period is planned for 5 years and the primary endpoint will be a further fall in

GFR of 20%. Questions such as who to treat and when will remain unanswered.

Conclusion

There is still much to be learned about the aetiological factor(s) and pathogenetic mechanism(s) in IHMN – it is by no means certain that a single agent (as yet unidentified) and a uniform pathogenetic process is responsible for causing this condition. Indeed the circumstantial evidence available would imply that this is not the case. Optimum treatment regimens almost certainly require a significant increase in knowledge and understanding of these phenomena. In the meantime, oedema, hypoalbuminaemia, hypertension, hypercholesterolaemia, and the hypercoagulable state associated with IHMN are at least partially treatable with conventional strategies. Proteinuria may respond to ACE inhibition or HMG Co-A reductase inhibition, and possibly to the relatively prolonged administration of corticosteroids and/or other immunosuppressive agents, although use of these potent compounds should be restricted to patients with a severe nephrotic syndrome. Finally, some evidence exists from randomized controlled trials on the potential to prevent the development of impaired renal function using combination corticosteroid and cytotoxic therapy. Very few data from controlled trials have yet been published to suggest that any readily available pharmaceutical agent has a significant effect on the progression of renal insufficiency once it has become manifest.

References

1. Tornroth T, Tallqvist G, Pasternack A *et al.* Non progressive, histologically mild membranous glomerulonephritis appearing in all evolutionary phases as histologically 'early' membranous glomerulonephritis. Kidney Int 1978;14:511–21.
2. Glassock RJ. Secondary membranous glomerulonephritis. Nephrol Dial Transplant 1992;7 (Suppl.1):64–71.
3. Wright NG, Nash AS, Thompson H, Fisher EW. Membranous nephropathy in the cat and dog: a renal biopsy and follow-up study of sixteen cases. Lab Invest 1981;45:269–77.
4. Fleuran GJ, van de Lee R, Greben HA *et al.* Experimental glomerulonephritis in the rat induced by antibodies directed against tubular antigens: IV. Investigations into the pathogenesis of the model. Lab Invest 1978;38:496–501.
5. Border WA, Ward HJ, Kamil ES, Cohen AH. Induction of membranous nephropathy in rabbits by administration of an exogenous cationic antigen. J Clin Invest 1982;69:451–61.
6. Kerjaschki D, Neale TJ. Molecular mechanisms of glomerular injury in rat experimental membranous nephropathy (Heymann nephritis). J Am Soc Nephrol 1996;7:2518–26.
7. Short CD, Mallick NP. Membranous glomerulopathy. In: Schrier RW, Gottschalk CW, editors. Diseases of the Kidney, 6th edn. Boston, MA: Little, Brown; 1997:269–99.
8. Gärtner HV, Fischbach H, Wehner H *et al.* Comparison of clinical and morphological features of peri-(epi-extra) membranous glomerulonephritis. Nephron 1974;13:288–301.

9. Rosen S, Tornroth T, Bernard DB. Membranous glomerulonephritis. In: Tischer CC, Brenner BM, editors. Renal Pathology. Philadelphia, PA: J.B. Lippincott; 1989:196–227.
10. Hunt LP. Statistical aspects of survival in membranous nephropathy. Nephrol Dial Transplant 1992;7(Suppl.1):55–9.
11. Manos J, Short CD, Acheson EJ *et al.* Relapsing idiopathic membranous nephropathy. Clin Nephrol 1982;18:286–90.
12. Franklin WA, Jennings RB, Earle DP. Membranous glomerulonephritis: long term serial observations on clinical course and morphology. Kidney Int 1973;4:36–56.
13. Tu WH, Petitti DB, Biava CG *et al.* Membranous nephropathy: predictors of terminal renal failure. Nephron 1984;36:118–24.
14. Murphy BF, Fairley KF, Kincaid-Smith PS. Idiopathic membranous glomerulonephritis: long term follow-up in 139 cases. Clin Nephrol 1988;30:175–81.
15. Honkanen E. Survival in idiopathic membranous glomerulonephritis. Clin Nephrol 1986;25: 122–8.
16. Hay MN, Bailey RR, Lynn KL *et al.* Membranous nephropathy: a 19 year prospective study in 51 patients. N Z Med J 1992;105:489–91.
17. Kida H, Asamoto T, Yokoyama H *et al.* Long term prognosis of idiopathic membranous nephropathy. Clin Nephrol 1986;25:64–9.
18. Abe S, Amagasaki Y, Konshi K *et al.* Idiopathic membranous glomerulonephritis: aspects of geographical differences. J Clin Pathol 1986;39:1193–8.
19. Cahen R, Francois B, Trolliet P *et al.* Aetiology of membranous glomeruonephritis: a prospective study of 82 adult patients. Nephrol Dial Transplant 1989;4:172–80.
20. Austin HA. Membranous Nephropathy. Ann Int Med 1992;116:672–82.
21. Short CD. Proteinuric glomerular disease. MD thesis, University of Manchester, 1990.
22. Davison AM. The United Kingdom Medical Research Council's Glomerulonephritis registry. In: Berlyne GM, Giovannetti SS, editors. Contributions to Nephrology. Basel: Karger; 1985: 24–35.
23. Preston RA, Stemmer CL, Materson BJ *et al.* Renal biopsy in patients 65 years of age or older. An analysis of the results of 334 biopsies. J Am Geriatr Soc 1990;38:669–74.
24. Collaborative study of the Adult Idiopathic Nephrotic Syndrome: a controlled study of short term prednisone treatment in adults with membranous nephropathy. N Engl J Med 1979;301: 1301–6.
25. Bone JM, Rustom R, Williams PS. Progressive versus indolent idiopathic membranous glomerulonephritis. Q J Med 1997;90:699–706.
26. Stirling CM, Simpson K, Boulton-Jones JM. Immunosuppression and outcome in idiopathic membranous nephropathy. Q J Med 1998;91:159–64.
27. Ramirez F, Brouhard BH, Travis LB *et al.* Idiopathic membranous nephropathy in children. J Pediatr 1982;5:677–81.
28. Trainin EB, Boichis H, Spitzer A *et al.* Idiopathic membranous nephropathy: clinical course in children. N Y State J Med 1976;76:357–60.
29. Forland M, Spargo BH. Clinicopathological correlations in idiopathic nephrotic syndrome with membranous nephropathy. Nephron 1969;6:498–525.
30. Honkanen E, Törnroth T, Grönhagen-Riska C. Natural history, clinical course and morphological evalution of membranous nephropathy. Nephrol Dial Transplant 1992;7(Suppl.1):35–41.
31. Flynn VJ, Roland AS. Nephrotic syndrome in a 92-year old woman. Geriatrics 1967;22:119–22.
32. Nauta J, de Heer E, Baldwin WM III *et al.* Transplacental induction of membranous nephropathy in a neonate. Pediatr Nephrol 1990;4:111–16.
33. Alpers CE, Cotran RS. Neoplasia and glomerular injury. Kidney Int 1986;30:465–73.
34. Berthoux FC, Berthoux P, Hassan AA *et al.* Immunogenetics of primary membranous glomerulonephritis. Presse Med 1990;19:990–3.
35. Klouda PT, Acheson EJ, Goldby FS *et al.* Strong association between idiopathic membranous nephropathy and HLA DRw3. Lancet 1979;ii:770–1.

36. Müller GA, Müller C, Liebow G *et al.* Strong association of idiopathic membranous nephropathy (MN) with HLA-DR3 and MT-2 without involvement of HLA-B18 and no association to BfF1. Tissue Antigens 1981;17:332–7.
37. Huang CC. Strong association of HLA-DR3 in Chinese patients with idiopathic membranous nephropathy. Tissue Antigens 1989;33:425–6.
38. Hiki Y, Kobayashi Y, Itoh I *et al.* Strong association of HLA-DR2 and MT1 with idiopathic membranous nephropathy in Japan. Kidney Int 1984;25:953–7.
39. Sacks SH, Nomura S, Warner C *et al.* Analysis of complement C4 loci in Caucasoids and Japanese with idiopathic membranous nephropathy. Kidney Int 1992;42:882–7.
40. Nishimukai H, Nakanishi I, Takeuchi Y *et al.* Complement C6 and C7 polymorphisms in Japanese patients with chronic glomerulonephritis. Hum Hered 1989;39:150–5.
41. Vaughan RW, Demaine AG, Welsh KI. A DQA1 allele is strongly associated with idiopathic membranous nephropathy. Tissue Antigens 1989;34:261–9.
42. Dyer PA, Short CD, Clarke EA *et al.* HLA antigen gene polymorphisms and haplotypes established by family studies in membranous nephropathy. Nephrol Dial Transplant 1992; 7(Suppl.1):42–7.
43. Brenchley P, Feehally J, Dore P *et al.* Gm allotypes in membranous nephropathy. N Engl J Med 1985;309:556.
44. Taube D, Brown Z, Williams DG. Impaired lymphocyte and suppressor cell function in minimal change nephropathy, membranous nephropathy and focal glomerulosclerosis. Clin Nephrol 1984;22:176–82.
45. Bannister KM, Hay J, Clarkson AR. Fc-specific reticulo-endothelial clearance in systemic lupus erythematosus and glomerulonephritis. Am J Kidney Dis 1984;3:287–92.
46. Matsumoto K. Increased release of tumor necrosis factor-alpha by monocytes from patients with glomerulonephritis. Clin Nephrol 1993;40:148–54.
47. Gamble CN, Reardan JB. Immunopathogenesis of syphilitic glomerulonephritis. Elution of antitreponemal antibody from glomerular immune complex deposits. N Engl J Med 1975;292: 449–54.
48. Edelwiss MI, Daudt HM, Goldstein HF *et al.* Hepatic hydatidosis with glomerular involvement: report of a case. Rev Assoc Med Bras 1992;38:31–2.
49. Couser WG, Wagonfeld JV, Spargo BH. Glomerular deposition of tumor antigen in membranous nephropathy associated with colonic carcinoma. Am J Med 1974;57:962–70.
50. Costanza ME, Pinn V, Schwartz RS *et al.* Carcinoembryonic antigen–antibody complexes in a patient with colonic carcinoma and nephrotic syndrome. N Engl J Med 1973;289:520–2.
51. Austin HA *et al.* Prognostic factors in lupus nephritis. Contribution of renal histological data. Am J Med 1983;75:382–91.
52. Adu D, Williams DG, Taube D *et al.* Late onset systemic lupus erythematosus and lupus-like disease in patients with apparent idiopathic glomerulonephritis. Q J Med 1983;52:471–87.
53. Jennette JC, Iskandar SS, Dalldorf FG. Pathologic differentiation between lupus and non-lupus membranous glomerulopathy. Kidney Int 1983;24:377–85.
54. Hall CL, Fothergill NJ, Blackwell MM *et al.* The natural course of gold nephropathy: long term study of 21 patients. Br Med J 1987;295:745–8.
55. Ross JH, McGinty F, Brewer DG. Penicillamine nephropathy. Nephron 1980;26:184–6.
56. Sellars L, Siamopoulos K, Wilkinson R *et al.* Renal biopsy appearances in rheumatoid disease. Clin Nephrol 1983;20:114–20.
57. Higuchi A, Suzuki Y, Okada T. Membranous glomerulonephritis in rheumatoid arthritis unassociated with gold or penicillamine treatment. Ann Rheum Dis 1987;46:488–90.
58. Hirose H, Udo K, Kojima M *et al.* Deposition of hepatitis B e antigen in membranous glomerulonephritis: identification by $F(ab')_2$ fragments of monoclonal antibody. Kidney Int 1984;26:338–41.
59. Stehman-Breen C, Alpers CE, Couser WG, Willson R, Johnson RJ. Hepatitis C virus associated membranous glomerulonephritis. Clin Nephrol 1995;44:141–7.
60. O'Regan S, Fong JSC, DeChadarevian JP *et al.* Treponemal antigens in congenital and acquired syphilitic nephritis. Ann Intern Med 1976;85:325–7.

61. Burstein DM, Korbet SM, Schwartz MM. Membranous glomerulonephritis and malignancy. Am J Kidney Dis 1993;22:5–10.
62. Eagen JW, Lewis EJ. Glomerulopathies of neoplasia. Kidney Int 1977;11:297–306.
63. Yamauchi H, Linsey MS, Biava CG *et al.* Cure of membranous nephropathy after resection of carcinoma. Arch Intern Med 1985;145:2061–3.
64. Hall CL. The natural history of gold and penicillamine nephropathy: a long term study of 54 patients. Adv Exp Med Biol 1989;252:247–56.
65. Campistol JM, Galofre J, Botey A *et al.* Reversible membranous nephritis associated with diclofenac. Nephrol Dial Transplant 1989;4:393–5.
66. Seedat YIC, Simjez AE, Naido DR. Nephrotic syndrome due to cosmetics containing mercury. S Afr Med J 1973;47:506.
67. Weetman AP, Pinching AJ, Pussel BA *et al.* Membranous glomerulonephritis and autoimmune thyroid disease. Clin Nephrol 1981;15:50–1.
68. Kobayashi K, Harada A, Onoyama K *et al.* Idiopathic membranous glomerulonephritis associated with diabetes mellitus: light, immunofluorescence and electron microscopic study. Nephron 1981;28:163–8.
69. Bonet Sol J, Teixido Planas J, Costa Pinel B *et al.* Sjögren's syndrome and membranous glomerulonephritis. Rev Clin Esp 1985;177:191–3.
70. Kleinknecht C, Levy M, Gagnadoux MF *et al.* Membranous glomerulonephritis with extrarenal disorders in children. Medicine 1979;58:219–28.
71. Khan IH, Simpson JG, Catto GR *et al.* Membranous nephropathy and granulomatous interstitial nephritis in sarcoidosis. Nephron 1994;66:459–61.
72. Reitsma D, Gratama S and Vroom TM. Clinical remission of membranous glomerulónephritis in primary biliary cirrhosis with cutaneous vasculitis. Br Med J 1984;288:27–8.
73. Davison AM, Johnston PA. Allograft membranous nephropathy. Nephrol Dial Transplant 1992;7(Suppl.1):114–18.
74. Briner J, Binswanger U, Largiader F. Recurrent and de novo membranous glomerulonephritis in renal cadaver allotransplants. Clin Nephrol 1980;13:189–96.
75. Mathew TH. Nephrotic syndrome in patients with transplanted kidneys. In: Cameron JS, Glassock RJ, editor. The Nephrotic Syndrome. New York: Marcel Dekker; 1988:805–47.
76. Hoitsma AJ, Kroon AA, Wetzels JFM *et al.* Association between ureteral obstruction and *de novo* membranous nephropathy in renal allografts. Transplant Proc 1990;22:1388–9.
77. Mallick NP, Short CD, Manos J. Clinical membranous nephropathy. Nephron 1983;34:209–19.
78. Kon SP, Coupes B, Short CD *et al.* Urinary C5b-9 excretion and clinical course in idiopathic human membranous nephropathy. Kidney Int 1995;48:1953–8.
79. Chan MK, Chan KW, Jones B. Immunoglobulins and complement components in nephrotic syndrome due to minimal change and other forms of glomerulonephritis: a clue for steroid therapy. Nephron 1987;47:125–30.
80. Llach F. Hypercoagulability, renal vein thrombosis, and other thrombotic complications of nephrotic syndrome. Kidney Int 1985;28:429–39.
81. Chopra JS,Mallick NP, Stone MC. Hyperlipoproteinaemia in nephrotic syndrome. Lancet 1971;i:317–21.
82. Short CD, Durrington PN, Mallick NP *et al.* Serum and urinary high density lipoproteins in glomerular disease with proteinuria. Kidney Int 1986;29:1224–8.
83. Short CD, Durrington PN, Mallick NP *et al.* Serum lipoprotein (a) in men with proteinuria due to idiopathic membranous nephropathy. Nephrol Dial Transplant 1992;7:109–13.
84. Coggins CH, Frommer JP, Glassock RJ. Membranous nephropathy. Semin Nephrol 1982;2: 264–73.
85. Kurki P, Helve T, von Bonsdorff M *et al.* Transformation of membranous glomerulonephritis into crescentic glomerulonephritis with glomerular basement membrane antibodies: serial determinations of anti-GBM before the transformation. Nephron 1984;38:134–6.
86. Tse WY, Howie AJ, Adu D *et al.* Association of vasculitic glomerulonephritis with membranous nephropathy: a report of 10 cases. Nephrol Dial Transplant 1997;12:1017–27.

87. Abe S, Amagasaki Y, Iyori S *et al.* Significance of tubulointerstitial lesion in biopsy specimens of glomerulonephritic patients. Am J Nephrol 1989;9:30–7.
88. Ehrenreich T, Churg J. Pathology of membranous nephropathy. In: Sommers SC, editor. Pathology Annual. New York: Appleton-Century-Crofts; 1968:145–86.
89. Zollinger HU, Mihatsch MJ. Epimembranous glomerulonephritis. In: Renal Pathology in Biopsy. Berlin: Springer-Verlag; 1978:261–78.
90. Gärtner HV, Watnabe T, Ott V *et al.* Correlations between morphologic and clinical features in idiopathic perimembranous glomerulonephritis. A study on 403 renal biopsies of 367 patients. Curr Top Pathol 1977;65:1–29.
91. Tornroth T, Skrifvars B. The development and resolution of glomerular basement membrane changes associated with subepithelial immune deposits. Am J Pathol 1975;79:219–36.
92. Couser WG. Mediation of immune glomerular injury. Clin Investig 1993;71:808–11.
93. Germuth FG, Taylor TJ, Siddiqui SY *et al.* Immune complex disease VI: some determinants of the varieties of glomerular lesions in the chronic bovine serum albumin–rabbit system. Lab Invest 1977;37:162–9.
94. Orlando RA, Kerjaschki D, Kurihara H *et al.* Gp330 associates with a 44 kDa protein in the rat kidney to form the Heymann nephritis antigenic complex. Proc Nat Acad Sci USA 1992; 89:6698–702.
95. Border WA, Ward HJ, Kamiz ES. Induction of membranous nephropathy in rabbits by administration of an exogenous cationic antigen. J Clin Invest 1982;69:451–61.
96. Oliveira DBG. Membranous nephropathy: an IgG4 mediated disease. Lancet 1998;351:670–1.
97. Bannister KM, Howarth GS, Clarkson AR *et al.* Glomerular IgG subclass distribution in human glomerulonephritis. Clin Nephrol 1983;19:161–5.
98. Passerini P, Pasquali S, Cesana B *et al.* Long-term outcome of patients with membranous nephropathy after complete remission of proteinuria. Nephrol Dial Transplant 1989;4:525–9.
99. Schieppati A, Mosconi L, Perna A *et al.* Prognosis of untreated patients with idiopathic membranous nephropathy. N Engl J Med 1993;329:85–9.
100. MacTier R, Boulton-Jones JM, Payton CD *et al.* The natural history of membranous nephropathy in the West of Scotland. Q J Med 1986;60:793–802.
101. Remuzzi G, Schieppati A, Garattini S. Treatment of idiopathic membranous glomerulopathy. Curr Opinion Nephrol Hypertens 1994;3:155–63.
102. Davison AM, Cameron JS, Kerr DNS *et al.* The natural history of renal function in untreated idiopathic membranous glomerulonephritis in adults. Clin Nephrol 1984;22:61–7.
103. Hopper JJ, Trew PA, Biava CG. Membranous nephropathy: its relative benignity in women. Nephron 1981;29:18–24.
104. Kauffman RH, Veltkamp JJ, Tilburg NHV *et al.* Acquired antithrombin III deficiency and thrombin in the nephrotic syndrome. Am J Med 1978;65:607–13.
105. Jennings M, Shortland JR, Maddocks JL. Interstitial nephritis associated with frusemide. J R Soc Med 1986;79:239–40.
106. Chamberlain MJ, Pringle A, Wrong OM. Oliguric renal failure in the nephrotic syndrome. Q J Med 1966;138:215–35.
107. Ordonez JD, Hiatt RA, Killebrew EJ *et al.* The increased risk of coronary heart disease associated with nephrotic syndrome. Kidney Int 1993;44:638–42.
108. Lai KN, Tam JS, Lin HJ *et al.* The therapeutic dilemma of usage of corticosteroids on patients with membranous nephropathy and peristent hepatitis B surface antigenemia. Nephron 1990; 54:12–17.
109. Johnston PA, Goode NP, Aparicio SR *et al.* Membranous allograft nephropathy. Remission of nephrotic syndrome with pulsed methylprednisolone and high-dose alternate-day steroids. Transplantation 1993;55:214–16.
110. Akcicek F, Yalniz T, Basci A *et al.* Diuretic effect of frusemide in patients with nephrotic syndrome: is it potentiated by intravenous albumin? Br Med J 1995;310:162–3.
111. Sarasin FP, Schifferli JA. Prophylactic oral anticoagulation in nephrotic patients with idiopathic membranous nephropathy. Kidney Int 1994;45:578–585.

112. Rostoker G, Durand-Zaleski I, Petit-Phar M *et al.* Prevention of thrombotic complications of the nephrotic syndrome by the low molecular weight heparin enoxaprin. Nephron 1995;69: 20–8.
113. Grundy SM. Management of hyperlipidaemia of kidney disease. Kidney Int 1990;37:847–53.
114. Kasiske BL, Velosa JA, Halstenson CE *et al.* The effects of lovastatin in hyperlipidaemic patients with the nephrotic syndrome. Am J Kidney Dis 1990;15:8–15.
115. Moorhead JF, Chan MK, El-Nahas M, Varghese Z. Lipid nephrotoxicity in chronic progressive glomerular and tubulo-interstitial disease. Lancet 1982;ii:1309–11.
116. Ramsay LE, Haq IU, Jackson PR, Yeo WW. The Sheffield table for primary prevention of coronary heart disease. Lancet 1996;348:1251–2.
117. Gansevoort RT, Heeg JE, Vriesendorp R, de Zeeuw D, de Jong PE. Antiproteinuric drugs in patients with idiopathic membranous nephropathy. Nephrol Dial Transplant 1992;7(Suppl.1): 91–6.
118. Rayner BL, Byrne MJ, van Zyl Smit R. A prospective clinical trial comparing the treatment of idiopathic membranous nephropathy and nephrotic syndrome with simvastatin and diet, versus diet alone. Clin Nephrol 1996;46:219–24.
119. Donker AJ, Brentjens JR, Van Der Hem GK *et al.* Treatment of the nephrotic syndrome with indomethacin. Nephron 1978;22:374.
120. Pollak VE. Treatment of membranous glomerulonephropathy. Am J Kidney Dis 1992;19:68–71.
121. Feldman HI, Madio MP. Cyclophosphamide in progressive membranous nephropathy: pro and con. Ann Intern Med 1992;117:696–7.
122. Glassock RJ. Treatment of immunologically mediated glomerular disease. Kidney Int 1992;42 (Suppl.38):121–6.
123. Lewis EJ. Idiopathic membranous nephropathy – to treat or not to treat? N Engl J Med 1993; 329:127–9.
124. Nieuhof CMG, Gaillard CA, van Brieda Vriesman PJC. Membranous glomerulonephritis – towards tailor made treatment? Neth J Med 1993;42:109–11.
125. Rostoker G. Idiopathic membranous nephropathy; new therapeutic trends. Eur J Med 1993;2: 106–16.
126. Glassock RJ. Therapy of idiopathic nephrotic syndrome in adults. Am J Nephrol 1993;13: 422–8.
127. Couchard C, Laville M, Boissel JP. Treatment of membranous nephropathy; a meta-analysis. Nephrol Dial Transplant 1994;9:469–70.
128. Piccoli A, Pillon L, Passerini P, Ponticelli C. Therapy for idiopathic membranous nephropathy; tailoring the choice by decision analysis. Kidney Int 1994;45:1193–202.
129. Hebert LA. Therapy of membranous nephropathy; what to do after (meta)analyses. J Am Soc Nephrol 1995;5:1543–5.
130. O'Callaghan CA, Cameron JS, Sacks SH. Early prediction of treatment outcome in idiopathic membranous nephropathy. Q J Med 1995;88:889–94.
131. Marx BE, Marx M. Prognosis of idiopathic membranous nephropathy: a methodologic meta-analysis. Kidney Int 1997;51:873–9.
132. Imperiale TF, Goldfarb S, Berns JS. Are cytotoxic agents beneficial in idiopathic membranous nephropathy? A meta-analysis of the controlled trials. J Am Soc Nephrol 1995;5:1553–8.
133. Miller RB, Harrington JT , Ramos CP. Long term results of steroid therapy in adults with idiopathic nephrotic syndrome. Am J Med 1969;46:919–29.
134. Ehrenreich T, Porush JG, Churg J *et al.* Treatment of idiopathic membranous nephropathy. N Engl J Med 1976;295:741–6.
135. Hopper J Jr, Biava LG, Tu WH. Membranous nephropathy: high-dose alternate-day therapy with prednisone. West J Med 1981;135:1–8.
136. Cameron JS. Pathogenesis and treatment of membranous nephropathy. Kidney Int 1979;15: 88–103.
137. Suki WN, Chavez A. Membranous nephropathy: response to steroids and immunosuppression. Am J Nephrol 1981;1:11–16.

138. Ponticelli C. Prognosis and treatment of membranous nephropathy. Kidney Int 1986;29:927–40.
139. Jensen H, Jensen E. Steroid treatment of the nephrotic syndrome in adults. Acta Med Scand 1967;182:741–54.
140. Rastogi SP, Hart-Mercer J, Kerr DNS. Idiopathic membranous glomerulonephritis in adults. Remission following steroid therapy. Q J Med 1969;38:335–50.
141. Bolton WK, Atuk NO, Sturgill BC *et al.* Therapy of the idiopathic nephrotic syndrome with alternate day steroids. Am J Med 1977;62:60–70.
142. Rotellar G, Rakowski T, Winchester JF. Short-term responsiveness of membranous glomerulopathy to cyclosporine. Am J Kidney Dis 1993;21:568–9.
143. Palla R, Cirami C, Panichi V *et al.* Intravenous immunoglobulin therapy of membranous nephropathy: efficacy and safety. Clin Nephrol 1991;35: 98–104.
144. Sugisaki T, Shimpo H, Boku T *et al.* High dose intravenous gammaglobulin for membranous nephropathy (MN), membranoproliferative glomerulonephritis (MPGN) and lupus nephritis (LN). Long term follow-up study. Abstracts, XIth Congress of the ISN, Tokyo, June 1990.
145. Nangaku M, Pippin J, Richardson CA *et al.* Beneficial effects of systemic immunoglobulin in experimental membranous nephropathy. Kidney Int 1996;50:2054–62.
146. Reichert LJ, Koene RA, Wetzels JF. Urinary excretion of beta 2 microglobulin predicts renal outcome in patients with idiopathic membranous nephropathy. J Am Soc Nephrol 1995;6: 1666–9.
147. Reichert LJ, Koene RA, Wetzels JF. Urinary IgG excretion as a prognostic factor in idiopathic membranous nephropathy. Clin Nephrol 1997;48:79–84.
148. Bazzi C, Petrini C, Rizza V, Arrigo G, Beltrame A, D'Amico G. Characterization of proteinuria in primary glomerulonephritides. Am J Kidney Dis 1997;29:27–35.
149. Zucchelli P, Pasquali S. Membranous nephropathy. In: Cameron JS, Davison AM, Grunfeld JP *et al.*, editors. Oxford Textbook of Clinical Nephrology. Oxford: Oxford University Press; 1992:370–88.
150. Cameron JS. Membranous nephropathy and its treatment. Nephrol Dial Transplant 1992;7 (Suppl.1):72–9.
151. Rostoker G, Belghiti D, Ben Maadi A *et al.* Long term cyclosporin A therapy for severe idiopathic membranous nephropathy. Nephron 1993;63:335–41.
152. Black DAK, Rose G, Brewer DB. Controlled trial of prednisone in adult patients with the nephrotic syndrome. Br Med J 1970;3:421–6.
153. Cameron JS, Healy MJR, Adu D. The Medical Research Council trial of short-term high-dose alternate-day prednisolone in idiopathic membranous nephropathy with nephrotic syndrome in adults. Q J Med 1990;74:133–56.
154. Cattran D, Delamore T, Roscoe J *et al.* A randomized controlled trial of prednisone in patients with idiopathic membranous nephropathy. N Engl J Med 1989;320:210–15.
155. Medical Research Council Working Party. Controlled trial of azathioprine and prednisone in chronic renal disease. Br Med J 1971;2:239–41.
156. Donadio JVJ, Holley KE, Anderson CF *et al.* Controlled trial of cyclophosphamide in idiopathic membranous nephropathy. Kidney Int 1974;6:431–9.
157. Canadian Medical Association. Controlled trial of azathioprine in the nephrotic syndrome secondary to idiopathic membranous glomerulonephritis. Can Med Assoc J 1976;115:1209–10.
158. Murphy BF, McDonald I, Fairley KF *et al.* Randomized controlled trial of cyclophosphamide, warfarin and dipyridamole in idiopathic membranous glomerulonephritis. Clin Nephrol 1992;37:229–34.
159. Lagrue G, Bernard D, Bariéty J *et al.* Treatment with chlorambucil and azathioprine in primary glomerulonephritis. Results of a controlled study. J Urol Nephrol Paris 1975;81:655–72.
160. Ponticelli C, Zuccelli P, Imbasciati E *et al.* Controlled trial of methylprednisolone and chlorambucil in idiopathic membranous nephropathy. N Engl J Med 1984;301:946–50.

161. Ponticelli C, Zucchelli P, Passerini P *et al.* A randomised trial of methylprednisolone and chlorambucil in idiopathic membranous nephropathy. N Engl J Med 1989;320:8–13.
162. Ponticelli C, Zucchelli P, Passerini P *et al.* A 10 year follow up of a randomised study with methylprednisolone and chlorambucil in membranous nephropathy. Kidney Int 1995;48: 1600–4.
163. Ponticelli C, Altieri P, Scolari F *et al.* A randomised study comparing methylprednisolone plus chlorambucil versus methylprednisolone plus cyclophosphamide in idiopathic membranous nephropathy. J Am Soc Nephrol 1998;9:444–50.
164. Short CD, Solomon LR, Gokal R, MallickNP. Methylprednisolone in patients with membranous nephropathy and declining renal function. Q J Med 1987;247:929–40.
165. Williams PS, Bone JM. Immunosuppression can arrest progressive renal failure due to idiopathic membranous glomerulonephritis. Nephrol Dial Transplant 1989;4:181–6.
166. Brown JH, Douglas AF, Murphy BG *et al.* Treatment of renal failure in idiopathic membranous nephropathy with azathioprine and prednisolone. Nephrol Dial Transplant 1998;13:443–8.
167. Mathieson PW, Turner AN, Maidment CGH *et al.* Prednisolone and chlorambucil treatment in idiopathic membranous nephropathy with deteriorating renal function. Lancet 1988;ii:869–72.
168. Brunkhorst R, Wrengger E, Koch KM. Low-dose prednisolone/chlorambucil therapy in patients with severe membranous glomerulonephritis. Clin Investig 1994;72:277–82.
169. Warwick GL, Geddes CG, Boulton-Jones JM. Prednisolone and chlorambucil therapy for idiopathic membranous nephropathy with progressive renal failure. Q J Med 1994;87:223–9.
170. Bruns FJ, Adler S, Fraley DS *et al.* Sustained remission of membranous glomerulonephritis after cyclophosphamide and prednisone. Ann Intern Med 1991;114:725–30.
171. Kibriya MG, Tishkov I, Nikolov D. Immunosuppressive therapy with cyclophosphamide and prednisolone in severe idiopathic membranous nephropathy. Nephrol Dial Transplant 1994;9:138–43.
172. Jindal K, West M, Bear R *et al.* Long-term benefits of therapy with cyclophosphamide and prednisone in patients with membranous glomerulonephritis and impaired renal function. Am J Kidney Dis 1992;19:61–7.
173. West ML, Jindal KK, Bear RA *et al.* A controlled trial of cyclophosphamide in patients with membranous glomerulonephritis. Kidney Int 1989;32:579–84.
174. Falk RJ, Hogan SL, Muller KE *et al.* Treatment of progressive membranous glomerulopathy. A randomized trial comparing cyclophosphamide and corticosteroids with corticosteroids alone. The Glomerular Disease Collaborative Network. Ann Intern Med 1992;116:438–45.
175. Cattran DC, Greenwood C, Ritchie S *et al.* A controlled trial of cyclosporine in patients with progressive membranous nephropathy. Kidney Int 1995;47:1130–5.

5 Mesangiocapillary glomerulonephritis

P.W. MATHIESON

Introduction

Throughout this chapter I will use the term mesangiocapillary glomerulonephritis (MCGN); identical morphological appearances are given the name (especially in the United States) of membranoproliferative glomerulonephritis (MPGN). As with other forms of glomerulonephritis, for example membranous nephropathy, the condition can occur as a 'secondary' consequence of a variety of extrarenal/systemic disorders or as a 'primary' (idiopathic) form, the renal lesion in these two situations being indistinguishable by light microscopy alone. As with membranous nephropathy, careful analysis of 'secondary' cases may give clues to the pathogenesis of the idiopathic form. Management of the 'secondary' forms is largely that of the underlying condition – if that condition can be eradicated the prognosis of the renal lesion is generally good. It is likely that the idiopathic form is not a single disease, resulting instead from a variety of possible conditions albeit with common features and probably with shared pathways leading to renal injury.

Further complexity is added by the fact that MCGN itself is not a single entity, and three subtypes (types I, II and III) are recognized. The light microscopic features of these three are similar, with diffuse thickening of the glomerular basement membrane (GBM) associated with increased cellularity, often giving a characteristic lobular appearance to the glomeruli. Using immunofluorescence and electron microscopy it is possible to subdivide further the morphological appearances. In type I MCGN there is typically IgG, IgM and complement C3 in mesangial areas and along the glomerular capillary loops in a subendothelial or intramembranous location. Electron microscopy shows discrete electron-dense deposits in these regions. In type II MCGN, immunoglobulins are typically absent but there is linear deposition of C3 along the capillary loops, sometimes also in tubular and vascular basement membranes. Electron microscopy shows thick linear deposition of electron-dense material along these basement membranes, giving rise to the synonym for type II MCGN, 'dense-deposit disease'. Type III MCGN is similar to type I except that there are subepithelial as well as subendothelial deposits, and there may be disruption of the GBM with accumulation of new basement membrane material in layers.

C.D. Pusey (ed.), The Treatment of Glomerulonephritis, 81–92.

Complement activation in MCGN

MCGN is the form of nephritis most closely associated with abnormalities of complement activation and/or regulation, and there is evidence, at least for some subtypes of MCGN, that complement dysregulation may directly cause the renal lesion. Although the morphological differences between types I, II and III MCGN are subtle, and only apparent at the ultrastructural level, the validity of this subdivision is greatly enhanced by the fact that the typical abnormalities of the complement system are different in the three types (Table 5.1). Type I is most commonly associated with classical pathway activation (depletion of both C3 and C4) and type II with alternative pathway activation (low C3, normal C4). In type III MCGN, low levels of terminal complement components, especially C5, are frequent, and in addition there may be variable (although usually mild) degrees of activation of the classical and alternative pathways, reflected respectively by depletion of both C3 and C4 or C3 alone [1]. The mechanisms of complement activation, and the implications for therapy, are considered further in the section on possible future therapeutic strategies.

Table 5.1 Typical patterns of complement activation in MCGN

MCGN type	Pathway predominantly activated	C3	C4	C5b-9
I	Classical	Low	Low	Normal
II	Alternative	Very low	Normal	Normal
III	Terminal (±classical, alternative)	Normal or slightly low	Normal or slightly low	Low

Problems with the assessment of therapy in MCGN

The subtle differences in patterns of glomerular injury, and more importantly the distinctive patterns of complement activation, in the three types of MCGN suggest that their pathogenesis may not be identical. Therefore the ideal forms of therapy, and the likelihood of success, may vary between the three subtypes. Herein lies the first problem in the assessment of the literature on treatment of MCGN: most studies include all three subtypes in varying proportions. This reflects the second problem: the relative rarity of MCGN, so that pooling of broadly similar patients has often been used to bolster numbers. Despite this, many of the studies are small and there is a dearth of randomized controlled trials. Another problem is that many studies in MCGN contain varying proportions of children, whose prognosis may be different from that of adults. Then there are the inevitable problems of patient heterogeneity, varying treatment regimens, variable duration of follow-up, etc., which bedevil so many small clinical trials. Nevertheless, the lack of any satisfactory animal model for MCGN means that these somewhat unsatisfactory clinical studies provide our only source of information on the current status of therapy for MCGN. Analysis of recent advances in the understanding of mechanisms of tissue injury in MCGN may allow us to speculate on novel forms of therapy which might prove useful in future, but the difficulties of adequately assessing these therapies will remain. There is an overwhelming need for multicentre, probably multinational, collaborations to mount studies of sufficient size and rigour to answer these important questions.

Natural history of MCGN

Knowledge of the natural history of the untreated condition is essential before the effects of therapy can be assessed for any condition, especially in the absence of large controlled trials. From the available literature, the following tentative conclusions can be drawn. Overall, the renal survival in MCGN at 10 years from diagnosis is of the order of 50%. Children tend to have a more acute presentation and a slower decline in renal function, although with lengthy follow-up the overall renal survival is similar to that in adults. The prognosis differs between the three subtypes of MCGN, with type II carrying the greatest risk of the development of end-stage renal failure (ESRF): in one recent study the median time to ESRF in types I, II and III was respectively 15.3 years, 8.7 years and 15.9 years [2]. Since presentation with the nephrotic syndrome carries a substantially increased risk of ESRF compared with other milder clinical syndromes [3], the adverse prognosis of type II MCGN may simply reflect the greater likelihood of nephrotic presentation with this histological type. In Japan, asymptomatic cases are ascertained by routine screening of the urine of normal schoolchildren followed by investigation of those found to have proteinuria [4]. Thus it is likely that mild and/or early cases will be included in Japanese series, explaining the apparently benign course of MCGN reported in one recent series [5]. Diffuse glomerular changes (the most common situation) carry a worse prognosis than focal lesions. As in many other forms of glomerular disease the presence of tubular atrophy and interstitial fibrosis indicates a worse prognosis, as does hypertension at the time of presentation.

Therapy of MCGN

The forms of therapy which have been applied to MCGN are familiar, being similar to those used in other forms of nephritis. Antiplatelet drugs, anticoagulants, corticosteroids and alkylating agents have been used alone or in various combinations. Reviews of the subject have usually concluded that there is no treatment of proven efficacy in MCGN [6–8]. Nevertheless, there are hints from some of the studies that certain drugs may have useful effects.

Cytotoxic therapy ± anticoagulants/dipyridamole

Initial enthusiasm for combination therapy was based on the report by Kincaid-Smith of the effects of cyclophosphamide, warfarin and dipyridamole in 16 patients with MCGN whose renal function was impaired: renal survival was substantially better than that in a retrospectively analysed group of 13 untreated patients [9]. However, the apparent benefits of therapy were magnified by the unexpectedly poor outcome in this 'control' group, in which all 13 patients progressed to ESRF. If the outcome in the treated patients is compared to that predicted from other studies of the natural history of MCGN the effects are less impressive. The Guy's group reported good results in six out of 10 patients with aggressive MCGN treated with a related regimen in which prednisolone plus azathioprine was substituted for cyclophosphamide [10]. Two subsequent controlled trials of 'triple therapy' (cyclophosphamide, anticoagulants and dipyridamole) in larger numbers of patients failed to show significant benefit, and highlighted some major adverse effects [11, 12]. Zimmerman *et al.* [13] used warfarin and dipyridamole together in a crossover trial in 18 patients, reporting a benefit between patients but not within patients; furthermore, there was a high rate of haemorrhagic complications. A recent uncontrolled study of 19 patients treated with a complex regimen of cyclophosphamide plus prednisone reported a high remission rate [14]. However, 38% of the patients relapsed and although some of those were successfully re-treated the long-term risk/benefit ratio of this treatment is uncertain. The cumulative doses of prednisone and cyclophosphamide used in this protocol were very high. Little information was given concerning adverse effects, but 40% of the patients had gonadal failure and, since MCGN is primarily a disease of the young, many nephrologists would be wary of this form of therapy without substantiation of its long-term benefits.

Antiplatelet therapy

The combination of aspirin plus dipyridamole was reported to have useful effects in a randomized, double-blind, placebo-controlled trial in 40 patients by Donadio *et al.* from the Mayo Clinic [15], and this resulted in this form of therapy being popular for some years for MCGN because of its relative safety. However, a later report by the same authors [7] indicated that the apparent benefits of therapy may have been spurious, arising because the patients were analysed from time of diagnosis rather than from initiation of therapy. This would artificially favour the treatment group since patients with the worst prognosis may not have survived to the start of treatment. Comparison of the two groups from the time of initiation of therapy showed no significant difference [7]. More recently, Zauner reported beneficial effects of aspirin plus dipyridamole on proteinuria in patients with nephrotic syndrome due to MCGN, but little effect on excretory renal function [16].

Corticosteroids

The Cincinnati group have published a series of reports advocating the long-term use of alternate-day high-dose prednisone [17–20]. Unfortunately, these have not been controlled trials, relying instead on comparisons with series published from other centres. Different dosage schedules have been used, some patients received daily rather than alternate-day doses and some patients received other immunosuppressive agents in addition. Nevertheless, the results do suggest that prednisone treatment alters the natural history: importantly this is the case whether the analysis is performed from the time of diagnosis or from the initiation of treatment [19]. Seventy-one prednisone-treated patients followed for a mean of over 10 years had a renal survival of 82% at 10 years from onset, and 75% from start of treatment, figures substantially better than would be predicted from the known natural history [19]. The recommended schedule involves oral administration of 2–2.5 mg/kg (approximately 60 mg/m^2, maximum dose 80 mg) of prednisone on alternate days, reducing slowly thereafter with average doses of 1.75, 1.5, 1.0 and 0.6 mg/kg in the 2nd, 3rd, 4th and 5th years respectively. These authors advocate continuation of treatment for several years, if not indefinitely. Relapse may occur when the prednisone is reduced or stopped, even after several years of treatment [20]. Clearly the long-term use of corticosteroids in young individuals has the potential to have major adverse effects on growth, metabolism and skeletal integrity. Alternate-day schedules probably reduce the adverse effects, but the price that may be paid for this 'successful' therapy remains so high that many nephrologists remain reluctant to adopt the Cincinnati approach.

The International Study of Kidney Disease in Children attempted to address the efficacy of alternate-day prednisone in a double-blind controlled trial [21]. The dose used was 40 mg/m^2, maximum dose 60 mg, smaller than that recommended by the Cincinnati group. Eighty patients were randomized (42 type I, 14 type II, 17 type III, seven not classified); 47 received prednisone and 33 received placebo (lactose). Mean duration of treatment was 41 months, and mean follow-up was 63 months. There was a modest overall difference in treatment failures (development of renal failure or withdrawal due to adverse effects): 40% in the prednisone group and 55% with placebo. The effect of treatment was more impressive when subjected to life-table analysis: at 130 months, renal survival was 61% in the prednisone group and 12% in the placebo group. However, this was still not statistically significant ($p = 0.07$). Also, had the analysis been performed at 110 months the difference would have been much smaller, since the Kaplan–Meier curve for the placebo group diverged at a late stage from that of the prednisone group. Another problem with the study was the significantly longer duration of disease prior to treatment in the placebo group (18.1 months vs. 8.9 months in the prednisone group), possibly indicating that the placebo group had more advanced disease. Thus the trial failed to resolve the question it addressed, despite a major international collaborative effort. Approximately twice the number of recruited patients would have been required for significance to have been demonstrated, illustrating the difficulties in analysis of the effects of treatment in such an uncommon and heterogeneous condition.

Others have modified the approach. Another US group [22] reported 16 patients with type I MCGN who received six alternate-day pulses of intravenous methylprednisolone, 30 mg/kg, maximum dose 1.5 g, followed by an alternate-day oral prednisone regimen similar to that proposed by the Cincinnati group. They reported substantial improvements in proteinuria and excretory renal function after mean follow-up of just over 4 years, and maintenance of improvement in 13 of the 16 whose therapy had been stopped for a mean of 20.8 months. Again, the total prednisone dosage administered to achieve this result seems unacceptably high to some observers. The group from Denver [23], using similar initial doses of corticosteroids, reported improvement in creatinine clearance and proteinuria in the majority of their 19 patients, with the improvement again being sustained after prednisone was stopped. However, in this study the majority of the patients were hypertensive at onset and antihypertensive agents were given contemporaneously with corticosteroids. Thus it is difficult to dissect the effects of prednisone therapy from the benefits of blood pressure control, which may have confounded the results. From Japan, Takeda *et al.* [24] reported 94% renal survival at 4–10 years in 18 children treated with prednisolone plus dipyridamole, but only three patients had heavy proteinuria at onset and, as mentioned earlier, Japanese series may include milder and/or earlier cases ascertained by screening. Somers *et al.* [3] reported 100% renal survival in 11 non-nephrotic children with MCGN, seven of whom did not receive prednisone, and recommended that such therapy should not be applied to all patients with MCGN, instead being targeted to those with nephrotic syndrome.

Other approaches

Long-term treatment with non-steroidal anti-inflammatory drugs (NSAID) has been advocated by Lagrue *et al.* [25] who reported observations in 53 patients, again without a control group. The effect of these agents on proteinuria, as seen in other conditions such as membranous nephropathy [26], may be explained by an effect on intrarenal haemodynamics. NSAID would not be expected to have sufficiently potent anti-inflammatory activity in the kidney to influence substantially the underlying immunopathology. Angiotensin-converting enzyme inhibitors (ACEI) have recently been shown to have useful renoprotective effects in patients with renal disease irrespective of the nature of the primary condition [27]. Of course, hypertension in patients with MCGN should be treated aggressively, and ACEI may be the agents of first choice; again they would not be expected to have potent effects on the underlying disease process.

Given the evidence for the presence of circulating factors causing complement activation in MCGN (considered further below), measures aimed at removal of these from the circulation would seem to offer a logical approach. Plasmapheresis has not been studied in a controlled manner, but one early report of its use in patients with MCGN whose renal function was deteriorating reported stabilization in some patients [28].

There is little information on the effects of cyclosporin in MCGN: anecdotal reports suggest beneficial effects (reviewed in reference 29). One recent study from Turkey included six patients with MCGN, and suggested that the majority of patients showed some improvement, at least in the short term [30]. Further information is awaited on the role of this agent in MCGN.

Analysis of subtypes of MCGN

In the analyses of the effects of therapy, I have not distinguished between the subtypes of MCGN since it is usually impossible to do so from the published information. Most of the trials contain predominantly patients with type I and type III, these being the more common forms, so that any conclusions regarding therapy can most safely be applied to those types. Type II MCGN is considered to carry the worst prognosis, and the available information is conflicting on whether this type is as responsive (or as unresponsive!) to treatment as the others. One analysis from the Cincinnati group reported clinical and histological improvement in a group of six patients with type II MCGN treated with alternate-day prednisone [31]. There was a suggestion in the ISKDC study [21] that patients with type II fared less well, there being little difference between prednisone and placebo in these individuals. However, the numbers were very small, only 14 of the 80 patients having type II. If the type II patients were excluded, and the 66 others analysed together, the effect of prednisone was greater than for the study group as a whole. In the uncontrolled study of plasmapheresis mentioned earlier [28], apparent benefit occurred only in patients with type I MCGN. Only two patients with hypocomplementaemic type II MCGN were included, but it is of interest that neither of these showed any response to plasmapheresis, especially since the evidence for a causative role of a circulating factor is strongest for this type of MCGN. There is one case report describing a patient with recurrent type II MCGN in a renal transplant who apparently improved after plasmapheresis [32].

Possible future therapeutic strategies

Rational design of specific forms of therapy for MCGN depends on careful analysis of the pathogenesis. As discussed earlier, drugs directed at platelets or at the coagulation cascade were used in early studies in MCGN, but since neither platelets nor fibrin are particularly prominent in the glomerular lesions seen in this condition perhaps it is not surprising that these therapies have proved ineffective. Anti-inflammatory agents such as corticosteroids may have useful effects in MCGN, but their non-specific nature and their adverse effects in other systems mean that a high price is paid for any beneficial effect on the renal lesion. More selective forms of anti-inflammatory therapy are becoming available, aimed at individual pro-inflammatory mediators such as tumour necrosis factor (which can be neutralized with specific monoclonal antibodies [33, 34]) or interleukin-1 (the effect of which can be abrogated using soluble IL-1 receptor antagonist [35]). Therapy aimed at selective neutralization of individual mediators is theoretically attractive because of the exquisite specificity of such an approach, but no single mediator has been shown to be primarily involved in MCGN (nor indeed in any other form of human nephritis).

Complement activation is frequently associated with MCGN, and one mode of action of anti-inflammatory agents in this condition may be via inhibition of complement-mediated injury. Complement activation in the glomerulus may mediate injury directly by leading to cell lysis, or indirectly by engaging other inflammatory mechanisms. C3a and C5a, by-products of cleavage of C3 and C5 respectively, are potent anaphylatoxins which can attract and activate leukocytes, recruiting them to the inflammatory focus. Therapies are becoming available which inhibit complement activation by both the classical and alternative pathways, for example the soluble complement receptor CR1 [36], and application of these forms of therapy may be practicable in the near future.

A variety of complement-activating factors in the serum of patients with MCGN has been described (reviewed in reference 37). In type I there may be circulating immune complexes, some patients have antibodies to Clq which probably directly activate the classical pathway, and some have so-called 'classical pathway nephritic factor', or 'C4 nephritic factor'. This is an unfortunate choice of names since it is distinct from the originally described nephritic factor (C3 nephritic factor, referred to as C3NeF, or more simply as NeF) which causes alternative pathway activation and is most closely associated with type II MCGN and partial lipodystrophy. In type II MCGN the alternative pathway activation is due to the presence of an IgG autoantibody (C3NeF, or NeF) which binds to a neoantigen formed when the alternative pathway C3 convertase enzyme, C3bBb, is assembled. The antibody stabilizes this enzyme and protects it from degradation by factor H. Thus the half-life of the enzyme is prolonged, and the normal regulatory mechanism is subverted. This type of nephritic factor has also been described in patients with type I and type III MCGN, but its presence is virtually a *sine qua non* in type II MCGN. In type III MCGN the presence of a circulating factor which activates complement slowly in a properdin-dependent manner has been postulated. The terminology is unfortunately confusing since this factor has also been labelled as a 'nephritic factor', but it is quite distinct from the NeF associated with type II MCGN and PLD, which causes rapid, properdin-independent complement activation. Why there should be preferential depletion of terminal pathway components, and what relationship this activation has to the renal injury, remain unanswered questions.

The best evidence for a causative role of complement activation in MCGN comes in type II. As mentioned above, most patients with type II MCGN have the IgG autoantibody known as nephritic factor (NeF) which allows unregulated alternative pathway activation. Two other situations in which there is similar overactivity of the alternative pathway, and an associated renal lesion with the appearances of type II MCGN, have recently been characterized. First, genetic deficiency of the regulatory protein known as factor H, which normally serves to degrade the alternative pathway C3 convertase, has been reported in a variety of in-bred pig [38] and also in rare human cases [39]. Second, there is a case report [40] of an individual whose serum contained a monoclonal lambda light chain which interacted with factor H *in vitro* and prevented its action, allowing unregulated alternative pathway activation. Therefore, in these three situations (the presence of NeF, genetic deficiency of factor H, or functional blocking of factor H), there is dysregulated alternative pathway activation, but due to completely different mechanisms. In each case the renal lesion is type II MCGN, strongly suggesting that it is the complement activation *per se* which leads to the renal injury. Thus therapy aimed at inhibiting this complement activation would be expected to be beneficial. Strategies to remove NeF (or other complement-activating factors found in the various types of MCGN) could include plasmapheresis or immunoadsorption, but these would only have short-term effects. Suppression of autoantibody synthesis with drugs which are relatively lymphocyte-specific, such as mycophenolate mofetil [41, 42], might be an attractive approach, offering greater specificity than alkylating agents. The therapy of autoimmune disease would be revolutionized if it were possible to restore tolerance to the autoantigen, for example with peptides, perhaps delivered by mucosal routes [43], and this would apply to NeF as well as to any other autoimmune condition. At present, however, such therapies are distant dreams.

Type II MCGN is often associated with partial lipodystrophy (PLD), in which there is permanent loss of adipose tissue from the face, arms and upper trunk. There is evidence that NeF-mediated alternative pathway complement activation may be directly responsible for the fat cell destruction in PLD and that a key factor in this is the local production of complement components by adipocytes [44, 45]. Since intrinsic renal cells also synthesize and secrete complement proteins, a similar mechanism may underlie type II MCGN [46]. Therapeutic measures aimed at down-regulating complement component expression, or up-regulating the expression of regulatory molecules such as factor H, would be potentially powerful, but at present such measures are not technically feasible.

Conclusions

The term MCGN covers a heterogeneous group of conditions in which, without treatment, the prognosis for renal survival is poor. The available literature does not provide convincing support for a beneficial effect of any form of therapy in MCGN. The best case exists for alternate-day prednisone. Nevertheless, high dosages are required for prolonged periods and the magnitude of benefit obtained may be too small to justify the risks of such treatment. Possibly by refining the dosage schedule, and by applying the treatment only to high-risk groups, such as those with severe nephrotic syndrome, the risk/benefit ratio may be more favourable. In the future, therapy aimed at the complement system may be rational, and could offer improvements over the generally disappointing results of current forms of treatment. Assessment of any novel forms of therapy can only meaningfully be achieved if international efforts to mount large trials are supported by the nephrological community.

References

1. Varade WS, Forristal J, West CD. Patterns of complement activation in idiopathic membranoproliferative glomerulonephritis, types I, II, III. Am J Kidney Dis 1990;16:196–206.
2. Schwertz R, de Jong R, Gretz N, Kirschfink M, Anders D, Scharer K. Outcome of idiopathic membranoproliferative glomerulonephritis in children. Acta Paediatr Scand 1996;85:308–12.
3. Somers M, Kertesz S, Rosen S *et al.* Non-nephrotic children with membranoproliferative glomerulonephritis: are steroids indicated? Pediatr Nephrol 1995;9:140–4.
4. Iitaka K, Igarashi S, Sakai T. Hypocomplementemia and membranoproliferative glomerulonephritis in school urinary screening in Japan. Pediatr Nephrol 1994;8:420–2.
5. Iitaka K, Ishidate T, Hojo M, Kuwao S, Kasai N, Sakai T. Idiopathic membranoproliferative glomerulonephritis in Japanese children. Pediatr Nephrol 1995;9:272–7.
6. Schena FP, Cameron JS. Treatment of proteinuric idiopathic glomerulonephritides in adults: a retrospective survey. Am J Med 1988;85:315–26.
7. Donadio JV, Offord KP. Reassessment of treatment results in membranoproliferative glomerulonephritis, with emphasis on life-table analysis. Am J Kidney Dis 1989;14:445–51.
8. Mathieson, PW, Rees AJ. Changing views on the treatment of glomerulonephritis. In: Andreucci VE, Fine LG, editors. International Yearbook of Nephrology 1991. Boston, MA: Kluwer; 1990:73–96.
9. Kincaid-Smith P. The treatment of chronic mesangiocapillary (membranoproliferative) glomerulonephritis with impaired renal function. Med J Aust 1979;2:587–92.
10. Chapman SJ, Cameron JS, Chantler C, Turner D. Treatment of mesangiocapillary glomerulonephritis in children with combined immunosuppression and anticoagulation. Arch Dis Child 1980;55:446–51.
11. Tiller DJ, Clarkson AR, Mathew T *et al.* A prospective randomized trial in the use of cyclophosphamide, dipyridamole and warfarin in membranous and mesangiocapillary glomerulonephritis. In: Zurukzoglu W, Papadimitriou M, Sion M *et al.*, editors. Eighth International Congress of Nephrology: Advances in Basic and Clinical Nephrology. Basel: Karger; 1981:345–51.
12. Cattran DC, Cardella CJ, Roscoe JH *et al.* Results of a controlled drug trial in membranoproliferative glomerulonephritis. Kidney Int 1985;27:436–41.
13. Zimmerman SW, Moorthy AV, Dreher WH, Friedman A, Varanasi U. Prospective trial of warfarin and dipyridamole in patients with membranoproliferative glomerulonephritis. Am J Med 1983;75:920–7.
14. Feadda R, Satta A, Tanda F, Pirisi M, Bartoli E. Immunosuppressive treatment of membranoproliferative glomerulonephritis. Nephron 1994;67:59–65.

15. Donadio JV, Anderson CF, Mitchell JCIII. Membranoproliferative glomerulonephritis: a prospective trial of platelet inhibitor therapy. N Engl J Med 1984;310:1421–6.
16. Zauner I, Bohler J, Braun N, Grupp C, Heering P, Schollmeyer P. Effect of aspirin and dipyridamole on proteinuria in idiopathic membranoproliferative glomerulonephritis: a multicentre prospective clinical trial. Nephrol Dial Transplant 1994;9:619–22.
17. McEnery PT, McAdams AJ, West CD. Membranoproliferative glomerulonephritis: improved survival with alternate day prednisone therapy. Clin Nephrol 1980;13:117–24.
18. McEnery PT, McAdams AJ, West CD. The effect of prednisone in a high-dose, alternate-day regime on the natural history of idiopathic membranoproliferative glomerulonephritis. Medicine 1986;64:401–24.
19. McEnery PT. Membranoproliferative glomerulonephritis: the Cincinnati experience - cumulative renal survival from 1957 to 1989. J Pediatr 1990;116:S109–14.
20. West CD. Idiopathic membranoproliferative glomerulonephritis in childhood. Pediatr Nephrol 1992;6:96–103.
21. Tarshish P, Bernstein J, Tobin JN, Edelmann CM. Treatment of mesangiocapillary glomerulonephritis with alternate-day prednisone – a report of the International Study of Kidney Disease in Children. Pediatr Nephrol 1992;6:123–36.
22. Bergstein JM, Andreoli SP. Response of type I membranoproliferative glomerulonephritis to pulse methylprednisolone and alternate-day prednisone therapy. Pediatr Nephrol 1995;9:268–71.
23. Ford DM, Briscoe DM, Shanley PF, Lum GM. Childhood membranoproliferative glomerulonephritis type I: limited steroid therapy. Kidney Int 1992;41:1606–12.
24. Takeda A, Niimura F, Matsutani H. Long-term corticosteroid and dipyridamole treatment of membranoproliferative glomerulonephritis type I in children. Jpn J Nephrol 1995;37:330–5.
25. Lagrue G, Laurent J, Belghiti D. Renal survival in membranoproliferative glomerulonephritis (MPGN): role of long-term treatment with non-steroid anti-inflammatory drugs (NSAID). Int Urol Nephrol 1988;20:669–77.
26. Velosa JA, Torres, VE, Donadio JV, Wagoner RD, Holley KE, Offord KP. Treatment of severe nephrotic syndrome with meclofenamate: an uncontrolled pilot study. Mayo Clin Proc 1985;60: 586–92.
27. The GISEN group. Randomised placebo-controlled trial of effect of ramipril on decline in glomerular filtration rate and risk of terminal renal failure in proteinuric, non-diabetic nephropathy. Lancet 1997;349:1857–63.
28. McGinley E, Watkins R, McLay A, Boulton-Jones JM. Plasma exchange in the treatment of mesangiocapillary glomerulonephritis. Nephron 1985;40:385–90.
29. Cattran DC. Current status of cyclosporin A in the treatment of membranous, IgA and membranoproliferative glomerulonephritis. Clin Nephrol 1991;35(Suppl.1):S43–7.
30. Noyan A, Anarat A, Tuncer I, Gonlusen G, Polat S. Efficacy and side effects of cyclosporin A in nephrotic syndrome of childhood. Nephron 1995;70:410–15.
31. McEnery PT, McAdams AJ. Regression of membranoproliferative glomerulonephritis type II (dense deposit disease): observations in six children. Am J Kidney Dis 1988;12:138–46.
32. Oberkircher OR, Enama M, West JC, Campbell P, Moran J. Regression of recurrent membranoproliferative glomerulonephritis type II in a transplanted kidney after plasmapheresis therapy. Transplant Proc 1988;20(Suppl.1):418–23.
33. Elliott MJ, Maini RN, Feldmann M *et al.* Randomised double-blind comparison of chimeric monoclonal antibody to tumour necrosis factor alpha (cA2) versus placebo in rheumatoid arthritis. Lancet 1994;344:1105–10.
34. Elliott MJ, Maini RN, Feldman M *et al.* Repeated therapy with monoclonal antibody to tumour necrosis factor alpha (cA2) in patients with rheumatoid arthritis. Lancet 1994;344:1125–7.
35. Weckmann AL, Alocer-Verela J. Cytokine inhibitors in autoimmune disease. Semin Arthritis Rheum 1996;26:539–57.
36. Fearon DT. Anti-inflammatory and immunosuppressive effects of recombinant soluble complement receptors. Clin Exp Immunol 1991;86(Suppl.1):43–6.

37. Mathieson PW, Peters KD. Deficiency and depletion of complement in the pathogenesis of nephritis and vasculitis. Kidney Int 1993;44(Suppl. 42):S13–18.
38. Hogasen K, Jansen JH, Mollnes TE, Hovdenes J, Harboe M. Hereditary porcine membranoproliferative glomerulonephritis type II is caused by factor H deficiency. J Clin Invest 1995;95: 1054–61.
39. Levy M, Halbwachs-Mecarelli L, Gubler M-C *et al.* H deficiency in two brothers with atypical dense intramembranous deposit disease. Kidney Int 1986;30:949–56.
40. Meri S, Koistinen V, Miettinen A, Tornroth T, Sepparla IJT. Activation of the alternative pathway of complement by monoclonal lambda light chains in membranoproliferative glomerulonephritis. J Exp Med 1992;175:939–50.
41. Lipsky JJ. Mycophenolate mofetil. Lancet 1996;348:1357–9.
42. Brazelton TR, Morris RE. Molecular mechanisms of action of new xenobiotic immunosuppressive drugs: tacrolimus (FK506), sirolimus (rapamycin), mycophenolate mofetil and leflunomide. Curr Opin Immunol 1996;8:710–20.
43. Wraith DC. Antigen-specific immunotherapy of autoimmune disease: a commentary. Clin Exp Immunol 1996;103:349–52.
44. Mathieson PW, Wurzner R, Oliveira DBG, Lachmann PJ, Peters DK. Complement-mediated adipocyte lysis by nephritic factor sera. J Exp Med 1993;177:1827–31.
45. Finn JE, Mathieson PW. Molecular analysis of C3 allotypes in patients with nephritic factor. Clin Exp Immunol 1993;91:410–14.
46. Mathieson PW, Peters DK. Are nephritic factors nephritogenic? Am J Kidney Dis 1994;24: 964–6.

6. IgA nephropathy and Henoch–Schönlein purpura

J. FEEHALLY

Introduction

IgA nephropathy

IgA nephropathy (IgAN) is a common pattern of glomerulonephritis defined by mesangial IgA deposition. It may occur at any age but most commonly presents in the second and third decades of life. Recurrent macroscopic haematuria is the most frequent clinical presentation but other patients present with microscopic haematuria, proteinuria or progressive renal failure. The apparent prevalence of the disease will increase if urine screening is widely used in any population in which renal biopsy is recommended for those with minor urine abnormalities. Hypertension is particularly common and usually predates renal impairment. Rapidly progressive renal failure is unusual; it may result from acute tubular necrosis as a consequence of macroscopic haematuria, or from superimposed crescentic nephritis. Recurrent IgA deposition after transplantation is common. IgA deposits are found in 50% of transplants, although structural glomerular injury is uncommon and the overall success of transplantation is not diminished.

Henoch–Schönlein nephritis

Henoch–Schönlein purpura (HSP) is a systemic vasculitis with characteristic rash, abdominal pain and arthralgia; it is particularly common in childhood but may occur at any age. Tissue IgA deposition is a hallmark of HSP. The nephritis which accompanies HSP (HS nephritis) may be histologically indistinguishable from IgAN. It is probable that IgAN is a monosymptomatic form of HSP. Recurrence of IgA deposits after transplantation is as common as in IgAN.

Natural history

IgA nephropathy
IgAN is slowly progressive: up to 25% of patients are said to reach end-stage

C.D. Pusey (ed.), The Treatment of Glomerulonephritis, 93–111.

renal disease (ESRD) within 25 years of diagnosis, but this depends upon the proportion of patients with isolated haematuria in any patient cohort since they have a very good prognosis. When proteinuria is trivial (<1 g/24 h) 98% 15-year renal survival is reported [1]. Clinical features predicting a poor prognosis are mostly those common to any chronic glomerular disease [2]: proteinuria, renal impairment and hypertension at presentation. Episodic macroscopic haematuria unexpectedly is associated in most series with good outcome, perhaps because such patients present earlier in the course of the disease because of overt symptoms. Pathological features defining poor prognosis are likewise common to any glomerular disease [2]: glomerular sclerosis, extensive crescent formation, tubular atrophy, interstitial fibrosis and arteriolosclerosis. The one specific unfavourable feature is deposition of IgA in capillary loops as well as the mesangium.

Henoch–Schönlein nephritis
The majority of HS nephritis is self-limiting: there is a transient urine abnormality which is never fully evaluated. Of those who undergo renal biopsy 40% eventually progress to ESRD. Prognostic markers are those described for IgAN.

Disease mechanisms in IgAN and HS nephritis

IgAN and HSP share many abnormalities of the IgA immune system [3]. Exaggerated polymeric IgA1 (pIgA1) responses are typical although increases in circulating IgA1 are modest. Because of the clinical association with mucosal infection the pIgA1 was thought to originate from the mucosal immune system, but evidence now indicates the bone marrow is the likely source [4]. However, a defect in mucosal IgA immunity may be present, increasing antigen penetration and challenge to the marrow. The mechanism of mesangial IgA deposition is not understood: IgAN and HS nephritis are often regarded as immune complex diseases although no specific antigen has consistently been identified in the deposits [5]. Altered glycosylation of IgA1 is a feature of IgAN and HSP and may promote mesangial IgA deposition and subsequent inflammation [6]. Mechanisms of ongoing inflammation and scarring are probably common to other chronic glomerulonephritis without IgA deposition.

Therapeutic strategies

In light of the disease mechanisms and natural history of IgAN the following approaches to treatment have been proposed:

1. reduce IgA production;

2. prevent glomerular IgA deposition or promote its removal;
3. alter early immune and inflammatory events which follow IgA deposition;
4. alter later non-specific events which promote progressive renal failure;
5. prevent recurrent disease after transplant.

Therapeutic endpoints

Haematuria
Reduction of episodes of macroscopic haematuria is a clear-cut goal but should not be taken to represent the loss of all disease activity. Controlled studies are needed since the natural history of IgAN is that macroscopic haematuria becomes less common with time without intervention.

Proteinuria
Reduction in proteinuria is an attractive short-term and long-term goal. Only a small minority of patients are nephrotic and in such patients the clinical benefits of reducing proteinuria and correcting serum albumin are unequivocal. However, treatment trial strategy often selects patients using non-nephrotic proteinuria as a marker of poor prognosis. The benefit of modest reductions in proteinuria, even if statistically significant, is uncertain unless accompanied by preservation of renal function.

Prevention of renal failure
Prevention of ESRD is the ultimate goal. However, IgAN is usually so slowly progressive that surrogate markers are required to provide data within an acceptable time frame. Doubling of serum creatinine or reduction in glomerular filtration rate (GFR) can be complemented by histological data from serial renal biopsy.

Study design

Study group heterogeneity
We cannot be certain that patients with mesangial IgA deposition always share a common disease process, but at present it remains the defining criterion for these studies. Renal histology can be useful in study recruitment to minimize heterogeneity, but this will be less useful if the interval between biopsy and recruitment is prolonged. Patients with HSP have been excluded from most available studies; it is therefore still uncertain whether any strategies developed for IgAN are indeed applicable to HS nephritis.

Risk versus benefit
In slowly progressive disease, the balance of risk against benefit when prolonged treatment is considered is often unfavourable. Acute immune interventions are not easy to plan. If there is crescentic nephritis with renal failure intensive treatment is justifiable; more often visible haematuria is clinically striking but transient and produces no functional renal impairment, weakening the justification for therapy. In any case clinically apparent haematuria is likely to represent the tip of an iceberg of ongoing injury, so that shaping and timing the intensity of therapy, even if rational treatments were available, is difficult.

The good prognosis for many patients, particularly those with isolated haematuria, argues against their involvement in prolonged studies of therapies with potential side-effects. On the other hand the selection of patients by proteinuria can introduce heterogeneity since proteinuria may reflect both active immune injury and fixed chronic damage. Any study using proteinuria alone as an entry criterion will provide therapeutic guidance for only a minority of patients with IgAN.

Randomized controlled trials
The need for randomized controlled trials (RCT) of adequate power to answer questions about the prevention of chronic renal failure in IgAN is pressing. It is disappointing, despite the prevalence of IgAN and consensus about its definition and natural history, that such studies are so few. Available studies are clearly defined in this chapter as RCT and shown in bold typeface in the tables.

Treatment of IgA nephropathy

Reduction of IgA production

Reduce mucosal antigen challenge
Dietary manipulation. Attempts have been made in uncontrolled studies to modify food antigen intake, particularly by modifying gluten intake (since circulating IgA antigliadin antibodies are reported in IgAN). There were reductions in proteinuria and haematuria after 6 months of gluten restriction but, despite this, renal impairment progressed [7]. A low-antigen diet has also been used in a preliminary study, with little benefit [8].

Altered mucosal permeability. Sodium cromoglycate and 5-aminosalicylic acid both alter mucosal permeability to food antigens. In IgAN they have each been shown to reduce proteinuria but have no other benefit [9, 10].

Antibiotics. A report of a controlled trial of tetracycline for 1 year showed a reduction in the magnitude of haematuria but no effect on proteinuria or renal impairment [11]. There is no other evidence for a role for prophylactic antibiotics.

Tonsillectomy. Tonsillectomy has been shown to reduce the frequency of episodic haematuria when tonsillitis is the provoking infection [12] but has not yet been shown to reduce the incidence of progressive renal failure. The one controlled trial showed reduction in proteinuria and haematuria 36 months after tonsillectomy, but only in those patients with initial serum creatinine <150 μmol/L [13].

Phenytoin

Phenytoin reduces serum IgA levels and has been given in two controlled trials [14, 15]. It produced no benefit to renal function or proteinuria, or to renal histology in repeat biopsies after treatment. In one study it did reduce the frequency of episodic macroscopic haematuria [15].

Other approaches to reduce IgA production

There are no other known strategies for reducing relevant IgA production. There is no evidence that any immunosuppressive treatment used in IgAN alters circulating IgA levels or modifies IgA1 glycosylation, although the possibility cannot be excluded that a number of immune manipulations may reduce a specific subset of nephritogenic pIgA1 molecules.

Prevention and removal of IgA deposits

The ideal treatment for IgAN would remove IgA from the glomerulus and prevent further IgA deposition. This remains a remote prospect while IgA deposition is so poorly understood. Such a treatment would also need to be extremely safe since it would require application to large numbers of patients with benign disease unless reliable early markers of progression risk were available. The prevalence of recurrent IgA deposition after transplantation suggests that conventional immunosuppression does not prevent IgA deposition even if it may alter subsequent inflammatory events.

Danazol. Danazol increases serum complement levels in those with complement deficiency such as hereditary angio-oedema. It could therefore assist complement-mediated solubilization of mesangial deposits. In a small uncontrolled trial [16] danazol did reduce proteinuria in patients with mild renal histology but there was no change in serum creatinine or haematuria. This has not been investigated further.

Altering immune and inflammatory events which follow IgA deposition

Rapidly progressive renal failure associated with crescentic IgA nephritis
In this uncommon situation the risk–benefit balance is most strongly placed in favour of intensive immunosuppressive therapy since, untreated, there will be rapid progression to ESRD. Unfortunately, available information is restricted to anecdotes. There are a number of case reports, of which nine are reviewed by Lai *et al.* [17]. The largest single experience is six cases treated by Roccattello *et al.* [18]. Treatment in the majority of cases has combined plasma exchange with prednisolone and cyclophosphamide. Early clinical response is favourable, as in other crescentic nephritis, but medium-term results are disappointing: nine of 15 treated patients reached ESRD by 12 months. The only report in children is of five cases [19], all of whom responded poorly, although treatment was less intensive (corticosteroids only in three cases, no patient given plasma exchange).

Small numbers of crescents are a relatively common finding in IgAN without renal failure. An aggressive regimen is justified only if there is rapidly progressive renal failure, particularly since the medium-term results are less favourable than in other crescentic nephritis. Crescentic IgAN is so uncommon that it is improbable that randomized controlled studies will ever be undertaken. It is not possible on present evidence to be certain which elements of the regimen (corticosteroids, cyclophosphamide, plasma exchange) are mandatory.

Early treatment with immunosuppressive/anti-inflammatory regimens
Interventions have been made in IgAN soon after diagnosis in those with active disease, even when renal function is still preserved. Treatments have included corticosteroids, cyclophosphamide, azathioprine and pooled human immunoglobulin. In some studies these have been combined with antiplatelet agents and warfarin.

Corticosteroids. The main studies are summarized in Table 6.1. There have been only two RCT of corticosteroids: one in nephrotic adults [20], the other in children with low-grade proteinuria [21]. Neither showed benefit. However, among the adults there was a minority with very minor histological changes who responded rapidly to treatment (see below: Nephrotic syndrome and IgAN).

Despite the negative outcome of these two short-term studies, corticosteroids have been widely used and there has been continuing interest in the influence of prolonged steroid treatment on outcome. Waldo *et al.* gave alternate-day prednisone (initial dose 60 mg/m^2) for 2–4 years to 13 children with preserved renal function and proteinuria >1g/24 h [22]. After 4–10 years of follow-up urinalysis had returned to normal in 12 out of 13, and there was preserved GFR and improved histology in those who were rebiopsied compared with historical controls. In adults with heavy proteinuria [24] corticosteroids appeared to preserve renal function if initial creatinine clearance was >70

Table 6.1 Corticosteroid treatment in IgA nephropathy

Authors [ref]	No. on active treatment	Treatment period (months)	Follow-up (months)	Proteinuria before treatment (mean, g/24 h)	Proteinuria after treatment (mean, g/24 h)	Benefit	Comment
Lai *et al.*, 1986 [20]	**17 (adults)**	**4**	**38 (12–106)**	**6.5**	**2.3**	**Remission of nephrotic syndrome in six of seven with minor histological changes**	**40% had steroid-related complications**
Welch *et al.*, 1992 [21]	**20 (children)**	**3**	**6**	**0.3**	**0.3**	**None**	**Low-grade proteinuria only**
Kobayashi *et al.*, 1988 [23]	29 (adults)	12–36	74 (34–102)	3.2	1.5	Proteinuria reduced; risk of renal failure reduced	Uncontrolled; bad prognosis in untreated cohort
Kobayashi *et al.*, 1996 [24] untreated	20 (adults)	18	120	1.4	0.8	Risk of renal failure reduced	Uncontrolled; 4/20 ESRD at 10 years, cf. 16/26
Waldo *et al.*, 1993 [22]	13 (children)	24–48	48–120	>1	Nil in 12/13	Resolution of haematuria and proteinuria; improved histology	Historical controls

Randomized controlled trials in **bold**. ESRD = end-stage renal disease.

ml/min, but there was no untreated control group in this study. In moderate proteinuria 10-year follow-up suggests reduced risk of ESRD with corticosteroids [25] but this was an uncontrolled study.

Immunosuppressive agents. The main studies are summarized in Table 6.2.

Cyclophosphamide. Cyclophosphamide has been used in combination with warfarin and dipyridamole in two RCT which are not consistent. The studies are of very similar design and both showed modest reduction in proteinuria [25, 26], but the preservation of renal function in one study [25] could not be confirmed [26]. Cyclophosphamide has not been used alone in IgAN. In any case many physicians regard the risk of cyclophosphamide as unacceptable in young adults with slowly progressive IgAN. Further studies have therefore assessed the combination of warfarin and dipyridamole without cyclophosphamide (see below: Antiplatelet agents).

Azathioprine. The only controlled trial of azathioprine (in combination with chlorambucil) showed no benefit [27]. In an open study of children with aggressive disease azathioprine with prednisolone appeared to preserve renal function [28]. In a large long-term retrospective study [29] azathioprine with low-dose prednisolone given to 66 patients preserved renal function compared with 48 untreated 'controls'. In this interesting study those who received azathioprine had more unfavourable initial features, yet a significant reduction in progression. A further prospective study of prednisolone/azathioprine would be most valuable.

Cyclosporin. Cyclosporin has been used in one RCT [30]. There was a reversible fall in proteinuria but this went in parallel with a fall in creatinine clearance, suggesting the changes were a haemodynamic effect of cyclosporin rather than an immune modulating effect.

Pooled human immunoglobulin. The immunomodulatory and anti-inflammatory effects of pooled human immunoglobulin are poorly defined, but they have some benefit in uncontrolled studies in systemic vasculitis and lupus. There is little short-term toxicity although long-term effects have not yet been well documented. Open studies of immunoglobulin have been reported in both 'severe' IgAN (heavy proteinuria with falling GFR) [31] and 'moderate' IgAN (persistent proteinuria with GFR >70 ml/min) [32]. Proteinuria lessened, deterioration in GFR slowed in the severe group, and histological activity scores lessened where repeat renal biopsies were available. No prospective controlled trial is yet available for this promising approach.

Nephrotic syndrome in IgAN

Nephrotic syndrome occurs in only 5% of IgAN. In many of these patients the heavy proteinuria is a manifestation of significant structural glomerular

Table 6.2 Immunosuppressive treatment in IgA nephropathy

Author [ref]	Agents	No. on active treatment	Treatment period (months)	Follow-up period (months)	Benefit	Comment
Woo *et al.*, 1991 [25]	**Cyclophosphamide+ dipyridamole/warfarin**	**27**	**36**	**60**	**Proteinuria reduced (mean 2.4–0.8 g/24 h)**	**Glomerulosclerosis prevented**
Walker *et al.*, 1990 [26]	**Cyclophosphamide**	**25**	**6**	**24**	**Proteinuria reduced (mean 1.7–1.2 g/24 h); renal function unchanged**	
Lagrue *et al.*, 1975 [27]	**Azathioprine+ chlorambucil**	**13**	**24**	**24**	**None**	
Andreoli and Bergstein, 1989 [28]	Azathioprine+ prednisolone	10	12	30 (9–90)	Proteinuria reduced (mean 4.1–1.7 g/24 h); renal function stabilized; disease activity less on repeat biopsy	Severe initial biopsy
Goumenos *et al.*, 1995 [29]	Azathioprine+ prednisolone	66	24 (12–98)	46 (12–180)	Proteinuria unchanged; renal function stabilized	
Lai *et al.*, 1987 [30]	**Cyclosporin**	**9**	**3**	**6**	**Transient reduction in proteinuria (mean 4.2–1.3 g/24 h)**	**Parallel fall in renal function reversed when cyclosporin withdrawn**

Randomized controlled trials in **bold**.

damage and progressive renal dysfunction. However a small minority, both adults and children, have nephrosis with minimal glomerular change on renal biopsy, although there are also IgA deposits and haematuria. In these cases proteinuria remits promptly in response to corticosteroids [20]. In these patients two common glomerular diseases may coincide – minimal change nephrotic syndrome and IgAN [33, 34]. This observation justifies a trial of corticosteroids in IgAN with nephrotic syndrome and preserved renal function when light microscopy shows minimal glomerular injury. However it does not justify prolonged exposure to corticosteroids if there is not a prompt response, nor their use in the presence of significant histological glomerular injury.

Treatment of slowly progressive IgAN

There is little to suggest that the events of progressive glomerular injury are unique to IgAN. The growing experimental evidence on mesangial injury and its resolution under the influence of growth factors and cytokines [35] seems to be applicable to mesangial glomerulonephritis whether or not there are IgA deposits. The adverse influence of hypertension and the likely role of proteinuria in progression likewise are common to all glomerular disease.

Treatments available are non-specific. They are reported as treatments for IgAN but it is more precise to regard them as treatments for chronic glomerular disease of which IgAN is the commonest and most easily defined. The immunosuppressive strategies reviewed above may equally be non-specific in their efficacy. The main approaches include treatment of hypertension and the use of antiplatelet agents, anticoagulants and fish oil.

Predicting risk of progression

The conventional clinical and histological criteria described at the beginning of this chapter predict at diagnosis those with a poor prognosis. More helpful would be the chance to identify those who will do badly even if they show none of the known adverse features at diagnosis. A role for ACE genotypes has recently been evaluated. A deletion allele (D) in the ACE gene is associated with increased serum and tissue ACE levels. Studies associate the DD genotype with susceptibility to IgAN but results are not entirely consistent [36]. The DD genotype may define risk of progression [37] even in patients who at presentation are normotensive with normal creatinine clearance [38]. However, it appears that the ACE genotype association is unlikely to be specific for IgAN: an association between increased rate of progression of chronic renal failure and DD genotype has been found in patients with all types of non-diabetic renal failure [39]. Even if the ACE gene polymorphism defines high-risk groups with IgAN, the extrapolation from a genetic abnormality in tissue ACE to a therapeutic role for ACE inhibitors requires caution. The ACE gene may be a marker rather than the susceptibility gene itself.

Anticoagulants and antiplatelet agents
Two studies of dipyridamole/warfarin in combination with cyclophosphamide give conflicting results [25, 26] (see Table 6.2). Likewise two RCT of dipyridamole/warfarin alone are inconsistent, with no benefit in one [40], and preservation of renal function in the other [41].

Urokinase has been used in view of the finding of fibrinogen deposits in the glomerulus in IgAN. A controlled trial [42] produced a short-term reduction in proteinuria and improvement in serum creatinine but these benefits were not sustained on longer follow-up.

Hypertension
There is compelling evidence for the benefit of lowering blood pressure in the treatment of chronic progressive glomerular disease. The question of the choice of hypotensive agent remains open. Angiotensin-converting enzyme inhibitors (ACE inhibitors) are favoured, but as yet evidence is incomplete (Table 6.3). ACE inhibitor therapy produced a very modest, though statistically significant, reduction in proteinuria in a short-term study in normotensive IgAN [43]. Two retrospective studies in IgAN suggest the benefit of using ACE inhibitors for hypertension compared with beta-blockers [44] or with a wide range of other agents [45]. The recent studies on ACE genotype distribution provide no direct data to inform the clinical value of ACE inhibitors. The only RCT of ACE inhibitors has reported interim data on 23 patients with proteinuria and GFR between 30 and 90 ml/min randomized to receive enalapril or nifedipine and followed for 12 months [46]. There was no significant difference in rate of deterioration in renal function, although proteinuria was reduced by enalapril but not by nifedipine.

Fish oil
Fish oil has been widely adopted for the treatment of IgAN in recent years. The available studies are summarized in Table 6.4.

The favourable effects of supplementing the diet with ω-3 fatty acids in the form of fish oil include reductions in eicosanoid and cytokine production, changes in membrane fluidity and rheology, and reduced platelet aggregability. These features should significantly reduce the adverse influence of many mechanisms thought to impact on progression of chronic glomerular disease.

The findings of the large study of Donadio *et al.* [47] provide convincing evidence of protection by 2 years treatment with fish oil (12 g daily). Doubling of serum creatinine, the major study end-point, occurred in only 6% of fish oil-treated patients, but 33% of controls; although it was surprising that fish oil did not significantly reduce proteinuria, which is a major risk factor for progression. The control group had progressive renal failure more rapid than usually expected in IgAN, but the treatment and control groups otherwise appeared well matched. Another small study also showed benefit from 1 year's treatment with fish oil [48]. However the study of Bennett *et al.* [49] showed no benefit, and that of Pettersson *et al.* [50] showed a small but significant decrease in renal

Table 6.3 Angiotensin-converting enzyne inhibitor treatment in IgA nephropathy

Authors [ref]	Type of study	Entry criterion	No. on ACE inhibitor	Follow-up (months)	Outcome	Comment
Maschio *et al.*, 1994 [43]	**Placebo-controlled cross-over**	**Proteinuria 1–2.5 g/24 h, normotensive**	**8**	**8**	**Proteinuria reduced (mean 1.8–1.4 g/24 h)**	**Short-term study; ? functional importance of minor reduction in proteinuria**
Cattran *et al.*, 1994 [45]	Retrospective	Proteinuria >1 g/24 h, hypertensive	27	19 (3–49)	Remission of proteinuria more frequent (18.5% cf. 2%)	ESRD 19% compared to 49% if other hypotensive agents used
Rekola *et al.*, 1991 [44]	Retrospective	Proteinuria (mean 1.8 g/24 h)	22	37	Proteinuria no different, reduction in GFR less on ACE inhibitor	Comparative group on beta-blockers
Bannister *et al.*, 1995 [46]	**RCT – enalapril vs. nifedipine**	**Hypertensive, GFR 30–90 ml/min**	**12**	**12**	**Proteinuria reduced (mean 2.0–1.2 g/24 h), renal function not different**	

Randomized controlled trials in **bold**. ESRD = end-stage renal disease.

Table 6.4 Fish oil treatment in IgA nephropathy

Authors [ref]	Entry criteria	No. on active treatment	Duration of treatment (months)	Outcome	Comment
Hamazaki *et al.* 1984 [48]	No details	10	12	Renal function stabilized	Randomization not described
Bennett *et al.*, 1989 [49]	**Proteinuria**	**17**	**24**	**No benefit**	
Cheng *et al.*, 1990 [51]	Creatinine 3.6 (2.0–6.0) mg/dl	11	10 (8–12)	No benefit	Advanced renal impairment at recruitment
Pettersson *et al.*, 1994 [50]	**Proteinuria >0.5 g/24 h, creatinine <2.8 mg/dl**	**15**	**6**	**No benefit**	
Donadio *et al.*, 1994 [47]	**Proteinuria >1 g/24 h, creatinine <3 mg/dl**	**55**	**24**	**Proteinuria unchanged, decline in renal function loss**	**Poor prognosis in control group**

Randomized controlled trials in **bold**.

function in those treated with fish oil for 6 months. The study of Cheng *et al.* [51] also showed no benefit, but renal impairment was so advanced that a favourable response to any treatment may not have been expected. A further confirmatory study of fish oil would be of great value.

Fish oil treatment does not have the drawbacks associated with immunosuppressive treatment. It is safe apart from a decrease in blood coagulability, which is not usually a practical problem, and an unpleasant taste with flatulence, which may make compliance difficult.

Post-transplant recurrence

Mesangial IgA deposition after transplantation is common, occurring in up to 50% of patients whose primary renal disease was IgAN [52]. Progressive glomerular injury following IgA deposition is relatively unusual and graft survival is no worse in registry data than for other primary renal disease. No treatment is known to reduce the risk of recurrent IgA deposits or to prevent any subsequent glomerular injury.

Treatment of Henoch–Schönlein nephritis

There are remarkably few published data to guide the treatment of HS nephritis: in particular there are no prospective randomized controlled trials. Most available data are in children. Most therapeutic studies of IgAN exclude those with HSP, so it is uncertain whether a number of potential treatments have a role in HS nephritis. Many patients have transient nephritis during the early phase of HSP which spontaneously remits and requires no treatment.

Rapidly progressive renal failure due to crescentic nephritis

Crescentic nephritis is more common than in IgAN, particularly early in the course of HSP. There is little information on treatment in adults. Regimens in children are variable and include corticosteroids and cyclophosphamide with the addition of plasma exchange or pulse methylprednisolone in some cases. Oner *et al.* [53] report optimistic experience: 11 of 12 children having normal GFR at 3 months, despite GFR <40 ml/min and >60% crescents at presentation. On the other hand, Jardim *et al.* [54] report four of nine children developing ESRD within 2 years. It is not possible to define the best regimen on available evidence.

Active HS nephritis without renal failure

In less aggressive HS nephritis there is little information. Corticosteroids alone have never been shown to be beneficial [55]. It has been proposed that early use of corticosteroids in HSP may prevent nephritis [56] but this has not been confirmed [57]. There are only very few patients with HS nephritis included in the promising studies of immunoglobulin [31, 32].

Slowly progressive renal failure

While the renal histology and clinical course of slowly progressive HS nephritis and IgAN may be indistinguishable, patients with HS nephritis have not been included in studies of ACE gene polymorphisms, ACE inhibitors or fish oil.

Transplant recurrence

Graft recurrence of HS nephritis is common. There is some evidence it is more common and more likely to cause graft loss in children receiving live related donor kidneys [58] than cadaver kidneys [59]. No treatment is known to reduce this risk.

Specific recommendations

IgA nephropathy

Recurrent macroscopic haematuria (preserved renal function)
No specific treatment (no role for antibiotics or tonsillectomy).

Macroscopic haematuria with acute renal failure

1. Renal biopsy mandatory.

2. Acute tubular necrosis – supportive measures only.

3. Crescentic nephritis
   (a) *Induction*: Prednisolone 0.5–1 mg/kg per day for up to 8 weeks.
   Cyclophosphamide 2.5 mg/kg per day for up to 8 weeks.
   (No evidence favouring oral or intravenous route – follow local practice)
   Daily plasma exchange for 7 days

   (b) *Maintenance*: Prednisolone in reducing dosage
   Azathioprine 2.5 mg/kg per day.

Proteinuria <1 g/24 h ($\pm$microscopic haematuria)
No specific treatment.

Nephrotic syndrome – with minimal change on light microscopy
Prednisolone 0.5–1 mg/kg per day (children 60 mg/m^2 per day) for up to 8 weeks.

Proteinuria >1 g/24 h ($\pm$microscopic haematuria) – including all other nephrotic syndrome
Consider fish oil – 12 g daily for 6 months.

Hypertension
1. Choice of agent according to physician's preference (superiority of ACE inhibitors unproven).

2. Conventional target blood pressure (no evidence for more aggressive control).

Transplantation
No special measures required.

Henoch–Schönlein nephritis

Crescentic nephritis
Regimen as above for crescentic IgA nephritis.

All other HS nephritis (including nephrotic syndrome)
No specific treatment – supportive measures only.

Hypertension
Choice of agent according to physician's preference.

Transplantation
Cadaveric donor may be preferrable to live related donor.

Future directions

Specific treatment to prevent mesangial IgA deposition is the ideal goal but remains a remote prospect until the fundamentals of the disease mechanisms are understood. It seems unlikely that controlled trials of crescentic IgAN or HS nephritis will ever be mounted. Prevention of slowly progressive renal failure remains the most promising field, particularly as this may inform the management of chronic glomerular disease other than that associated with IgA deposition. A study confirming the value of fish oil is required. Other low-risk strategies need to be developed from an understanding of the mechanisms of progressive renal scarring.

The value of ACE inhibitors requires formal confirmation in prospective studies. ACE gene polymorphisms or other genetic markers of progression may be particularly valuable in designing future studies of progression, allowing restriction of therapy to those at highest risk.

References

1. Bailey RR, Lynn KL, Robson RA, Smith AH, Wells JE. Long term follow up of patients with IgA nephropathy. N Z Med J 1994;107:142–4.
2. Ibels LS, Gyorgy AZ. IgA nephropathy: analysis of the natural history, important factors in the progression of renal disease, and a review of the literature. Medicine (Baltimore) 1994;73:79–102.
3. Feehally J. Immune mechanisms in glomerular IgA deposition. Nephrol Dial Transplant 1988; 3:361–78.
4. van Es LA, de Fijter JW, Daha MR. Pathogenesis of IgA nephropathy. Nephrology 1997;3:3–12.
5. Galla JH. IgA nephropathy. Kidney Int 1995;47:377.
6. Allen AC. Abnormal glycosylation of IgA: is it related to the pathogenesis of IgA nephropathy? Nephrol Dial Transplant 1995;10:1121–4.
7. Coppo R, Roccatello D, Amore A *et al.* Effects of a gluten-free diet on primary IgA nephropathy. Clin Nephrol 1990;33:72–86.
8. Ferri C, Puccini R, Paleologo G *et al.* IgA nephropathy: preliminary results of low-antigen content diet. Arch Intern Med 1992;152:429–38.
9. Sato M, Takayama K, Kojima H *et al.* Sodium cromoglycate therapy in IgA nephropathy: a preliminary short-term trial. Am J Kidney Dis 1990;15:141–6.
10. Bazzi C, Sinico RA, Petrini C *et al.* Low doses of drug able to alter intestinal mucosal permeability to food antigens (5-aminosalicylic acid and sodium cromoglycate) do not reduce proteinuria in patients with IgA nephropathy: a preliminary non-controlled trial. Nephron 1992;61:192–5.
11. Kincaid-Smith P, Nicholls K. Mesangial IgA nephropathy. Am J Kidney Dis 1983;3:90–102.
12. Clarkson AR, Woodroffe AJ. Therapeutic perspectives in mesangial IgA nephropathy. Contrib Nephrol 1984;40:187–94.
13. Iino Y, Ambe K, Kato Y *et al.* Chronic tonsillitis and IgA nephropathy. Acta Laryngol 1993;508 (Suppl.):29–35.
14. Clarkson AR, Seymour AE, Woodroffe AJ *et al.* Controlled trial of phenytoin therapy in IgA nephropathy. Clin Nephrol 1980;13:215–18.
15. Egido J, Rivera F, Sancho J *et al.* Phenytoin in IgA nephropathy: a long-term controlled trial. Nephron 1984;38:30–9.
16. Tomino Y, Sakai H, Miura M *et al.* Effect of danazol on solubilization of immune deposits in patients with IgA nephropathy. Am J Kidney Dis 1984;4:135–40.
17. Lai KN, MacMoune Lai F, Leung ACT *et al.* Plasma exchange in patients with rapidly progressive idiopathic IgA nephropathy: a report of two cases and review of the literature. Am J Kidney Dis 1987;10:66–70.
18. Roccatello D, Ferro M, Coppo R *et al.* Report on intensive treatment of extracapillary glomerulonephritis with focus on crescentic IgA nephropathy. Nephrol Dial Transplant 1995; 10:2054–9.
19. Welch TR, McAdams AJ, Berry A. Rapidly progressive IgA nephropathy. Am J Dis Child 1988;142:789–93.

20. Lai KN, Lai FM, Ho CP *et al.* Corticosteroid therapy in IgA nephropathy with nephrotic syndrome: a long-term controlled trial. Clin Nephrol 1986;26:174–80.
21. Welch TR, Fryer C, Shely E *et al.* Double blind controlled trial of short term prednisone therapy in immunoglobulin A glomerulonephritis. J Pediatrics 1992;121:474–7.
22. Waldo FB, Wyatt R, Kelly DR *et al.* Treatment of IgA nephropathy in children: efficacy of alternate-day oral prednisone. Pediatr Nephrol 1993;7:529–32.
23. Kobayashi Y, Fujii K, Hiki Y *et al.* Steroid therapy in IgA nephropathy: a retrospective study in heavy proteinuric cases. Nephron 1988;48:12–17.
24. Kobayashi Y,Hiki Y, Kokubo T *et al.* Steroid therapy during the early stage of progressive IgA nephropathy. Nephron 1996;72:237–42.
25. Woo KT, Lee GSL, Lau YK *et al.* Effects of triple therapy in IgA nephritis: a follow-up study 5 years later. Clin Nephrol 1991;36:60–6.
26. Walker RG, Yu SH, Owen JE *et al.* The treatment of mesangial IgA nephropathy with cyclophosphamide, dipyridamole amd warfarin: a two-year prospective trial. Clin Nephrol 1990;34:103–7.
27. Lagrue G, Bernard D, Bariety J *et al.* Traitment par la chlorambucil et azathioprine dans les glomerulonephrites primitives. Resultats d'une etude 'controlee'. J Urol Nephrol 1975;9:655–72.
28. Andreoli SP, Bergstein JM. Treatment of severe IgA nephropathy in children. Pediatr Nephrol 1989;3:248–53.
29. Goumenos D, Ahuja M, Shortland JR *et al.* Can immunosuppressive drugs slow the progression of IgA nephropathy? Nephrol Dial Transplant 1995;10:1173–81.
30. Lai KN, Mac-Moune Lai F, Li PKT *et al.* Cyclosporin treatment of IgA nephropathy: a short term controlled trial. Br Med J 1987;295:1165–8.
31. Rostoker G, Desvaux-Belghiti D, Pilatte Y *et al.* High–dose immunoglobulin therapy for severe IgA nephropathy and Henoch–Schönlein purpura. Ann Intern Med 1994;120:476–84.
32. Rostoker G, Desvaux–Belghiti D, Pilatte Y *et al.* Immunomodulation with low–dose immunoglobulins for moderate IgA nephropathy and Henoch–Schönlein purpura. Preliminary results of a prospective uncontrolled trial. Nephron 1995;69:327–34.
33. Furuse A, Hiramatsu M, Adachi N *et al.* Dramatic response to corticosteroid therapy of nephrotic syndrome associated with IgA nephropathy. Int J Pediatr Nephrol 1985;6:205–6.
34. Clive DM, Galvanek DG, Silva FG. Mesangial immunoglobulin A deposits in minimal change nephrotic syndrome: a report of an older patient and a review of the literature. Am J Nephrol 1990;10:31–6.
35. Johnson RJ. The glomerular response to injury. Mechanisms of progression or resolution. Kidney Int 1994;45:1769–82
36. Feehally J. Immunoglobulin A nephropathy: fish oils and beyond. Curr Opin Nephrol Hypertens 1996;5:442–6.
37. Hunley TE, Julian BA, Phillips JA *et al.* Angiotensin converting enzyme gene polymorphism: potential silencer motif and impact on progression in IgA nephropathy. Kidney Int 1996;49: 571–7.
38. Yoshida H, Mitari T, Kawamura T *et al.* Role of the deletion polymorphism of the angiotensin converting enzyme gene in the progression and therapeutic responsiveness of IgA nephropathy. J Clin Invest 1995;96:2162–9.
39. van Essen GG, Rensma PL, de Zeeuw D *et al.* Association between angiotensin-converting enzyme gene polymorphism and failure of renoprotective therapy. Lancet 1996;347:94–5
40. Chan MK, Kwan SYL, Chan KW *et al.* Controlled trial of antiplatelet agents in mesangial IgA glomerulonephritis. Am J Kidney Dis 1987;9:417–21.
41. Lee GS, Choong HL, Chiang GSC, Woo KT. 3 year randomised controlled trial of dipyridamole and low-dose warfarin in patients with IgA nephropathy with renal impairment. Nephrology 1997;3:117–21.
42. Miura M, Endoh M, Nomoto Y *et al.* Long-term effect of urokinase therapy in IgA nephropathy. Clin Nephrol 1989;32:209–16.

43. Maschio G, Cagnoli L, Claroni F *et al.* ACE inhibition reduces proteinuria in normotensive patients with IgA nephropathy: a multicentre, randomised placebo–controlled trial. Nephrol Dial Transplant 1994;9:265–9.
44. Rekola S, Bergstrand A, Bucht H *et al.* Deterioration rate in hypertensive IgA nephropathy: comparison of a converting enzyme inhibitor and β–blocking agents. Nephron 1991;59:57–60.
45. Cattran D, Greenwood C, Ritchie S. Long-term benefits of angiotensin–converting enzyme inhibitor therapy in patients with severe immunoglobulin A nephropathy: a comparison to patients receiving treatment with other antihypertensive agents and to those receiving no therapy. Am J Kidney Dis 1994;23:247–54.
46. Bannister KM, Weaver A, Clarkson AR, Woodroffe AJ. Effect of angiotensin-converting enzyme and calcium channel inhibition on progression of IgA nephropathy. Contrib Nephrol 1995;111:184–93.
47. Donadio JV, Bergstalh EJ, Offord KP *et al.* A controlled trial of fish oil in IgA nephropathy. N Engl J Med 1994;331:1194–9.
48. Hamazaki T, Tateno S, Shishido H. Eicosapentanoic acid and IgA nephropathy. Lancet 1984;i: 1017–18.
49. Bennett WM, Walker RG, Kincaid-Smith P. Treatment of IgA nephropathy with eicosapentanoic acid (EPA): a two–year prospective trial. Clin Nephrol 1989;31:128–9.
50. Pettersson EE, Rekola S, Berglund L *et al.* Treatment of IgA nephropathy with omega-3-polyunsaturated fatty acids:a prospective, double-blind, randomised study. Clin Nephrol 1994; 41:183–90.
51. Cheng IKP, Chan PCK, Chan MK. The effects of fish-oil dietary supplementation on the progression of mesangial IgA glomerulonephritis. Nephrol Dial Transplant 1990;5:241–6.
52. Odum J, Peh CA, Clarkson AR *et al.* Recurrent mesangial IgA nephritis following renal transplantation. Nephrol Dial Transplant 1994;9:309–12.
53. Oner A, Tinaztepe K, Erdogan O. The effect of triple therapy on rapidly progressive type of Henoch–Schönlein nephritis. Pediatr Nephrol 1995;9:6–10.
54. Jardim H, Leake J, Risdon RA *et al.* Crescentic glomerulonephritis in children. Pediatr Nephrol 1992;6:231–5.
55. Haycock GB. The nephritis of Henoch–Schönlein purpura. In: Cameron S, Davison AM, Grunfeld J-P, Kerr D, Ritz E, editors. Oxford Textbook of Clinical Nephrology. Oxford: Oxford University Press; 1992:595–612.
56. Mollica F, LiVolti S, Garozzo R, Russo G. Effectiveness of early prednisone treatment in preventing the development of nephropathy in anaphylactoid purpura. Eur J Pediatr 1992;151: 140–4.
57. Saulsbury FT. Corticosteroid therapy does not prevent nephritis in Henoch–Schönlein purpura. Pediatr Nephrol 1993;7:69–71.
58. Hasegawa A. Fate of renal grafts with recurrent Henoch–Schönlein purpura nephritis in children. Transplant Proc 1989;21:2130.
59. Habib R. Purpura rheumatoide. In: Royer P, Habib R, Mathieu H, Broyer M, editors. Nephrologie Pediatrique. Paris: Flammarion; 1983:342–68.

7. Crescentic glomerulonephritis and systemic vasculitis

G. GASKIN AND C.D. PUSEY

Causes and classification of crescentic glomerulonephritis

Crescentic glomerulonephritis was first recognized in the autopsy studies of Volhard and Fahr [1], who described cells amassed within Bowman's capsule around severely damaged glomerular tufts, and termed the appearance 'extra-capillary proliferation'. The more graphic term 'crescent' was later introduced, and is to be preferred, as it does not imply a particular origin for the cells found in Bowman's space. The pathogenesis of crescentic glomerulonephritis is discussed more fully below. Figure 7.1 illustrates the characteristic histological appearance of crescentic glomerulonephritis. With time, it was appreciated that glomerular crescents were associated with progression to renal failure over a matter of weeks or months, and the clinical term 'rapidly progressive glomerulonephritis' (RPGN) was coined [2]. Initially attributed solely to post-streptococcal glomerulonephritis, the crescentic lesion was later recognized in small vessel vasculitis [3], Wegener's granulomatosis [4] and antiglomerular basement membrane antibody-mediated disease [5], in addition to other primary glomerular and systemic inflammatory diseases [6–8]. With the accumulation of clinical data and the advent of immunohistology, three broad categories of crescentic nephritis came to be recognized:

1. *Crescentic glomerulonephritis with linear immunoglobulin deposition on the glomerular basement membrane.* This corresponds to antiglomerular basement antibody-mediated (anti-GBM) disease or Goodpasture's disease, which is a discrete, but rare, syndrome associated with circulating antibodies directed against the non-collagenous (NC1) domain of the $\alpha 3$ chain of type IV collagen [9–12], a component of selected basement membranes [13]. When the anti-GBM immune response also targets the alveolar basement membrane, lung haemorrhage results. However, access of antibodies and other immune reactants to the alveolar basement membrane may require a degree of lung injury, for example from exposure to industrial or other environmental toxins [14], or perhaps as a result of certain cytokines during infection [15]. Lung haemorrhage is therefore not an invariable occurrence, but appears to be associated with cigarette smoking [16, 17] or hydrocarbon exposure [18].

C.D. Pusey (ed.), The Treatment of Glomerulonephritis, 113–142.

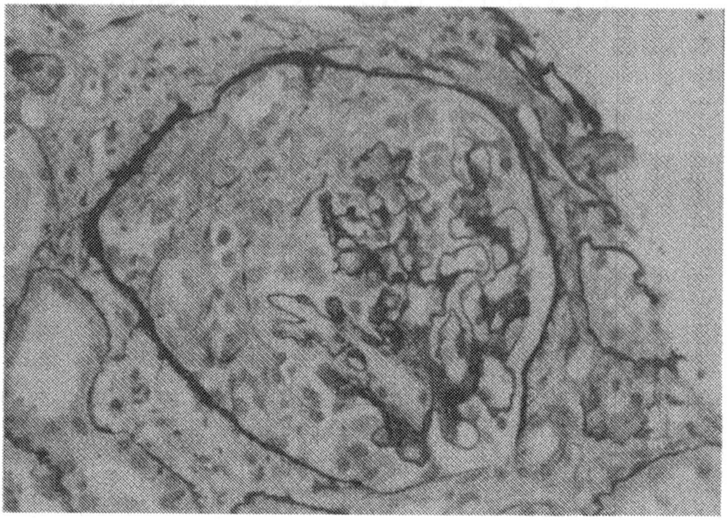

Figure 7.1 ANCA-associated crescentic glomerulonephritis. A large cellular crescent surrounds the remains of the glomerular tuft (silver methenamine; original magnification × 500). Courtesy of Dr Terry Cook

One variant of anti-GBM disease merits particular mention. A proportion of patients with end-stage renal failure due to Alport's syndrome develop anti-GBM immunity following transplantation, usually without significant glomerular injury [19, 20]. These anti-GBM alloantibodies are predominantly directed against the chain of type IV collagen in which the patient's collagen mutation resides – which is the α5 chain in the majority [21].

2. *Crescentic glomerulonephritis in which immune deposits are scanty or absent.* The second category, pauci-immune crescentic glomerulonephritis, is now recognized as the renal lesion of primary small vessel vasculitis. This group of diseases is associated with circulating ANCA specific for one of two neutrophil granule enzymes: proteinase 3 and myeloperoxidase. *In vitro*, these autoantibodies have numerous effects which suggest a possible role in injury to the vascular endothelium [22]. Mounting evidence suggests that pauci-immune crescentic glomerulonephritis without extrarenal vasculitis is also part of the ANCA-associated vasculitis spectrum. This evidence includes: the coexistence of vasculitic lesions in the kidney [23], the potential for developing vasculitic lesions later in the disease course [24], and the consistent association with ANCA [25, 26]. Thus it seems unlikely that there is a residual category of pauci-immune 'idiopathic RPGN' unrelated to vasculitis [27], particularly if necrotizing lesions are considered to be part of the typical picture [28].

3. *Crescentic glomerulonephritis with prominent granular immune deposits.* This third category is heterogeneous. It includes nephritis associated with systemic illnesses such as Henoch–Schönlein purpura, mixed essential cryoglobulinaemia and systemic lupus erythematosus, nephritis associated with or following infection, and primary glomerular diseases such as IgA nephropathy and mesangiocapillary glomerulonephritis in a crescentic phase.

Numerous studies have attempted to define the relative incidence of these three categories of crescentic glomerulonephritis. The recent study of Anganco *et al.* [27], reviewing all biopsies containing crescentic glomerulonephritis from a single region in the UK, confirms the pattern in older series (Figure 7.2). ANCA-associated pauci-immune glomerulonephritis was the most common diagnosis, while anti-GBM disease was rarer, though probably still over-represented due to the referral practice of the reporting centre. The remaining cases were divided between acute post-infectious glomerulonephritis, primary glomerulonephritis and other immune complex nephritides associated with systemic inflammatory diseases. These conditions are discussed in other sections; this chapter will focus on treatment of anti-GBM disease and vasculitis-associated glomerulonephritis.

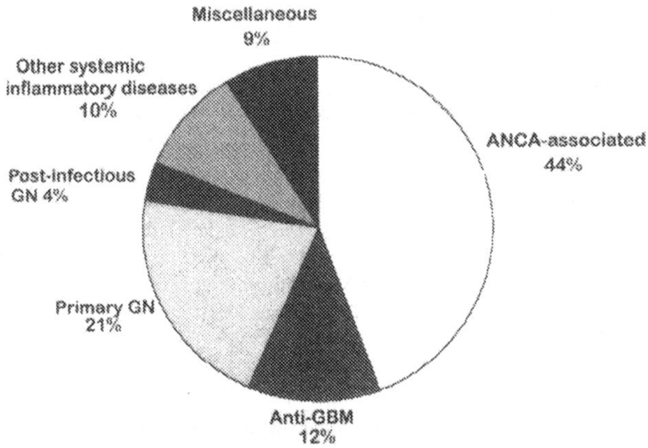

Figure 7.2 Relative frequency of causes of crescentic glomerulonephritis (GN). From Angangco *et al.* [27]

It is worth noting that ANCA-associated vasculitis is not only the most common cause of crescentic glomerulonephritis, but also the most common cause of immune-mediated pulmonary haemorrhage [29–32]. Thus, while Goodpasture's syndrome is classically associated with anti-GBM disease, it is actually more commonly due to vasculitis. Anti-GBM disease affects only 0.5–1 per million of the population per year in the United Kingdom [33], while the incidence of ANCA-associated vasculitis is nearer 20 per million per year [34] and appears to be increasing [35].

Clinical presentation of crescentic glomerulonephritis

Occasionally the patient has loin pain and tenderness, due to renal swelling and capsular distension in a severely destructive glomerulonephritis, or symptoms of uraemia when the renal lesion is advanced. More commonly, however, other constitutional and/or organ-specific symptoms alert the patient, and the physician, to the presence of a systemic illness. Up to two-thirds of patients with anti-GBM disease have alveolar haemorrhage [17, 36–38], which may be sufficient to cause symptomatic iron-deficiency anaemia. The systemic vasculitis syndromes most commonly associated with a crescentic glomerulonephritis are Wegener's granulomatosis, a small vessel vasculitis with characteristic granulomatous involvement of the upper and lower respiratory tracts, and microscopic polyangiitis, a small vessel vasculitis without these granulomatous features [39]. Churg–Strauss syndrome was recognized from the first description to encompass glomerular lesions, though rapidly progressive renal failure due to crescentic glomerulonephritis is uncommon [40]. All three of these vasculitis syndromes are associated with ANCA [25, 41]. Table 7.1 lists typical clinical features of ANCA-associated vasculitis.

Table 7.1 Organ involvement in Wegener's granulomatosis and microscopic polyangiitis

	Wegener's granulomatosis	Microscopic polyangiitis
Kidney	90% – Necrotizing and crescentic glomerulonephritis	100% – Necrotizing and crescentic glomerulonephritis
Lung	90% – Granulomas, alveolar haemorrhage, pleural effusion	40% – Alveolar haemorrhage, pleural effusion
Ear, nose and throat	95% – Epistaxis, nasal bridge collapse, sinusitis, deafness, subglottic stenosis	–
Skin	55% – purpura, ulceration, digital ischaemia	
Nervous system	55% – Mononeuritis multiplex, distal neuropathy, altered consciousness, focal signs	
Eye	55% – Episcleritis, retinal vasculitis, orbital granuloma	30% – Episcleritis, retinal vasculitis
Musculoskeletal	70% – Arthralgia, myalgia	
Gut	10% – Bleeding, perforation, abdominal pain	40% – Bleeding, perforation, abdominal pain
Heart	5% – Pericarditis, valvular lesions	5% – Pericarditis
Mouth	15% – Oral ulceration	

Renal involvement should be sought during the initial assessment of these diseases by dipstick-testing of the urine for blood and protein, and examination of the urine for red cell casts, which are generally indicative of severe glomerular inflammation. Renal dysfunction is an unreliable guide to the presence of nephritis in its early stages. Confirmation of the presence of crescentic glomerulonephritis will require renal biopsy, which may also be necessary to define the underlying disease. While certain underlying conditions have characteristic extrarenal features – such as the respiratory granulomas of Wegener's granulomatosis – other illnesses may look superficially similar. For example, microscopic polyangiitis, mixed essential cryoglobulinaemia and infectious endocarditis may all cause a febrile illness with vasculitic skin lesions and glomerulonephritis, both vasculitis and anti-GBM disease may present with pulmonary haemorrhage and RPGN, and both may present without extrarenal disease. Numerous serological investigations are useful in pointing to, or away from, the diagnosis of anti-GBM disease or vasculitis, and may be available to guide treatment before a renal biopsy can be obtained. These tests are summarized in Table 7.2.

A small subgroup of patients has features of both anti-GBM disease (linear IgG on biopsy, circulating anti-GBM antibodies) and vasculitis with detectable ANCA [42]. Their ANCA are typically specific for myeloperoxidase [43–45], though not exclusively so [46], while their anti-GBM antibodies are indistinguishable from those detected in patients with typical anti-GBM disease [47], once non-specific binding has been excluded [48]. These 'double-positive' patients are more likely to have extrarenal vasculitis and systemic symptoms, and perhaps to run a relapsing course, than those with anti-GBM antibodies alone [42, 44]. It is attractive to speculate that tissue injury from one disease releases antigens which triggers the other, but the sequence of antibody detection is not consistent [49, 50]. Although there are no therapeutic trials in this subgroup of patients, most authors believe that it is important to identify them in order to ensure that treatment is appropriately designed.

Histological features

Anti-GBM disease

On light microscopy, the earliest glomerular changes comprise segmental mesangial matrix expansion and hypercellularity, progressing to a more generalized but still focal and segmental proliferative glomerulonephritis, with increased numbers of neutrophils in the glomeruli. Later, glomeruli show a diffuse nephritis with segmental or total necrosis and extensive crescent formation. Interstitial inflammation is common, and in occasional cases there are granulomatous changes around glomeruli [51, 52]. This sequence of changes may occur extremely rapidly, with corresponding loss of renal function over days. Immunohistology reveals the characteristic linear binding of IgG to

Table 7.2 Blood tests of value in crescentic glomerulonephritis

Test	Associated condition
Specific	
Antiglomerular basement membrane antibodies	Anti-GBM disease
Antineutrophil cytoplasmic antibodies	Systemic vasculitis
Antiproteinase 3, antimyeloperoxidase antibodies	Systemic vasculitis
Anti-dsDNA antibodies, anti-Sm antibodies	Systemic lupus erythematosus
Cryoglobulins	Essential mixed cryoglobulinaemia type II
C3 nephritic factor	Mesangiocapillary glomerulonephritis type II
Raised ASOT	Poststreptococcal glomerulonephritis
Non-specific	
Complement (typical findings)	
Low C4, normal C3	Essential mixed cryoglobulinaemia type II
Low C4 + C3	Systemic lupus erythematosus
Low C3, normal C4	Mesangiocapillary glomerulonephritis type II
Low C3 + C4	Postinfectious glomerulonephritis, mesangiocapillary glomerulonephritis type I
Raised C3, C4	Systemic vasculitis
Immunoglobulins	
Raised IgG, IgM	Systemic lupus erythematosus, systemic vasculitis, postinfectious glomerulonephritis
Raised IgE	Churg–Strauss syndrome
Raised IgA	IgA nephropathy, Henoch–Schönlein purpura
Paraprotein (usually IgM)	Essential mixed cryoglobulinaemia type II
Acute-phase response	
Raised C-reactive protein + ESR	Systemic vasculitis
Raised ESR	Systemic lupus erythematosus
Raised alkaline phosphatase, low albumin	Systemic vasculitis
Haematology	
Neutrophilia, thrombocytosis	Systemic vasculitis
Eosinophilia	Churg–Strauss syndrome
Leukopenia, thrombocytopenia	Systemic lupus erythematosus
Severe anaemia	Anti-GBM disease
Moderate anaemia	Systemic vasculitis, systemic lupus erythematosus, essential mixed cryoglobulinaemia
Microbiology	
Blood cultures positive	Infective endocarditis Ventriculoatrial shunt nephritis

ASOT, anti-streptolysin O titre; ESR, erythrocyte sedimentation rate

the glomerular basement membrane (Figure 7.3), and sometimes to the distal convoluted tubule; other immunoglobulins are also present in up to a third of cases (but very rarely alone) and linear C3 is present in around 60% [52, 53]. Renal biopsy findings are the same in those with isolated glomerulonephritis and those with Goodpasture's syndrome.

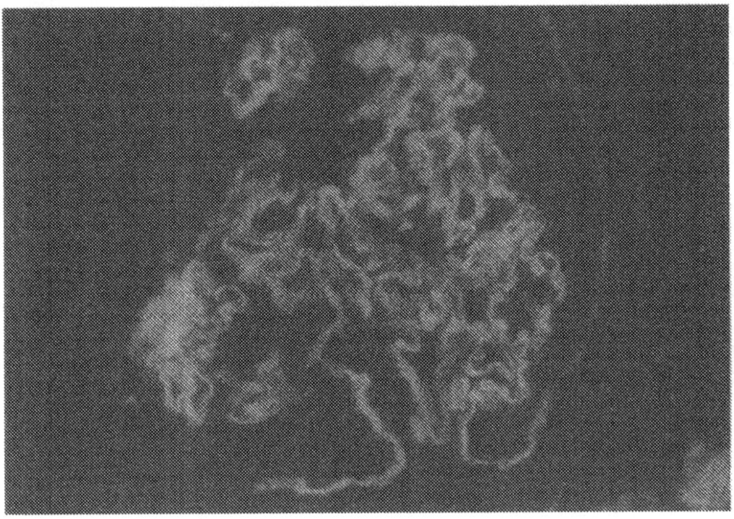

Figure 7.3 Anti-GBM disease. Direct immunofluorescence showing linear deposition of IgG along the basement membrane. Courtesy of Dr Mary Thompson

ANCA-associated vasculitis and glomerulonephritis

On light microscopy the earliest findings are an increase in glomerular neutrophils and focal, segmental areas of necrosis (Figure 7.4). As the disease progresses, the necrosis becomes more extensive and crescents develop. However, in contrast to anti-GBM disease, the lesions are often of widely differing ages, with some glomeruli normal, some with new segmental necrosis, others with marked crescent formation, and yet others sclerosed. This distinction can be helpful when faced with the need for urgent treatment before immunohistology or circulating antibody assays are available. Associated renal arteritis is detected infrequently: it was present in 18/40 biopsies reported by Bindi *et al.* [54] and only 10/81 reported by Jennette *et al.* [26]. Renal granulomas in Wegener's granulomatosis are rare [55]; granulomatous inflammation around severely damaged glomeruli is not specific to Wegener's granulomatosis. There is often a pronounced interstitial infiltrate, and both necrotizing lesions [56] and leukocytoclastic peritubular capillaritis [26] have been reported in the renal medulla. Immunohistology in ANCA-associated crescentic glomerulonephritis reveals few or no immune deposits [26, 57].

One recent report suggests that there may be differences in renal histology according to ANCA specificity, with more chronicity seen in biopsies from patients with antimyeloperoxidase ANCA, associated with a slower rate of progression of renal dysfunction [58]. These interesting data are yet to be widely confirmed.

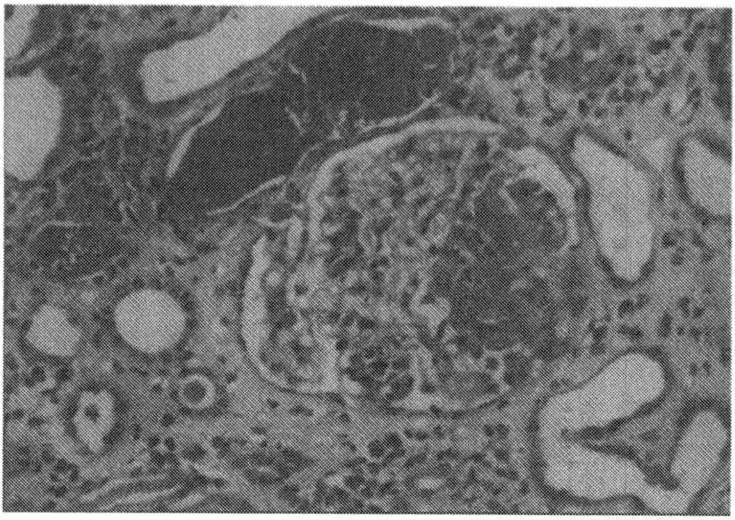

Figure 7.4 Wegener's granulomatosis. The glomerulus shows segmental fibrinoid necrosis (H&E; original magnification ×400). Courtesy of Dr Terry Cook

Treatment

Initial treatment

Crescentic glomerulonephritis requires urgent intervention, particularly in anti-GBM disease where the pace of renal damage can be extremely fast. There are similarities in the treatment of ANCA-associated and anti-GBM-mediated crescentic nephritis, which are sufficient to allow empirical initial therapy to cover both eventualities. However, there are also differences in the need for, and type of, adjunctive therapies, and in the optimal duration of immunosuppressive therapy. For this reason the two diseases will be considered separately.

Treatment of crescentic glomerulonephritis due to anti-GBM disease
This is a rare disease in which treatment has developed empirically. Current treatment regimens are derived from observations of the beneficial effect of corticosteroids [52] and immunosuppressive agents [59, 60] and application of the knowledge that anti-GBM antibodies eluted from the kidney are nephritogenic when transferred into squirrel monkeys [61]. On theoretical grounds, therefore, an effective treatment might encompass removal of pathogenic antibody, prevention of its resynthesis and suppression of renal inflammation. The combination of corticosteroids, cyclophosphamide, azathioprine and daily plasma exchange reported by Lockwood *et al.* [62] was designed on this basis,

Table 7.3 Treatment of anti-GBM disease

Prednisolone 60 mg daily, reducing to 20 mg daily by 6 weeks and more slowly thereafter
Cyclophosphamide 2–3 mg/kg daily (lower dose if >55 years); discontinued if white cell count $<4.0 \times 10^9$/L or in presence of severe infection
Plasma exchange 4 L daily for 5% albumin; continued for 14 days or until anti-GBM antibody levels controlled; fresh frozen plasma 400 ml given at end of exchange in presence of lung haemorrhage or within 3 days of invasive procedure

and led to an improvement in outcome [63], as has been demonstrated by others [59, 64–67]. One small trial indicated that nine patients treated with plasma exchange in conjunction with immunosuppression fared better than eight treated with immunosuppression alone [68], though renal function at commencement of treatment was a more powerful predictor of outcome than treatment modality. A large randomized study of plasma exchange has not been performed and is perhaps unlikely. There are isolated case reports of the use of protein A immunoadsorption instead of plasma exchange to remove circulating anti-GBM antibodies [69]. The use of pulsed high-dose steroids has also been proposed [69], although not widely adopted, in lieu of plasma exchange; some reports suggest that it is not of benefit [70]. The details of our current treatment policy (which no longer includes azathioprine) are given in Table 7.3. This therapeutic strategy is directed at rapid initial control of disease, removing circulating antibodies with daily plasma exchange until the level is within the normal range, and suppressing their recrudescence with a 3 month course of cyclophosphamide. Corticosteroids are tailed down and stopped by about 6 months. In the very unlikely event of clinical relapse [71], therapy is the same as in the presenting illness.

In certain cases a decision must be made whether to treat at all. All patients with pulmonary haemorrhage, a life-threatening complication, should be treated, irrespective of the likelihood of renal recovery. In patients without pulmonary haemorrhage, the decision to treat is influenced by the severity of renal failure at presentation, since the risks of aggressive immunosuppression may not be justified by the likely benefit. A presenting creatinine >600 μmol/L has been consistently associated with a poorer outcome [17, 29, 37, 63] and complete anuria is particularly ominous [67]. Recovery from dialysis-dependence, while reported [60, 65, 67], is rare. The biopsy appearances may also help; poor outcomes are associated with a high percentage of glomeruli affected by circumferential crescents [17, 36, 37]. In patients with severe isolated renal disease we are prompted to treat by: young age, recent onset of renal failure, and a biopsy showing active inflammation without excessive scarring. Similar considerations apply to the issue of how long to continue immunosuppression if there is no recovery of renal function, in the absence of pulmonary haemorrhage; one strategy might be to assess renal viability by repeat biopsy and to tail off the steroids and cyclophosphamide early if damage is deemed irreversible. We have seen recovery at up to a month, and rarely 3 months. Even without intensive immunosuppression, anti-GBM antibody levels will tend to fall gradually over a period of 18–24 months in most cases, permitting consideration of renal transplantation [72].

Treatment of ANCA-associated pauci-immune crescentic glomerulonephritis
Treatment of ANCA-associated crescentic glomerulonephritis is a more complex issue, as therapeutic approaches have evolved in a number ways. Firstly, regimens have been derived from rheumatologists' treatment of patients with vasculitis with variable severity of renal disease [73–75]. Secondly, regimens for severe nephritis in vasculitis have been designed by nephrologists by analogy with anti-GBM disease [76]. Finally, regimens have been designed for isolated crescentic glomerulonephritis as a distinct entity [69, 70]. The first approach has brought the use of cyclophosphamide to the fore, the second has introduced the use of plasma exchange and the third has illustrated the value of high-dose corticosteroids. All three modalities have a place in the current management of pauci-immune glomerulonephritis, with an increasing tendency to apply the same therapies irrespective of the presence of extrarenal vasculitis [77].

Oral corticosteroids
Oral corticosteroids were the first agents to make an impact on the outcome of Wegener's granulomatosis [78, 79], though this benefit could not be sustained long-term [80]. Similarly, the earliest attempts to treat microscopic polyangiitis and classical polyarteritis used oral corticosteroids alone, with an improvement in overall survival from 13% at 5 years in untreated patients to around 50% [81, 82]. However, over the years which followed, there was an increasing realization that additional treatment was needed to improve the outcome in severe renal or extrarenal vasculitis.

Cyclophosphamide
The most important change in the treatment of generalized necrotizing vasculitis, irrespective of the severity of the associated renal disease, was the introduction of cytotoxic agents, initially in Wegener's granulomatosis [73, 80, 83, 84] and later in microscopic polyangiitis and classical polyarteritis [74, 85, 86] and in vasculitis patients with prominent necrotizing glomerulonephritis [23, 87–89]. Cyclophosphamide was the agent of choice in most series, though Leib *et al.* (74] reported good outcomes with azathioprine.

Fauci's initial therapy for Wegener's granulomatosis at the NIH [73] comprised daily oral cyclophosphamide (2 mg/kg) together with daily oral prednisolone (1 mg/kg). After 1–2 weeks the daily steroids were converted to an alternate-day regimen and slowly tailed off, reaching a dose of 20 mg on alternate days by 6–12 months. Cyclophosphamide was continued at the starting dose until the patient had been in complete remission for at least 1 year. The dose was then reduced by 25 mg every 2–3 months until either the drug was stopped, or a dose reached below which the patient relapsed. Patients with fulminant disease received higher initial doses of both prednisolone (2 mg/kg for a few days) and cyclophosphamide (4–5 mg/kg). Fauci's treatment rapidly became the 'gold standard'. However, long-term follow-up of patients treated with the regimen revealed a high level of morbidity from both the disease and its treatment [90].

During the past 20 years we have employed an induction regimen with similarities to the NIH protocol. An important difference is that we discontinue cyclophosphamide after approximately 3 months, substituting azathioprine, to reduce the risk of cyclophosphamide toxicity. We use this as the basic drug regimen for all patients with ANCA- or vasculitis-associated glomerulonephritis, adding plasma exchange for patients with severe renal failure (see below). Other British groups have used a similar approach [23, 87–89]. It is worth noting that we also reduce the dose of cyclophosphamide in older patients, who appear to be especially prone to leukopaenia.

Pulsed intravenous methylprednisolone

Treatment has been intensified by the addition of bolus doses of intravenous methylprednisolone in groups of patients with pauci-immune crescentic nephritis, with and without extrarenal vasculitis [69, 70, 77, 87, 89, 91, 92]. The published doses of methylprednisolone and renal outcomes vary. Bolton and Sturgill [69] used three pulses of 30 mg/kg in addition to oral prednisolone, in patients who were dialysis-dependent due to isolated crescentic glomerulonephritis. In their study, 16/23 survivors came off dialysis, in contrast to 0/9 treated instead with varying combinations of oral steroids and other agents. Falk *et al.* [77] used lower doses (7 mg/kg) with varying regimens of prednisolone and cyclophosphamide; 6/12 patients discontinued dialysis. Andrassy *et al.* [93] used even lower doses (250 mg pulses administered on days 1–3) as one component of a variety of protocols for the treatment of Wegener's granulomatosis with renal involvement, which achieved excellent results. Other series report selected use of methylprednisolone, typically at doses of 1 g daily.

Pulsed cyclophosphamide

The success of pulsed intravenous cyclophosphamide in lupus nephritis [94], the potential reduction in total dose and the ease of use of concomitant mesna to prevent bladder toxicity has led to a number of studies in systemic vasculitis, and even to its routine adoption in some centres. Published studies include two completed controlled trials [95, 96] and preliminary results of a third trial have also been presented [97]. There are, in addition, uncontrolled studies in patients with a variety of vasculitic disorders with and without renal disease, reporting differing success rates with pulse therapy. In these reports, cyclophosphamide pulses were usually, but not invariably, given intravenously; Adu *et al.* [95] used oral pulses after the first month. The doses used varied from 0.375 g/m^2 to

1 g/m^2 and there were also differences in dose frequency (2 weekly to 4 weekly), in adjustments made for renal failure, age and leukopenia, and in concurrent therapy. Given these differences, it is unsurprising that the outcomes were rather heterogeneous. However, several trends can perhaps be identified.

Pulsed cyclophosphamide can achieve initial remission rates which are comparable to continuous cyclophosphamide [95–97] and with less toxicity. Haubitz *et al.* [97] recorded a lower rate of leukopenia and Guillevin *et al.* [96] noted a lower incidence of opportunist infections, though the oral therapy was deliberately adjusted to achieve a leukocyte count less than 3×10^9/L. However, pulsed therapy may not achieve induction of remission after relapse [98, 99], even if the dose is escalated [98], and appears to be less effective in predominantly non-renal Wegener's granulomatosis [99]. Furthermore, remission may be harder to sustain using pulsed therapy; in Guillevin *et al.*'s study [96] relapse occurred in 12/23 patients treated with pulses (of whom four died and three developed end-stage renal failure), compared with 3/17 treated with continuous cyclophosphamide. In the trial by Adu *et al.* [95] there were no significant differences in outcome, relapse rates or adverse effects between the pulse and continuous cyclophosphamide-treated limbs, but it should be noted that the steroid protocol also differed in the two groups, and that the pulsed therapy was more prolonged than the course of oral cyclophosphamide.

The number of patients with severe renal failure due to crescentic glomerulonephritis in the published studies is small. In the interim report from Haubitz *et al.* [97] the rate of recovery from dialysis dependence was lower in the pulsed group than in those treated with continuous oral cyclophosphamide [1/7 vs. 4/6], despite the routine addition of pulsed methylprednisolone. Bearing in mind these negative results, we would be reluctant to recommend pulsed rather than oral therapy in patients with severe renal failure on the basis of current evidence. Further data are required.

Plasma exchange

Although the pathogenesis of vasculitis is unknown, it is compelling to speculate that plasma exchange treatment could be beneficial by removing critical immune or inflammatory mediators. Indeed, the removal of ANCA may be itself valuable, since *in vitro* these autoantibodies have effects which could contribute to vascular injury [22]. Thus there may be a parallel with the application of plasma exchange to remove pathogenic autoantibodies in anti-GBM disease. The clinical evidence for its usefulness in vasculitis has been debated since early reports in the 1970s [76]. It is hard to assess its contribution to the treatment response in uncontrolled studies [76, 89, 100, 101] and one study which claimed to distinguish the benefit of plasma exchange from the benefit of immunosuppressive drugs was hampered by the sequential use of the therapies [102].

Data from randomized controlled trials are potentially more valuable. The first to be published, a multicentre study reported by Glockner *et al.* [103], was weakened by infrequent (three times a week) plasma exchange, inclusion of patients with other diseases and late addition of plasma exchange therapy in the 'control' groups. It failed to show a benefit from the addition of plasma exchange. Pusey *et al.* [104], and Cole *et al.* [105] subsequently published more rigorous randomized controlled trials.

Pusey *et al.* [104], at Hammersmith Hospital, used oral steroids, cyclophosphamide and, in the earlier years of the study only, azathioprine as baseline drug therapy. Forty-eight patients with vasculitis-associated or isolated necrotizing glomerulonephritis were randomized to receive a minimum of five plasma exchanges of 4 L in addition to drug therapy. Plasma exchange did not improve outcome in patients with only mild or moderate renal involvement, but was associated with a significantly greater renal recovery rate in patients presenting with dialysis-dependent renal failure [10/11 vs. 3/8]. This result has been confirmed by our own more recent analysis of 74 consecutive patients presenting with a creatinine over 500 μmol/L and treated with five or more plasma exchanges; 74% were alive with improved renal function 2 months after presentation [106].

Cole *et al.* [105] reported a study by the Canadian apheresis group in patients with isolated pauci-immune glomerulonephritis. Baseline therapy was pulsed followed by oral steroids, and azathioprine. Patients were randomized to receive at least 10 plasma exchange treatments, each of one plasma volume, within the first 16 days. In the patients as a whole there was no benefit from the addition of plasma exchange. The number of dialysis-requiring patients was small; 3/4 treated with plasma exchange but only 2/7 without recovered renal function.

A recent analysis of 32 patients with glomerulonephritis associated with microscopic polyangiitis and Churg–Strauss syndrome,by Guillevin *et al.* [107], suggested that there was no benefit from the routine addition of plasma exchange. The majority of the patients did not have severe renal impairment. However, 4/6 dialysis-dependent patients treated with plasma exchange recovered renal function.

Together, these studies lead us to believe that the place of adjunctive plasma exchange lies in the treatment of vasculitis-associated crescentic nephritis with severe renal dysfunction [108], and that earlier and milder disease can be satisfactorily treated with drugs alone. One exception to this is the group of patients with both ANCA and anti-GBM antibodies, where it seems prudent (in the absence of outcome data) to add plasma exchange to remove the anti-GBM antibodies. There are also anecdotal reports of benefit from plasma exchange in other life-threatening complications of vasculitis, including lung haemorrhage and cerebral involvement.

If removal of IgG ANCA is the mechanism whereby plasma exchange confers its benefit, protein A immunoadsorption should be similarly efficacious. A small, uncontrolled study by Esnault *et al.* [109] showed that ANCA could be effectively removed by this form of therapy, in parallel with clinical recovery. Palmer *et al.* [110] used protein A immunoadsorption in conjunction with pulsed methylprednisolone, oral prednisolone and cyclophosphamide, in seven patients with dialysis-dependent ANCA-associated RPGN. Six recovered renal function, although most were left with significant renal impairment. Unfortunately, in the absence of a controlled comparison, the contribution of the immunoadsorption to the improvement, and to the high incidence of infectious complications reported, is unclear.

The optimum induction regimen

This consideration of individual treatment modalities in crescentic glomerulonephritis associated with ANCA and vasculitis begs the question of which components form the optimum initial regimen. Most nephrologists would consider that it should contain oral prednisolone (typically starting at 60 mg/day) and cyclophosphamide, though there is less agreement on whether the latter drug should be given continuously or intermittently. We still favour continuous oral therapy where there is significant renal impairment, commencing at 2–3 mg/kg daily. The next issue is whether, and when, to add in an additional therapy, and which to choose. Extensive uncontrolled experience and data from the control limb of Pusey *et al.*'s trial [104] suggest that additional therapy is unnecessary in the absence of severe renal impairment. This was also the consensus view of experts in vasculitis designing a European controlled trial for patients with creatinine <500 μmol/L [111]. While some nephrologists would advocate the routine addition of pulsed steroid, in view of its cheapness and simplicity, we are mindful of its potential adverse effects, including osteoporotic fractures, avascular necrosis and cataract. These were prominent in the study of Bolton and Sturgill [69]. Furthermore, total steroid dose is the most important risk factor for infectious complications [112].

If, then, one reserves adjunctive therapy for those with severe renal impairment, which agent should one choose – pulsed steroid or plasma exchange? Both treatments have disadvantages; plasma exchange is expensive, and carries the risks of allergic reactions, transfer of infection, and bleeding due to anticoagulation and depletion of clotting factors. It also requires vascular access, though this will already be in place in dialysis-requiring patients. Suggestions from early studies that plasma exchange is associated with increased infection risk have not been confirmed [113]. Methylprednisolone is cheaper, but may be associated with significant adverse effects, as noted above. The best results reported with each type of adjunctive therapy are similar [92, 114, 115], although probably best of all in the trial reported by Pusey *et al.* [104]. A randomized controlled trial coordinated by the ECSYSVASTRIAL group seeks to resolve the issue [111]. In the absence of data the choice lies between methylprednisolone (usually three pulses of 7–15 mg/kg) and plasma exchange (five to 10 exchanges of 1–1.5 plasma volumes).

Finally, should pulsed methylprednisolone and plasma exchange be used together? Levy and Winearls [92] combined the treatments successfully, while others [88, 116] have drawn attention to the risk of sepsis in patients in whom multiple immunosuppressive strategies are combined.

Other induction therapies
A number of treatments which have been used in vasculitis with well-preserved renal function are not appropriate for the treatment of crescentic glomerulonephritis. These include cotrimoxazole, which may have a place in the treatment of the respiratory manifestations of Wegener's granulomatosis [117–119]. Methotrexate has also gained some popularity in patients with Wegener's granulomatosis as a possible alternative to daily cyclophosphamide [120–122]. However, in these studies moderate renal impairment was considered a contraindication to use of methotrexate, due to the increased risk of adverse effects in the face of renal impairment. Intravenous immunoglobulin is another immunomodulatory treatment which has been used with some success in vasculitis [123, 124], though as yet precise indications for its use are unclear. Unfortunately, the risk of nephrotoxicity becomes increasingly likely as renal function deteriorates.

Maintenance and long-term therapy

Anti-GBM disease
Anti-GBM disease is usually a one-hit disease. Although early exacerbations of disease in the presence of persisting antibody are well-recognized, and may follow infection [125], late relapses are unusual; there are only infrequent reports of reappearance of anti-GBM antibody [126] or overt clinical relapse [71, 127]. Therefore, after an intensive course of immunosuppression to reduce circulating antibody levels to the normal range, treatment is tailed off. Typically, cyclophosphamide is discontinued after 3 months and corticosteroids are tailed down and stopped between 3 and 6 months. Treatment may be curtailed sooner if there is no recovery of renal function and pulmonary haemorrhage has not occurred.

Vasculitis
While there is broad agreement that a regimen including corticosteroids and cyclophosphamide is appropriate for induction therapy, there is little agreement about how to maintain remission thereafter. For example, a recent survey of the policies currently adopted by units in Europe participating in the ECSYSVASTRIAL studies showed wide variations in approach [111]. Long-term data from the NIH indicate that simply continuing with the same standard induction agents carries excessive risk [90]. Alternative strategies include early cessation of therapy and conversion to safer agents, of which azathioprine is best established.

Is maintenance therapy necessary? We believe so. In the 1970s the policy of our unit was to discontinue therapy in most patients during the first year; 25% of patients relapsed by 1 year. Following the introduction of maintenance therapy continuing to and beyond 12 months, the proportion of patients relapsing by 1 year reduced to 11%. Similarly, as our treatment progressively lengthened, relapse rate fell from 53% at 5 years to 22% [128]. Data from other groups reinforce the view that relapse is a major problem during follow-up [129–131], and that early discontinuation of therapy is associated with recurrence of disease [87]. Of particular concern is the tendency for recurrent nephritis to precipitate an inexorable progression to end-stage renal failure in patients with residual renal impairment after previous crescentic nephritis.

Our approach to continuing therapy is common to many British units, for example see reference [89]. Oral prednisolone dose is progressively reduced from a typical starting dose of 60 mg daily, to 20 mg daily by 6 weeks, and 10 mg daily by 6 months, reducing subsequently to a maintenance dose of around 5 mg daily in the second year. We substitute azathioprine dose-for-dose for oral cyclophosphamide, at 3 months, assuming remission has been achieved, and then progressively reduce to a maintenance dose of 1 mg/kg or less. Azathioprine is usually well tolerated, safer than cyclophosphamide and maintains remission in many patients. Some patients relapse and require reversion to cyclophosphamide; however, such relapse is rarely severe and permanent renal damage is unusual if diagnosed promptly.

We would also tend to use maintenance therapy for patients with both ANCA and anti-GBM antibodies, unlike those with anti-GBM antibodies alone, since they appear to mirror vasculitis patients in their potential to relapse.

Other agents being used for maintenance therapy include intravenous immunoglobulin and methotrexate, but these have not been formally compared with the more widely used combination of low-dose steroids and azathioprine. Furthermore, residual renal impairment after crescentic nephritis may preclude their use. Mycophenolate mofetil can replace azathioprine in renal transplantation regimens, with a reduction in rejection rates [132] which suggests greater potency. A pilot study is under way to examine its potential as a vasculitis maintenance agent [133], though whether it will prove sufficiently superior to azathioprine to justify its cost remains to be established.

The optimal duration of therapy is unknown. Relapse can occur years after initial presentation, and can have devastating consequences. However, it is likely that the risk of toxicity of treatment will outweigh the benefits if it is indiscriminately continued in every patient. Our current impression is that patients with persisting ANCA, irrespective of specificity, and patients whose disease was initially associated with proteinase 3-specific ANCA, are at greatest risk of relapse [128].

An alternative approach to maintenance of remission without undue treatment risk is to use non-immunosuppressive therapies. This is a possibility in patients with Wegener's granulomatosis. Stegeman *et al.* [134] tested cotrimoxazole as an adjunctive agent to maintain remission in Wegener's granulomatosis, in a placebo-controlled prospective study. Although 19% of the patients discontinued cotrimoxazole due to adverse effects, a significant reduction in relapses was achieved in the treated group, predominantly due to a reduction in relapse affecting the respiratory tract. Patients who are nasal carriers of *Staphylococcus aureus* appear to be at particular risk of relapse [135] and it is possible that the beneficial effect of cotrimoxazole is mediated through the eradication of this organism.

Therapy for refractory vasculitis

Despite the use of combinations of oral and pulsed corticosteroids, cyclophosphamide and plasma exchange, a minority of patients with vasculitis will show relentless progression of disease, or will continue to show disease activity for such prolonged periods that toxicity of conventional treatment becomes limiting. Two groups have recently used anti-T lymphocyte antibodies to treat such patients. Following success with one patient [136], Lockwood *et al.* [137, 138] went on to use a combination of two humanized monoclonal antibodies, CAMPATH 1H, directed against CDw52, and an anti-CD4 antibody, more widely, with some success and surprisingly few adverse effects, despite the production of marked and prolonged lymphopenia. Polyclonal anti-T cell antibodies, in the form of rabbit antithymocyte globulin, were used by Hagen *et al.* [139] to treat five patients with Wegener's granulomatosis; four showed a favourable response.

Prophylaxis against adverse effects

The treatments described above for both anti-GBM disease and systemic vasculitis have the potential for significant toxicity, both immediate and late. Patients are at increased risk of opportunist infections, which include *Pneumocystis carinii* [96], and many units now routinely use prophylaxis with low-dose cotrimoxazole. Tuberculosis is reported [54], and isoniazid prophylaxis should be considered in any patient at risk of reactivation. Cytomegalovirus, nocardia, aspergillus and other fungal infections are also well recognized. Herpes zoster is common [90] and may occasionally be fatal [54]. Presentation of opportunist infection may occasionally mimic manifestations of the original disease, and thorough and speedy investigation is mandatory.

Bacterial infections, with a variety of organisms and at a variety of sites, may also lead to death. A policy for early cessation of cytotoxic agents if the leukocyte count begins to fall is vital. The use of G-CSF can limit the risk of overwhelming sepsis due to neutropenia, although there are anecdotal reports that its use may be associated with a rapid recurrence of vasculitis disease activity; in other contexts it has been associated with the development of vasculitis.

Urinary excretion of a toxic metabolite of cyclophosphamide, acrolein, has the potential to cause haemorrhagic cystitis in the short term and bladder carcinoma in the longer term [140, 141], and cyclophosphamide treatment should be combined with a high fluid intake (renal function permitting). Mesna should be administered when high-dose, pulsed, therapy is used. Immunosuppressive therapy also increases the risk of malignancies other than bladder cancer [90, 130]. These include skin cancer [130] and it seems prudent to advise all patients of measures to reduce sun exposure.

Patients should also be warned about the risk of infertility after cyclophosphamide. The precise risk associated with the doses used to treat nephritis is uncertain, but is probably small if cyclophosphamide courses are kept short [142], increasing with duration of therapy and increasing age in females [143]. The pulsed cyclophosphamide regimens for vasculitis described to date have not avoided the induction of amenorrhoea [96]. In treatment of crescentic nephritis there is rarely time for storage of sperm or oocyte collection before commencement of therapy.

The principal hazard of plasma exchange is the risk of bleeding due to depletion of clotting factors, which should be replaced to normal levels in patients at particular risk of bleeding, for example after a renal biopsy or in the presence of pulmonary haemorrhage. Routine exchange for fresh frozen plasma is not advisable in view of the risk of severe allergic reactions; in one study of 7538 plasma exchanges in 887 patients, performed for a variety of indications, there were three deaths, all related to the administration of fresh frozen plasma [144].

Finally, prophylaxis should be considered against steroid-induced osteoporosis. Since the use of biphosphonates is precluded by severe renal dysfunction, initial prophylaxis depends chiefly on calcium supplementation and appropriate formulations of vitamin D. Hormone replacement may be considered in postmenopausal females, though the increased thrombotic tendency of vasculitis patients should be borne in mind.

Outcome

Anti-GBM disease

Historically, Goodpasture's syndrome was fatal in the majority of cases, either as a result of overwhelming pulmonary haemorrhage or renal failure [145], though with hindsight not all cases were attributable to anti-GBM disease. Bilateral nephrectomy was performed in desperate cases in an attempt to turn off the immune response. With the introduction of therapeutic regimens containing plasma exchange and cytotoxic drugs, and as a result of improvements in supportive care for renal and respiratory failure, 1-year mortality has reduced to 10–20% [17, 37, 38].

Renal outcome remains unsatisfactory in many patients, largely because renal impairment is often advanced at presentation. Few patients presenting with a creatinine higher than 500 or 600 μmol/L avoid long-term dialysis [17, 36, 37, 67, 146], though occasional patients recover renal function after an initial requirement for dialysis [60, 65, 66]. The experience from our own unit, using an intensive plasma exchange schedule, is similar; only 11% of patients with a creatinine greater than 600 μmol/L had independent renal function at 1 year, in contrast to 90% with a presenting creatinine below this figure [33]. Early referral is therefore critical, but rarely achieved [146], perhaps because the renal injury progresses so rapidly.

Anti-GBM antibodies have the potential to cause nephritis in a transplanted kidney. It is prudent to wait until circulating antibodies have been undetectable in a sensitive solid-phase assay for at least 6 months before proceeding to transplantation; under such circumstances the risk of recurrent anti-GBM disease in the graft is very low [147].

Outcome in ANCA-associated disease

Data on outcome in ANCA-associated renal disease are far more extensive, although different series report patients with widely varying degrees of renal dysfunction, depending on the specialty and referral practice of the authors. This section concentrates on patients with severe renal dysfunction at presentation.

Patient survival

Early mortality in vasculitis patients with severe renal disease varies from around 10% to over 30% in published series. This is mainly from uncontrolled disease, particularly pulmonary haemorrhage [148], although there are also deaths due to treatment complications and a few due to unrelated events in a predominantly elderly population. A small number of deaths occur later in the first year, with a significant contribution from opportunist infections. Levy and Winearls [92] reported a 1-year survival of 86%. Survivals in other similar series were 81% [87], 78% [149] and 62% [88].

Late deaths include a small number due to relapse and a proportion due to the adverse effects of therapy, including haematological malignancies in patients with prolonged exposure to cyclophosphamide. The remainder are attributable to unrelated causes. Prognosis appears to have improved with early recognition of disease activity and the more judicious use of immuno-suppression. Data from Guy's Hospital indicate a marked improvement in actuarial survival at 5 years, from 38% [23] to 77% [89]. Indeed, 5-year survivals of 55–75% are now the norm [87, 129, 149] even when many of the patients present with advanced renal impairment. Our current data indicate an overall 5-year survival of 63% in small vessel vasculitis; this is reduced to 50% by 10 years, but it is worth remembering that patients tend to present in later life.

Survival is similar in Wegener's granulomatosis and microscopic polyangiitis [150]. ANCA specificity for proteinase 3 was associated with a higher mortality in one series [148], but this has not been confirmed by others [150]. A more consistent message emerges from the literature on the effect of age at presentation: older patients are at greater risk of death [54, 88, 89, 116, 130, 151, 152] and excess deaths are usually due to infective complications. Our experience is that these can be minimized by modification of immunosuppressive regimens, and satisfactory outcomes achieved [153].

Mortality is higher in vasculitis patients with renal disease than in those without. Furthermore, the severity of renal impairment is highly relevant. Oliguria and advanced renal failure at presentation have been highlighted as risk factors for high mortality in many series [23, 154]. Failure to recover independent renal function with therapy also carries an increased mortality, although this is no higher than that of patients with end-stage renal failure due to other causes [155, 156].

Whether the presence of extrarenal vasculitis alters mortality is open to debate. Weiss and Crissman [157] found no difference in outcome, while Croker *et al.* [158] found a higher morbidity in patients without systemic disease. They attributed the difference to later presentation with more advanced renal damage where medical help was not sought for systemic symptoms. This is also our experience; of 22 patients without extrarenal vasculitis, 15 patients required dialysis at presentation. Velosa [159] suggested that the presence of vasculitis might imply a better prognosis independently of other variables, but the conclusions were drawn from a study in which presenting renal function and treatment administered were quite different in the two groups [160]. Indeed, in general, cytotoxic drugs have been used less frequently in isolated RPGN than in systemic vasculitis. Bindi *et al.* [54] found that a smaller number of extrarenal organs involved was associated with a better prognosis when differences in treatment were excluded. One systemic manifestation clearly associated with a high early mortality is the presence of lung haemorrhage [26, 54, 148].

Renal function

Table 7.4 summarizes renal outcome data from a number of series, including our own. The results vary substantially, perhaps reflecting the variation of treatment policies between, and even within, centres. However, it is important to note that recovery from dialysis dependence is common, even when the biopsy shows a high percentage of crescents [93], and immunosuppressive therapy should not be withheld due to pessimism about renal outcome. Sometimes renal recovery is delayed; Coward *et al.* [87] described renal recovery as late as 4 months after presentation.

A proportion of the patients with independent renal function after initial therapy later progress to end-stage renal failure. This was particularly notable in the North Carolina series [148]. Some of these patients had an incomplete response to initial therapy, either due to extensive glomerular sclerosis and interstitial damage at presentation, or due to insufficiently aggressive initial therapy; Hogan *et al.* noted a poorer renal outcome in patients treated with steroids alone [148]. Other patients sustain further renal damage during relapse. Our experience suggests that patients who make a good response to initial therapy, and who remain in remission, usually maintain stable and independent renal function during long-term follow-up; 5-year renal survival

Table 7.4 Renal outcome in advanced ANCA-associated crescentic glomerulonephritis

Reference (no. of patients)	Type of patient	Treatment	Initial response: % alive with independent renal function
Coward *et al.* (1986) [87] (*n* = 18)	WG, MP Dialysis	Mix of MP, P, C, A, PE	50
Fuiano *et al.* (1988) [89] (*n* = 5)	WG, MP Creatinine >600 μmol/L	Mix of MP, P C, A, PE	60
Falk *et al.* (1990) [77] (*n* = 12)	ANCA + GN Dialysis	Mix of MP, P, i.v. or oral C	50
Andrassy *et al.* (1991) [93] (*n* = 14)	WG Dialysis	P, i.v. C, MP PE in 2	93
Garrett *et al.* (1992) [152] (*n* = 19)	ANCA + GN Dialysis	Mix of P, C, A, MP, PE	41
Cole *et al.* (1992) [105] (*n* = 11)	RLV Dialysis	MP, P, A MP, P, A, PE	29 75
Bindi *et al.* (1993) [54] (*n* = 17)	ANCA + GN, Creatinine >600 μmol/L	P and/or MP, C, PE in 6	47
Levy and Winearls (1994) [92] (*n* = 20)	WG, MP, RLV Dialysis	P, C, PE and/or MP	70
Haubitz *et al.* (1995) [97] (*n* = 13)	WG, MP Dialysis	MP, P, oral C MP, P, i.v. C	66 14
Hammersmith data (*n* = 80)	WG, MP, RLV, Creatinine >500 μmol/L	P, C, PE	73

A = azathioprine; C = cyclophosphamide; GN = glomerulonephritis; MP = methylprednisolone; P = prednisolone; PE = plasma exchange; WG = Wegener's granulomatosis; i.v. = intravenous; RLV = renal-limited vasculitis

is 83% in those improving with initial therapy [106]. This experience is shared by other groups [87, 88, 93, 101].

Oliguria [23], severe renal impairment [160] and an initial requirement for dialysis [93] have been highlighted as presenting features increasing the likelihood of permanent renal failure. This may reflect the contribution of patients with irreversible renal damage, as indicated by sclerosed glomeruli and interstitial scarring and atrophy, since these independently predict a poorer prognosis [54, 93]. Arterial sclerosis was also associated with a worse outcome in one series [148]. A low percentage of normal glomeruli also suggests a poorer prognosis, but this is not simply a function of the crescent score, which alone does not predict outcome [161]. In general, histological parameters are an unreliable predictor of outcome in individual patients, and should not be used to decide whether to withhold immunosuppressive therapy.

Further prognostic information is yielded by the response to initial therapy. Grotz *et al.* [101] found creatinine at 2 weeks to be predictive of long-term renal outcome and, in general, patients who make a good response to initial therapy, and who remain in remission, maintain stable renal function [87, 88, 93].

Control of disease
When patients have significant extrarenal vasculitis, its control is an equally important goal of therapy. Recent studies suggest that complete control of disease activity can be achieved with first-line therapy in 70–80% of vasculitis patients [90, 96, 129]. However, over 90% show improvement, and the residual symptoms are infrequently life-threatening. Unfortunately, irreversible tissue damage often occurs before the disease activity is quelled [162]. Furthermore, published experience suggests that, despite initial control of disease, between one-third and one-half of patients with generalized small vessel vasculitis will relapse during follow-up, whether the diagnosis is Wegener's granulomatosis or microscopic polyangiitis [86, 87, 90, 129]; preliminary data suggest that patients with proteinase 3-specific ANCA are at particular risk [128, 135]. The characteristics of relapse are not necessarily those of the original presentation [129], and disease which was confined to the kidney at presentation may become more generalized.

Relapse has been reported from 3 months to 16 years after induction of complete remission [90]; our experience is similar. Relapse may occur during reduction of immunosuppressive therapy or following discontinuation [73, 87, 128, 150]. Withdrawal of treatment should therefore be gradual, performed only when there is no evidence of disease activity and accompanied by close monitoring for early signs of disease recurrence. Assays for ANCA may assist the identification of patients at particular risk of relapse.

Future directions

Although the outcome for patients with crescentic glomerulonephritis and vasculitis has improved dramatically in the past 30 years, there is still much scope for improvement. Early recognition and referral are critical, and the increasing availability of specific and sensitive immunoassays for anti-GBM antibodies and ANCA [41, 163], coupled with a high index of suspicion and readiness to investigate in primary care [164], should help. Even after prompt diagnosis, outcome in some patients is unsatisfactory due to the failure or toxicity of non-specific immunotherapy. Safer and more effective approaches may be facilitated in the future by an increasing understanding of pathogenetic mechanisms [11, 22]. Therapeutic avenues being explored include specific immunoadsorption for the removal of pathogenic antibodies [165] and are likely to call upon the increasing range of new therapies being introduced in transplantation. Meanwhile, there is a need to define the best regimens using current agents, and the EUVAS study group is conducting international randomized controlled trials [111] in vasculitis to improve the evidence base.

References

1. Volhard F, Fahr T. Die Brightsche Nierenkrankheit. Berlin: Springer; 1914.
2. Ellis A. Natural history of Bright's disease. Clinical, histological and experimental observations. Lancet 1942;i:34–6.
3. Davson J, Ball J, Platt R. The kidney in periarteritis nodosa. Q J Med 1948;17:175–202.
4. Godman GC, Churg J. Wegener's granulomatosis: pathology and review of the literature. Arch Pathol 1954;58:533–53.
5. Scheer RL, Grossman MA. Immune aspects of glomerulonephritis associated with pulmonary haemorrhage. Ann Intern Med 1964;60:1009–21.
6. Whitworth JA, Morel-Maroger L, Mignon F, Richet G. The significance of extracapillary proliferation. Clinicopathological review of 60 patients. Nephron 1976;16:1–19.
7. Stilmant M, Bolton WK, Sturgill BC, Schmitt G, Couser WG. Crescentic glomerulonephritis without immune deposits: clinicopathological features. Kidney Int 1979;15:184–95.
8. Neild GH, Cameron JS, Ogg CS *et al.* Rapidly progressive glomerulonephritis with extensive glomerular crescent formation. Q J Med 1983;52:395–416.
9. Morrison KE, Germino G, Reeders ST. Use of the polymerase chain reaction to clone and sequence a cDNA encoding the bovine alpha 3 chain of type IV collagen. J Biol Chem 1991; 266:34–9.
10. Turner AN, Mason PJ, Brown R *et al.* Molecular cloning of the human Goodpasture antigen demonstrates it to be the alpha 3 chain of type IV collagen. J Clin Invest 1992;89:592–601.
11. Hudson BG, Kalluri R, Gunwar S, Noelken ME, Mariyama M, Reeders ST. Molecular characteristics of the Goodpasture autoantigen. Kidney Int 1993;43:135–9.
12. Kalluri R, Wilson CB, Weber M *et al.* Identification of the alpha 3 chain of type IV collagen as the common autoantigen in antibasement membrane disease and Goodpasture syndrome. J Am Soc Nephrol 1995;6:1178–85.
13. Derry CJ, Pusey CD. Tissue-specific distribution of the Goodpasture antigen demonstrated by 2-D electrophoresis and western blotting. Nephrol Dial Transplant 1994;9:355–61.
14. Yamamoto T, Wilson CB. Binding of anti–basement membrane antibody to alveolar basement membrane after intratracheal gasoline installation in rabbits. Am J Pathol 1987;126:497–505.
15. Queluz TH, Pawlowski I, Brunda MJ, Brentjens JR, Vladutiu AO, Andres G. Pathogenesis of an experimental model of Goodpasture's hemorrhagic pneumonitis. J Clin Invest 1990;85: 1507–15.
16. Donaghy M, Rees AJ. Cigarette smoking and lung haemorrhage in glomerulonephritis caused by autoantibodies to glomerular basement membrane. Lancet 1983;ii:1390–3.
17. Herody M, Bobrie G, Gouarin C, Grunfeld J-P, Noel L-H. Anti-GBM disease: predictive value of clinical, histological and serological data. Clin Nephrol 1993;40:249–55.
18. Bombassei JH, Kaplan AA. The association between hydrocarbon exposure and anti-glomerular basement membrane antibody-mediated disease (Goodpasture's syndrome). Am J Ind Med 1992;21:141–53.
19. Peten E, Pirson Y, Cosyns J–P *et al.* Outcome of thirty patients with Alport's syndrome after renal transplantation. Transplantation 1991;52:823–6.
20. Gobel J, Olbricht CJ, Offner G *et al.* Kidney transplantation in Alport's syndrome: long-term outcome and allograft anti-GBM nephritis. Clin Nephrol 1992;38:299–304.

21. Brainwood D, Kashtan C, Gubler MC, Turner AN. Targets of alloantibodies in Alport anti-glomerular basement membrane disease after renal transplantation. Kidney Int 1998;53:762–6.
22. Kallenberg CG, Brouwer E, Weening JJ, Tervaert JW. Anti-neutrophil cytoplasmic antibodies: current diagnostic and pathophysiological potential. Kidney Int. 1994;46:1–15.
23. Serra A, Cameron JS, Turner DR *et al.* Vasculitis affecting the kidney: presentation, histopathology and long-term outcome. Q J Med 1984;53:181–207.
24. Woodworth TG, Abuelo JG, Austin HA, Esparza A. Severe glomerulonephritis with late emergence of classic Wegener's granulomatosis: report of 4 cases and review of the literature. Medicine 1987;66:181–91.
25. Cohen Tervaert JW, Goldschmeding R, Elema JD *et al.* Autoantibodies against myeloid lysosomal enzymes in crescentic glomerulonephritis. Kidney Int 1990;37:799–806.
26. Jennette JC, Wilkman AS, Falk RJ. Anti-neutrophil cytoplasmic autoantibody-associated glomerulonephritis and vasculitis. Am J Pathol 1989;135:921–30.
27. Angangco R, Thiru S, Esnault VL, Short AK, Lockwood CM, Oliveira DB. Does truly 'idiopathic' crescentic glomerulonephritis exist? Nephrol Dial Transplant 1994;9:630–6.
28. Ferrario F, Tadros MT, Napodano P, Sinico RA, Fellin G, D'Amico G. Critical re-evaluation of 41 cases of 'idiopathic' crescentic glomerulonephritis. Clin Nephrol 1994;41:1–9.
29. Holdsworth S, Boyce N, Thomson NM, Atkins RC. The clinical spectrum of acute glomerulonephritis and lung haemorrhage (Goodpasture's syndrome). Q J Med 1985;55:75–86.
30. Bosch X, Mirapeix E, Font J *et al.* Anti-myeloperoxidase autoantibodies in patients with necrotizing glomerular and alveolar capillaritis. Am J Kidney Dis 1992;20:231–9.
31. Travis WD, Colby TV, Lombard C, Carpenter HA. A clinicopathologic study of 34 cases of diffuse pulmonary haemorrhage with lung biopsy confirmation. Am J Surg Pathol 1990;14: 1112–25.
32. Niles JL, Bottinger EP, Saurina GR *et al.* The syndrome of lung haemorrhage and nephritis is usually an ANCA-associated condition. Arch Intern Med 1996;156:440–5.
33. Turner AN, Rees AJ. Antiglomerular basement membrane disease. In: Davison AM, Cameron JS, Grunfeld J-P, Kerr DNS, Ritz E, Winearls CG, editors. Oxford Textbook of Clinical Nephrology, 2nd edn. Oxford: Oxford University Press; 1998:647–66.
34. Watts RA, Carruthers DM, Scott DGI. Epidemiology of systemic vasculitis: changing incidence or definition? Semin Arthritis Rheum 1995;25:28–34.
35. Andrews M, Edmunds M, Campbell A, Walls J, Feehally J. Systemic vasculitis in the 1980s – is there an increasing incidence of Wegener's granulomatosis and microscopic polyarteritis? J R Coll Phys Lond 1990;24:284–8.
36. Daly C, Conlon PJ, Medwar W, Walshe JJ. Characteristics and outcome of anti-glomerular basement membrane disease: a single center experience. Renal Failure 1996;18:105–12.
37. Merkel F, Pullig O, Marx M, Netzer KO, Weber M. Course and prognosis of anti-basement membrane antibody (anti-BM-ab)-mediated disease: report of 35 cases. Nephrol Dial Transplant 1994;9:372–6.
38. Savage CO, Pusey CD, Bowman C, Rees AJ, Lockwood CM. Antiglomerular basement membrane antibody mediated disease in the British Isles 1980–4. Br Med J 1986;292:301–4.
39. Jennette JC, Falk RJ, Andrassy K *et al.* Nomenclature of systemic vasculitides. Proposal of an international consensus conference. Arthritis Rheum 1994;37:187–92.
40. Clutterbuck EJ, Evans DJ, Pusey CD. Renal involvement in Churg–Strauss syndrome. Nephrol Dial Transplant 1990;5:161–7.
41. Hagen EC, Daha MR, Hermans J *et al.* Diagnostic value of standardized assays for anti-neutrophil cytoplasmic antibodies in idiopathic systemic vasculitis. EC/BCR project for ANCA assay standardization. Kidney Int 1998;53:743–53.
42. Jayne DRW, Marshall PD, Jones SJ, Lockwood CM. Autoantibodies to GBM and neutrophil cytoplasm in rapidly progressive glomerulonephritis. Kidney Int 1990;37:965–70.

43. Short AK, Esnault VL, Lockwood CM. Anti-neutrophil cytoplasm antibodies and anti-glomerular basement membrane antibodies: two coexisting distinct autoreactivities detectable in patients with rapidly progressive glomerulonephritis. Am J Kidney Dis 1995;26:439–45.
44. Bosch X, Mirapeix E, Font J *et al.* Prognostic implication of anti-neutrophil cytoplasmic autoantibodies with myeloperoxidase specificity in anti-glomerular basement membrane disease. Clin Nephrol 1991;36:107–13.
45. Weber MF, Andrassy K, Pullig O, Koderisch J, Netzer K. Antineutrophil cytoplasmic antibodies and antiglomerular basement membrane antibodies in Goodpasture's syndrome and in Wegener's granulomatosis. J Am Soc Nephrol 1992;2:1227–34.
46. Kalluri R, Meyers K, Mogyorosi A, Madaio MP, Neilson EG. Goodpasture syndrome involving overlap with Wegener's granulomatosis and anti-glomerular basement membrane disease. J Am Soc Nephrol 1997;8:1795–800.
47. Hellmark T, Niles JL, Collins AB, McCluskey RT, Brunmark C. Comparison of anti-GBM antibodies in sera with or without ANCA. J Am Soc Nephrol 1997;8:376–85.
48. Pusey CD, Turner AN, Gaskin G *et al.* Specificity of anti-GBM antibodies found in patients with ANCA. Am J Kidney Dis 1991;18:210–11 (abstract).
49. Wahls TL, Bonsib SM, Schuster VL. Coexistent Wegener's granulomatosis and anti-glomerular basement membrane disease. Human Pathol 1987;18:202–5.
50. O'Donaghue DJ, Short CD, Brenchley PEC, Lawler W, Ballardie FW. Sequential development of systemic vasculitis with anti-neutrophil cytoplasmic antibodies complicating anti-glomerular basement membrane disease. Clin Nephrol 1989;32:251–5.
51. Ferrario F, Rastaldi MP. Pathology of rapidly progressive glomerulonephritis. In: Pusey CD, Rees AJ, editors. Rapidly Progressive Glomerulonephritis. Oxford: Oxford University Press; 1998:59–107.
52. Wilson CB, Dixon FJ. Anti-glomerular basement membrane antibody-induced glomerulonephritis. Kidney Int 1973;3:74–89.
53. Salant DJ. Immunopathogenesis of crescentic glomerulonephritis and lung purpura. Kidney Int 1987;32:408–25.
54. Bindi P, Mougenot B, Mentre F *et al.* Necrotizing crescentic glomerulonephritis without significant immune deposits: a clinical and serological study. Q J Med 1993;86:55–68.
55. Bajema IM, Hagen EC, Ferrario F *et al.* Renal granulomas in systemic vasculitis. EC/BCR project for ANCA-assay standardization. Clin Nephrol 1997;48:16–21.
56. Bonsib SM, Goeken JA, Fandel T, Houghton DC. Necrotizing medullary lesions in patients with ANCA associated renal disease. Mod Pathol 1994;7:181–5.
57. Ronco P, Verroust P, Mignon F *et al.* Immunopathological studies of polyarteritis nodosa and Wegener's granulomatosis: a report of 43 patients with 51 renal biopsies. Q J Med 1983;52: 212–23.
58. Franssen CF, Gans RO, Arends B *et al.* Differences between anti-myeloperoxidase and anti-proteinase 3-associated renal disease. Kidney Int 1995;47:193–9.
59. Briggs WA, Johnson JP, Teichman S, Yeager HC, Wilson CB. Antiglomerular basement membrane antibody-mediated glomerulonephritis and Goodpasture's syndrome. Medicine 1979;58:348–61.
60. Cohen LH, Wilson CB, Freeman RM. Goodpasture syndrome: recovery after severe renal insufficiency. Arch Intern Med 1976;136:835–7.
61. Lerner RA, Glassock RJ, Dixon FJ. The role of anti-glomerular basement membrane antibody in the pathogenesis of human glomerulonephritis. J Exp Med 1967;126:989–1004.
62. Lockwood CM, Rees AJ, Pearson TA, Evans DJ, Peters DK. Immunosuppression and plasma exchange in the treatment of Goodpasture's syndrome. Lancet 1976;i:711–15.
63. Pusey CD, Lockwood CM, Peters DK. Plasma exchange and immunosuppressive drugs in the treatment of glomerulonephritis due to antibodies to the glomerular basement membrane. Int J Artif Organs 1983;6(Suppl.1):15–18.
64. Bruns FJ, Stachura I, Adler S, Segel DP. Effect of early plasmapheresis and immunosuppressive therapy on natural history of anti-glomerular basement membrane glomerulonephritis: report of a 22-month follow-up. Arch Intern Med 1979;139:372–4.

65. Johnson JP, Whitman W, Briggs WA, Wilson CB. Plasmapheresis and immunosuppressive agents in antibasement membrane antibody-induced Goodpasture's syndrome. Am J Med 1978;64:354–9.
66. Simpson IJ, Doak PB, Williams LC *et al.* Plasma exchange in Goodpasture's syndrome. Am J Nephrol 1982;2:301–11.
67. Walker RG, Scheinkestel C, Becker GJ, Owen JE, Dowling JP, Kincaid-Smith P. Clinical and morphological aspects of the management of crescentic anti-glomerular basement membrane antibody (anti-GBM) nephritis/Goodpasture's syndrome. Q J Med 1985;54:75–89.
68. Johnson JP, Moore J Jr, Austin HA III, Balow JE, Antonovych TT, Wilson CB. Therapy of anti-glomerular basement membrane antibody disease: analysis of prognostic significance of clinical, pathologic and treatment factors. Medicine 1985;64:219–27.
69. Bolton WK, Sturgill BC. Methylprednisolone therapy for acute crescentic rapidly progressive glomerulonephritis. Am J Nephrol 1989;9:368–75.
70. Bygren P, Freiburghaus C, Lindholm T, Stimonsen O, Thysell H, Wieslander J. Goodpasture's syndrome treated with staphylococcal protein A immunoadsorption. Lancet 1985;ii:1295–6.
71. Levy JB, Lachmann RH, Pusey CD. Recurrent Goodpasture's disease. Am J Kidney Dis 1996;27:573–8.
72. Flores JC, Taube D, Savage CO *et al.* Clinical and immunological evolution of oligoanuric anti-GBM nephritis treated by haemodialysis. Lancet 1986;i:5–8.
73. Fauci AS, Haynes BF, Katz P, Wolff S. Wegener's granulomatosis: prospective clinical and therapeutic experience with 85 patients over 21 years. Ann Intern Med 1983;98:76–85.
74. Leib ES, Restivo C, Paulus HE. Immunosuppressive and corticosteroid therapy of polyarteritis nodosa. Am J Med 1979;67:941–5.
75. Fauci AS, Doppman JL, Wolff SM. Cyclophosphamide-induced remissions in polyarteritis nodosa. Am J Med 1978;64:890–4.
76. Lockwood CM, Rees AJ, Pinching AJ *et al.* Plasma-exchange and immunosuppression in the treatment of fulminant immune-complex crescentic nephritis. Lancet 1977;i:63–7.
77. Falk RJ, Hogan S, Carey TS, Jennette JC. Clinical course of anti-neutrophil cytoplasmic autoantibody-associated glomerulonephritis and systemic vasculitis. Ann Intern Med 1990; 113:656–63.
78. Fahey JL, Leonard E, Churg J, Godman G. Wegener's granulomatosis. Am J Med 1954;17: 168–79.
79. Walton EW. Giant-cell granuloma of the respiratory tract (Wegener's granulomatosis). Br Med J 1958;ii:265–70.
80. Hollander D, Manning RT. The use of alkylating agents in the treatment of Wegener's granulomatosis. Ann Intern Med 1967;67:393–8.
81. Frohnert PP, Sheps SG. Long-term follow-up study of periarteritis nodosa. Am J Med 1967; 43:8–14.
82. Sack M, Cassidy JT, Bole GG. Prognostic factors in polyarteritis. J Rheumatol 1975;2:411–20.
83. Novack S, Pearson CM. Cyclophosphamide therapy in Wegener's granulomatosis. N Engl J Med 1971;284:938–41.
84. Fauci AS, Wolff S, Johnson JS. Effect of cyclophosphamide upon the immune response in Wegener's granulomatosis. N Engl J Med 1971;285:1493–6.
85. Fauci AS, Katz P, Haynes BF, Wolff SM. Cyclophosphamide therapy of severe necrotizing vasculitis. N Engl J Med 1979;301:235–8.
86. Savage COS, Winearls CG, Evans DJ, Rees AJ, Lockwood CM. Microscopic polyarteritis: presentation, pathology and prognosis. Q J Med 1985;56:467–83.
87. Coward RA, Hamdy NAT, Shortland JS, Brown CB. Renal micropolyarteritis: a treatable condition. Nephrol Dial Transplant 1986;1:31–7.
88. Adu D, Howie AJ, Scott DGI, Bacon PA, McGonigle RJS, Michael J. Polyarteritis and the kidney. Q.J Med 1987;62:221–37.
89. Fuiano G, Cameron JS, Raftery M, Hartley BH, Williams DG, Ogg CS. Improved prognosis of renal microscopic polyarteritis in recent years. Nephrol Dial Transplant 1988;3:383–91.

90. Hoffman GS, Kerr GS, Leavitt RY *et al.* Wegener granulomatosis: an analysis of 158 patients. Ann Intern Med 1992;116:488–98.
91. Stevens ME, McConnell M, Bone JM. Aggressive treatment with pulse methylprednisolone or plasma exchange is justified in rapidly progressive glomerulonephritis. Proc Eur Dial Transplant Assoc 1982;19:724–31.
92. Levy JB, Winearls CG. Rapidly progressive glomerulonephritis: what should be first-line therapy? Nephron 1994;67:402–7.
93. Andrassy K, Erb A, Koderisch J, Waldherr R, Ritz E. Wegener's granulomatosis with renal involvement: patient survival and correlations between initial renal function, renal histology, therapy and renal outcome. Clin Nephrol 1991;35:139–47.
94. Austin HA III, Klippel JH, Balow JE *et al.* Therapy of lupus nephritis. Controlled trial of prednisone and cytotoxic drugs. N Engl J Med 1986;314:614–19.
95. Adu D, Pall A, Luqmani RA *et al.* Controlled trial of pulse versus continuous prednisolone and cyclophosphamide in the treatment of systemic vasculitis. Q J Med 1997;90:401–9.
96. Guillevin L, Cordier J-F, Lhote F *et al.* A prospective, multicenter, randomized trial comparing steroids and pulse cyclophosphamide versus steroids and oral cyclophosphamide in the treatment of generalized Wegener's granulomatosis. Arthritis Rheum. 1997;40:2187–98.
97. Haubitz M, Brunkhorst R, Schellong S *et al.* A prospective randomised study comparing daily oral versus monthly i.v. cyclophosphamide application in patients with ANCA-associated vasculitis and renal involvement (preliminary results). Clin Exp Immunol 1995;101(Suppl.1): 43.
98. Hoffman GS, Leavitt RY, Fleisher TA, Minor JR, Fauci AS. Treatment of Wegener's granulomatosis with intermittent high-dose intravenous cyclophosphamide. Am J Med 1990; 89:403–10.
99. Reinhold Keller E, Kekow J, Schnabel A *et al.* Influence of disease manifestation and antineutrophil cytoplasmic antibody titer on the response to pulse cyclophosphamide therapy in patients with Wegener's granulomatosis. Arthritis Rheum 1994;37:919–24.
100. Szpirt W, Rasmussen N, Thomsen B. Plasma exchange in patients with antineutrophil cytoplasmic antibodies (ANCA) and acute renal failure. APMIS 1990;98(Suppl.19):63–4.
101. Grotz W, Wanner C, Keller E *et al.* Crescentic glomerulonephritis in Wegener's granulomatosis: morphology, therapy, outcome. Clin Nephrol 1991;35:243–51.
102. Thysell H, Bygren P, Bengtsson U *et al.* Immunosuppression and the additive effect of plasma exchange in treatment of rapidly progressive glomerulonephritis. Acta Med Scand 1982;212: 107–14.
103. Glockner W, Sieberth HG, Wichmann HE *et al.* Plasma exchange and immunosuppression in rapidly progressive glomerulonephritis: a controlled multi-centre study. Clin Nephrol 1988; 29:1–88.
104. Pusey CD, Rees AJ, Evans DJ, Peters DK, Lockwood CM. Plasma exchange in focal necrotizing glomerulonephritis without anti-GBM antibodies. Kidney Int 1991;40:757–63.
105. Cole E, Cattran D, Magil A *et al.* A prospective randomized trial of plasma exchange as additive therapy in idiopathic crescentic glomerulonephritis. Am J Kidney Dis 1992;20:261–9.
106. Gaskin G, Pusey CD. Long-term outcome after plasma exchange for severe nephritis in ANCA-associated vasculitis. Clin Exp Immunol 1998;112(Suppl.1):57 (abstract).
107. Guillevin L, Cevallos R, Durand-Gasselin *et al.* Treatment of glomerulonephritis in microscopic polyangiitis and Churg–Strauss syndrome. Indications of plasma exchanges, meta-analysis of 2 randomized studies on 140 patients, 32 with glomerulonephritis. Ann Med Interne Paris 1997;148:198–204.
108. Gaskin G, Pusey CD. Plasma exchange is not excluded as a useful treatment for vasculitis-associated glomerulonephritis. Ann Med Interne Paris 1997;148:196–7.
109. Esnault VL, Testa A, Jayne DR, Soulillou JP, Guenel J. Influence of immunoadsorption on the removal of immunoglobulin G autoantibodies in crescentic glomerulonephritis. Nephron 1993;65:180–4.

110. Palmer A, Cairns T, Dische F *et al.* Treatment of rapidly progressive glomerulonephritis by extracorporeal immunoadsorption, prednisolone and cyclophosphamide. Nephrol Dial Transplant 1991;6:536–42.
111. Rasmussen N, Jayne DRW, Abramowicz D *et al.* European therapeutic trials in ANCA-associated systemic vasculitis: disease scoring, consensus regimens and proposed clinical trials. Clin Exp Immunol 1995;101(Suppl.1):29–34.
112. Cohen J, Pinching AJ, Rees AJ, Peters DK. Infection and immunosuppression. A study of the infective complications of 75 patients with immunologically-mediated renal disease. Q J Med 1982;51:1–15.
113. Pohl M, Lan S, Berl T and the Lupus Nephritis Collaborative Study Group. Plasmapheresis does not increase the risk for infection in immunosuppressed patients with severe lupus nephritis. Ann Intern Med 1991;114:924–9.
114. McLelland P, Williams PS, Stevens ME, Bone JM. Letter. Nephrol Dial Transplant 1989;4: 917.
115. Bruns FJ, Adler S, Fraley DS, Segel DP. Long-term follow-up of aggressively treated idiopathic rapidly progressive glomerulonephritis. Am J Med 1989;86:400–6.
116. Rondeau E, Levy M, Dosquet P *et al.* Plasma exchange and immunosuppression for rapidly progressive glomerulonephritis: prognosis and complications. Nephrol Dial Transplant 1989; 4:196–200.
117. DeRemee RA. The treatment of Wegener's granulomatosis with trimethoprim/sulfamethoxazole: illusion or vision? Arthritis Rheum 1988;31:1068–72.
118. Israel H. Sulfamethoxazole–trimethoprim therapy for Wegener's granulomatosis. Arch Intern Med 1988;148:2293–5.
119. Reinhold–Keller E, Beigel A, Duncker G *et al.* Trimethoprim–sulphamethoxazole (T/S) in the long–term treatment of Wegener's granulomatosis. Clin Exp Immunol 1993;93:(Suppl.1):38.
120. Hoffman GS, Leavitt RY, Kerr GS, Fauci AS. The treatment of Wegener's granulomatosis with glucocorticoids and methotrexate. Arthritis Rheum 1992;35:1322–9.
121. Sneller MC, Hoffman GS, Talar-Williams C, Kerr GS, Hallahan CW, Fauci AS. An analysis of forty-two Wegener's granulomatosis patients treated with methotrexate and prednisone. Arthritis Rheum 1995;38:608–13.
122. de Groot K, Muhler M, Reinhold-Keller E, Paulsen J, Gross WL. Induction of remission in Wegener's granulomatosis with low dose methotrexate. J Rheumatol 1998;25:492–5.
123. Jayne DR, Davies MJ, Fox CJ, Black CM, Lockwood CM. Treatment of systemic vasculitis with pooled intravenous immunoglobulin. Lancet 1991;337:1137–9.
124. Richter C, Schnabel A, Csernok E *et al.* Treatment of Wegener's granulomatosis with intravenous immunoglobulin. In: Gross WL, editor. ANCA-Associated Vasculitides: Immunological and Clinical Aspects. New York: Plenum Press; 1993:487–9.
125. Rees AJ, Lockwood CM, Peters DK. Enhanced allergic tissue injury in Goodpasture's syndrome by intercurrent bacterial infection. Br Med J 1977;ii:723–6.
126. Hind CR, Bowman C, Winearls CG, Lockwood CM. Recurrence of circulating anti-glomerular basement membrane antibody three years after immunosuppressive treatment and plasma exchange. Clin Nephrol 1984;21:244–6.
127. Mehler PS, Brunvand MW, Hutt MP, Anderson RJ. Chronic recurrent Goodpasture's syndrome. Am J Med 1987;82:833.
128. Gaskin G, Pusey CD. Prevention of relapse in systemic vasculitis. J Am Soc Nephrol 1995;6: 921 (abstract).
129. Gordon M, Luqmani RA, Adu D *et al.* Relapses in patients with a systemic vasculitis. Q J Med 1993;86:779–89.
130. Westman KW, Bygren PG, Olsson H, Ranstam J, Wieslander J. Relapse rate, renal survival, and cancer morbidity in patients with Wegener's granulomatosis or microscopic polyangiitis with renal involvement. J Am Soc Nephrol 1998;9:842–52.
131. Nachman PH, Hogan SL, Jennette JC, Falk RJ. Treatment response and relapse in antineutrophil cytoplasmic autoantibody-associated microscopic polyangiitis and glomerulonephritis. J Am Soc Nephrol 1996;7:33–9.

132. Halloran P, Mathew T, Tomlanovitch S, Groth C, Hooftman L, Barker C. Mycophenolate mofetil in renal allograft recipients: a pooled efficacy analysis of three randomized, double-blind, clinical studies in prevention of rejection. The International Mycophenolate Mofetil Renal Transplant Study Groups. Transplantation 1997;63:39–47.
133. Nowack R, Birck R, van der Woude FJ. Mycophenolate mofetil for systemic vasculitis and IgA nephropathy. Lancet 1997;349:774.
134. Stegeman C, Cohen Tervaert JW, de Jong PE, Kallenberg CGM, the Dutch Co–trimoxazole Wegener study group. Trimethoprim–sulphamethoxazole (co–trimoxazole) for the prevention of relapses in Wegener's granulomatosis. N Engl J Med 1996;335:16–20.
135. Stegeman CA, Tervaert JW, Sluiter WJ, Manson WL, de Jong PE, Kallenberg CG. Association of chronic nasal carriage of *Staphylococcus aureus* and higher relapse rates in Wegener granulomatosis. Ann Intern Med 1994;120:12–17.
136. Mathieson PW, Cobbold SP, Hale G *et al.* Monoclonal antibody therapy in systemic vasculitis. N Engl J Med 1990;323:250–4.
137. Lockwood CM, Thiru S, Isaacs JD, Hale G, Waldmann H. Long-term remission of intractable systemic vasculitis with monoclonal antibody therapy. Lancet 1993;341:1620–2.
138. Lockwood CM, Thiru S, Stewart S *et al.* Treatment of Wegener's granulomatosis with humanized monoclonal antibodies. Q J Med 1996;89:903–12.
139. Hagen EC, de Keizer RJW, Andrassy K *et al.* Compassionate treatment of Wegener's granulomatosis with rabbit anti-thymocyte globulin. Clin Nephrol 1995;43:351–9.
140. Stillwell TJ, Benson RC, DeRemee RA, McDonald TJ, Weiland LH. Cyclophosphamide-induced bladder toxicity in Wegener's granulomatosis. Arthritis Rheum 1988;31:465–70.
141. Talar-Williams C, Hijazi YM, Walther MM *et al.* Cyclophosphamide-induced cystitis and bladder cancer in patients with Wegener granulomatosis. Ann Intern Med 1996;124:477–84.
142. Trompeter RS, Evans PR, Barratt TM. Gonadal function in boys with steroid-responsive nephrotic syndrome treated with cyclophosphamide for short periods. Lancet 1981;i:1177–9.
143. Boumpas DT, Austin HA, Vaughan EM, Yarboro CH, Klippel JH, Balow JE. Risk for sustained amenorrhea in patients with systemic lupus erythematosus receiving intermittent pulse cyclophosphamide therapy. Ann Intern Med 1993;119:366–9.
144. Bussel A, Jais JP. Side effects and mortality associated with plasma exchange: a three year experience with a regional register. Life Support Systems 1987;5:353–8.
145. Benoit FL, Rulon DB, Theil GB, Dooland PD, Watten RH. Goodpasture's syndrome. A clinicopathological entity. Am J Med 1964;37:424–44.
146. Andrews PA, Sheerin NS, Hicks JA, Williams DG, Sacks SH. Unusual presentations of anti-glomerular basement membrane antibody mediated disease are associated with delayed diagnosis and poor outcome. Clin Nephrol 1995;44:262–5.
147. Kotanko P, Pusey CD, Levy JB. Recurrent glomerulonephritis following renal transplantation. Transplantation 1997;63:1045–52.
148. Hogan SL, Nachman PH, Wilkman AS, Jennette JC, Falk RJ, and the glomerular disease collaborative network. Prognostic markers in patients with anti-neutrophil cytoplasmic autoantibody-associated microscopic polyangiitis and glomerulonephritis. J Am Soc Nephrol 1996;7:23–32.
149. Cohen Tervaert JW, Stegeman CA, de Jong PE *et al.* Long-term follow-up of anti-neutrophil cytoplasmic antibodies (ANCA)-associated glomerulonephritis (GN). Clin Exp Immunol 1995;101(Suppl.1):66.
150. Geffriaud Ricouard C, Noel LH, Chauveau D, Houhou S, Grunfeld JP, Lesavre P. Clinical spectrum associated with ANCA of defined antigen specificities in 98 selected patients. Clin Nephrol 1993;39:125–36.
151. Wilkowski MJ, Velosa J, Holley KE *et al.* Risk factors in idiopathic renal vasculitis and glomerulonephritis. Kidney Int 1989;36:1133–41.
152. Garrett PJ, Dewhurst AG, Morgan LS, Mason JC, Dathan JR. Renal disease associated with circulating antineutrophil antibody. Q J Med 1992;85:731–49.
153. Gaskin G, Pusey CD. ANCA-associated renal disease [letter; comment]. Q J Med 1993;86: 138–9.

154. ten Berge IJM, Wilmink JM, Meyer CJLM *et al.* Clinical and immunological follow-up of patients with severe renal disease in Wegener's granulomatosis. Am J Nephrol 1985;5:21–9.
155. Nissensen AR, Port FK. Outcome of end-stage renal disease in patients with rare causes of renal failure. III: systemic/vascular disorders. Q J Med 1990;74:65–74.
156. Allen AR, Pusey CD, Gaskin G. Outcome of renal replacement therapy in ANCA-associated systemic vasculitis. J Am Soc Nephrol 1998;9:1258–63.
157. Weiss MA, Crissman JD. Segmental necrotizing glomerulonephritis: diagnostic, prognostic and therapeutic significance. Am J Kidney Dis 1985;6:199–211.
158. Croker PB, Lee T, Gunnells JC. Clinical and pathological features of polyarteritis nodosa and its renal-limited variant: primary crescentic and necrotizing glomerulonephritis. Human Pathol 1987;18:38–44.
159. Velosa JA. Idiopathic crescentic glomerulonephritis or systemic vasculitis? Mayo Clin Proc 1987;62:145–7.
160. Heilman RL, Offord KP, Holley KE, Velosa JA. Analysis of risk factors for patient and renal survival in crescentic glomerulonephritis. Am J Kidney Dis 1987;9:98–107.
161. Bajema IM, Hagen EC, Hermans J *et al.* Assessing the severity of renal disease in systemic vasculitis: how do the histopathological data predict the renal outcome? J Am Soc Nephrol 1995;6:918 (abstract).
162. Exley AR, Carruthers DM, Luqmani RA *et al.* Damage occurs early in systemic vasculitis and is an index of outcome. Q J Med 1997;90:391–9.
163. Niles JL, Pan GL, Collins AB *et al.* Antigen-specific radioimmunoassays for anti-neutrophil cytoplasmic antibodies in the diagnosis of rapidly progressive glomerulonephritis. J Am Soc Nephrol 1991;2:27–36.
164. Cassidy MJD, Gaskin G, Savill J, Pusey CD, Rees AJ. Towards an earlier diagnosis of rapidly progressive glomerulonephritis. Br Med J 1990;301:329–31.
165. Boutaud AA, Kalluri R, Kahsai TZ, Noelken ME, Hudson BG. Goodpasture syndrome: selective removal of anti-alpha 3 (IV) collagen autoantibodies. A potential therapeutic alternative to plasmapheresis. Exp Nephrol 1996;4:205–12.

8. Treatment of glomerulonephritis in systemic disease

WAI Y. TSE and D. ADU

TREATMENT OF LUPUS NEPHRITIS

Introduction

The overall survival of patients with systemic lupus erythematosus (SLE) and nephritis has improved considerably over the past few decades [1–8] (Table 8.1). This improved survival is probably due to a combination of the wider use of corticosteroids and immunosuppressants, together with the availability of more effective antihypertensive drugs and antibiotics. Thus early deaths from extrarenal lupus and infection are now uncommon, and renal failure and cardiovascular disease have emerged as important determinants of morbidity and mortality [9–12].

Clinically apparent nephritis develops in about 40–75% of patients with SLE [13]. The renal manifestations of lupus nephritis are heterogeneous both in clinical presentation and histology. Pollak *et al.* [1] and Baldwin *et al.* [2] defined three major patterns of lupus nephritis based on renal histology: focal proliferative, diffuse proliferative and membranous glomerulonephritis. This classification was subsequently expanded by a World Health Organization (WHO) committee (Table 8.2) [14].

Patients with minimal changes or mesangial glomerulonephritis (WHO class I and II lesions) usually have an inherently low rate of progressive renal failure [12, 15–18]. Patients with membranous nephropathy (WHO class V) have an intermediate prognosis for renal function [12, 15–18]. In contrast, patients with focal or diffuse proliferative glomerulonephritis (WHO class III and IV) have a

Table 8.1 Overall patient survival (%) in patients with lupus glomerulonephritis

Reference	3 years	5 years	10 years	15 years	20 years
Pollak *et al.* (1964) [1]	51				
Baldwin *et al.* (1970) [2]	48				
Ponticelli *et al.* (1987) [3]		98	87		
Nossent *et al.* (1990) [4]		84	71		
Cameron (1994) [5]		85	85		
Neumann *et al.* (1995) [7]		97	92	84	
Moroni *et al.* (1996) [8]		100	100		86

C.D. Pusey (ed.), The Treatment of Glomerulonephritis, 143–176.

Table 8.2 The World Health Organization classification of lupus nephritis

Class I	Normal or minimal change disease (1–4%) (a) Nil (by all techniques) (b) Normal by light microscopy but deposits by electron or immunofluorescence microscopy
Class II	Mesangial glomerulonephritis (20%) (a) Mesangial widening and/or mild hypercellularity (b) Moderate hypercellularity
Class III	Focal proliferative glomerulonephritis (25%) (a) 'Active' necrotizing lesions (b) 'Active' and sclerosing lesions (c) Sclerosing lesions
Class IV	Diffuse proliferative glomerulonephritis (37%) (a) Without segmental lesions (b) With 'active' necrotizing lesions (c) With 'active' and sclerosing lesions (d) With sclerosing lesions
Class V	Membranous glomerulonephritis (13%) (a) Pure membranous glomerulonephritis (b) Associated with lesions of category II (a or b) (c) Associated with lesions of category III (a–c)* (d) Associated with lesions of category IV (a–d)*

*Alternatively cases in these subcategories may be classified under category IV.

high risk of progressive renal failure [12, 15–18]. Thus, histological classification of lupus nephritis allows identification of disease subsets with differing risks of developing renal failure and provides a basis for planning therapy. Therapeutic measures which can prevent progressive renal damage are obviously important in the management of the higher-risk groups of patients. Despite numerous studies, no consensus has been reached on the optimal treatment for patients with lupus nephritis. The purpose of this section is to review the available literature, in an attempt to define the most effective and least toxic ways of treating lupus nephritis. The difficulties in defining the best treatment of lupus nephritis are fuelled by the scarcity of randomized controlled trials.

Clinical presentation

In almost all patients, lupus nephritis develops in those with evident systemic lupus erythematosus, and extrarenal symptoms such as rash, arthralgia, Raynaud's phenomenon and pleuro-pericarditis. Rarely, renal disease may be the presenting feature of SLE and we have seen 11 such patients who subsequently, after a period of months to years, developed extrarenal signs [13].

Renal presentation

This is usually with proteinuria which is often accompanied by the nephrotic syndrome. Microscopic haematuria is common but an acute nephritic syndrome is not. A few patients present with rapidly progressive glomerulonephritis which may be severe enough to lead to acute renal failure. In such patients diffuse crescentic nephritis, often with intracapillary glomerular thrombi, may be seen (Figure 8.1).

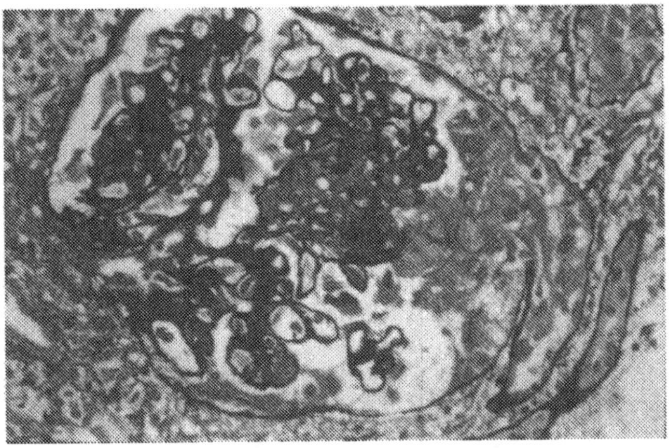

Figure 8.1 Diffuse proliferative lupus glomerulonephritis (WHO class IV), with segmental glomerular thrombosis and extracapillary proliferation (PA-silver; original magnification × 100)

Renal histology

The histology of lupus nephritis has been previously reviewed [13, 19, 20]. A distinctive feature of lupus nephritis on light microscopy is the variability of the glomerular changes seen in a single biopsy and at times within the same glomerulus. This makes classification of renal histology difficult. The classification most widely used is the modified WHO classification which is shown in Table 8.2. Segmental glomerular thrombosis, necrosis and extracapillary proliferation (crescents) are frequently found in association with the proliferative type lesions (WHO class III and IV). On immunofluorescence microscopy, there is often florid deposition of IgG, IgA, and IgM as well as C3, C4 and C1q.

Treatment

There are several considerations in the approach to the treatment of patients with lupus nephritis. The first is based on the histological severity of the renal lesion. The second is based on the severity of the clinical presentation. The third consideration is the choice of therapy for inducing remission of acute disease and for maintaining remission and treating relapses. The heterogeneity of the clinical course of lupus nephritis and the relatively few randomized controlled trials make choice of treatment difficult. Thus there are substantial disagreements on the optimum treatment of lupus nephritis. We discuss treatment options in this section and examine the evidence for this in the next section.

Mesangial proliferative glomerulonephritis (WHO class II)

Most such patients present with proteinuria and microscopic haematuria, often with little in the way of renal impairment. The biopsy findings are illustrated in Figure 8.2. There are no controlled trials to guide treatment. We treat such patients with corticosteroids in the hope that this will prevent progression to a more severe glomerulonephritis, although that is not certain.

Membranous nephropathy (WHO class V)

In patients with lupus nephritis, the frequency of membranous nephropathy is approximately 12% when the definition of the renal histology is confined to

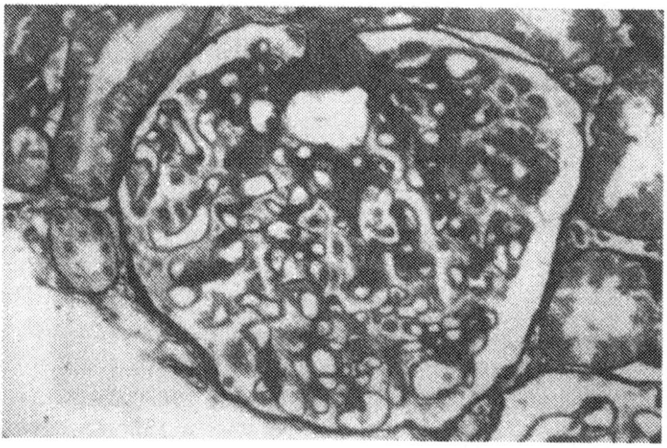

Figure 8.2 Mesangial lupus glomerulonephritis (WHO class II) (PA-silver; original magnification ×125)

pure membranous nephropathy or membranous nephropathy with mild mesangial hypercellularity, expansion and scattered deposits (WHO classes Va and Vb). The frequency increases to approximately 26% when there is, in addition, a focal segmental proliferative (WHO class Vc) or diffuse proliferative glomerulonephritis (WHO class Vd) [21]. The clinical presentation is with proteinuria and in about 50% of cases a nephrotic syndrome [22]. Patients with WHO class Va and Vb lesions have a low rate of progressive renal failure whilst patients with WHO class Vc or Vd lesions have higher risk of progressive renal failure, comparable to that of patients with proliferative glomerulonephritis. Here again there are no controlled trials of treatment and thus there is no consensus on treatment. In some studies patients with WHO class Va and Vb have been treated with prednisolone and a smaller proportion also received methylprednisolone pulses or oral cyclophosphamide and azathioprine [22, 23]. By contrast most patients with WHO class Vc and Vd have been treated with cyclophosphamide or azathioprine in addition to prednisolone [22, 23]. With these approaches to treatment the 10-year survival free of death and renal failure in WHO class Va and Vb was 72–92% and in WHO class Vc and Vd was 35–81% [22, 23] (Table 8.3).

Table 8.3 Patient survival (%) in lupus membranous nephropathy (LMN) showing the 5- and 10-year survival rates without reaching death or end-stage renal disease

Reference	Pure LMN (WHO Va+Vb)		LMN with proliferative lesions (WHO Vc+Vd)	
	5 years	10 years	5 years	10 years
Pasquali *et al.* (1993) [22]	96	92	88	81
Sloan *et al.* (1996) [23]	86	72	60	35

It seems reasonable to treat patients with membranous nephropathy and proliferative glomerulonephritis with cyclophosphamide as well as prednisolone because of the proven efficacy of this regimen in patients with proliferative lupus glomerulonephritis. Our practice is to treat patients with pure lupus membranous nephropathy, with or without minor mesangial proliferation, with prednisolone and to consider adding azathioprine as a corticosteroid-sparing agent.

Focal and diffuse proliferative glomerulonephritis (WHO class III and IV)

Because the prognosis of patients with these types of lupus nephritis was much poorer than that of patients with mesangial proliferative glomerulonephritis and membranous nephropathy [24], these patients have been the focus of most of the clinical trials of treatment. In patients with severe focal proliferative or diffuse proliferative glomerulonephritis, corticosteroids alone will reduce the extrarenal manifestations, but are less effective in preserving renal function [25–40]. There is now overwhelming evidence that the addition of cyclophosphamide to prednisolone confers benefit when compared with prednisolone alone [35–40]. The evidence that azathioprine confers such benefit is less good although we feel that this agent has a role in maintaining remission. A series of clinical trials from the National Institutes of Health (NIH) provided evidence for the effectiveness of intermittent intravenous cyclophosphamide together with oral prednisolone in preserving renal function in patients with severe lupus nephritis [36–38] (reviewed later). This regimen is preferable to continuous oral cyclophosphamide as it has less bladder toxicity, although the frequency of gonadal toxicity is unaffected. It is not yet known whether pulse cyclophosphamide is less carcinogenic than continuous oral therapy. From the NIH data, pulse cyclophosphamide (0.5–0.75 g/m^2), adjusted for the glomerular filtration rate and leukocyte count at 10–14 days, is given monthly for the first 6 months, then quarterly for 18–24 months. The longer course of cyclophosphamide was associated with fewer relapses than a shorter 6-month course [38]. Preliminary studies with pulse oral cyclophosphamide have shown encouraging results, and if validated will minimize the inconvenience associated with intravenous therapy. To reduce the bladder toxicity of intravenous cyclophosphamide, patients should be hydrated either with oral or intravenous fluid, and mesna given concomitantly. Prednisolone is given in conjunction with the cyclophosphamide at an initial dose of 0.5–1 mg/kg per day for 6–8 weeks with gradual tapering, preferably to an alternate-day regimen to minimize toxicity. This regimen has been reported in detail [19, 20, 41], and these reports should be referred to prior to its use.

In other uncontrolled but extensive observations, treatment with intravenous methylprednisolone followed by combined prednisolone and azathioprine or oral cyclophosphamide gave long-term results comparable with those of the NIH studies [3, 42]. The results of controlled trials do not, however, indicate that the combination of azathioprine and prednisolone confers a renal protective effect. Azathioprine is less toxic than cyclophosphamide, but is also less effective at inducing remission [25, 28, 36]. A number of studies have demonstrated that azathioprine may prevent relapse and may also have a steroid-sparing effect [25, 43, 44]. An alternative regimen to the NIH one is to use oral prednisolone at an initial dose of 60 mg/day and tapering, together with oral cyclophosphamide 2 mg/kg per day, and then to change from cyclophosphamide to azathioprine 2 mg/kg per day at 8–12 weeks.

On the basis of these randomized controlled studies, we feel that the NIH regimen is a reasonable initial treatment for severe lupus nephritis. Much of the toxicity of that approach results from the prolonged maintenance course of pulse cyclophosphamide. Whether conversion after 6 months to azathioprine is as effective in maintaining remission as continued pulse cyclophosphamide remains to be established.

The use of plasmapheresis in the treatment of severe diffuse crescentic glomerulonephritis has not been formally examined in a controlled trial. The controlled trials of plasmapheresis were in patients with all types of proliferative glomerulonephritis and showed no benefit over treatment with prednisolone and immunosuppressants alone [45–47]. Whether synchronization of plasmapheresis with the administration of pulse cyclophosphamide will be effective in treating severe lupus nephritis is under investigation in a prospective, controlled study by the international Lupus Plasmapheresis Study Group [48–50]. We currently use plasmapheresis only in patients with a severe diffuse proliferative glomerulonephritis whose disease does not respond to prednisolone and cyclophosphamide.

A key feature of the care of patients with lupus nephritis is the close monitoring of the white cell count and renal function, and detailed surveillance and management of infection, extrarenal lupus and hypertension. A summary of the treatment strategies for lupus nephritis is shown in Table 8.4.

The major treatments used for lupus nephritis

Corticosteroids

It is accepted that patients with significant lupus nephritis (WHO II–V) should be treated with corticosteroids. Although treatment with corticosteroids yielded a clear improvement of the prognosis in patients with lupus nephritis, especially when relatively high doses were used [1, 51], no prospective trial comparing a corticosteroid-treated group with a placebo group has been performed in such patients. However, since the majority of patients with renal disease have, in addition, extrarenal manifestations, treatment with corticosteroids is necessary. In contrast, numerous prospective studies have compared a corticosteroid regimen with an immunosuppressive regimen plus cortico-

Table 8.4 Summary of treatment strategies for lupus glomerulonephritis

Renal history	Treatment
Mesangial glomerulonephritis (WHO class II)	Prednisolone
Focal/diffuse proliferative glomerulonephritis (WHO class III/IV)	Oral prednisolone + intermittent intravenous cyclophosphamide (NIH regimen)
Membranous glomerulonephritis (WHO class Va/Vb)	Prednisolone + azathioprine as a steroid-sparing agent
Membranous glomerulonephritis with proliferative glomerulonephritis (WHO class Vc/Vd)	Prednisolone + cyclophosphamide

steroids [25–40] The efficacy of corticosteroids in renal preservation will be discussed (see below).

Azathioprine

Azathioprine was effective in combination with corticosteroids in the NZB/NZW mouse model of SLE [52]. In patients with lupus nephritis, a number of controlled studies have compared the effect of azathioprine or azathioprine plus prednisolone versus the effect of prednisolone alone, with conflicting results [25–37].

Donadio *et al.* examined the effect of prednisolone alone versus prednisolone and azathioprine in a controlled trial of 16 patients, most of whom had diffuse proliferative glomerulonephritis [27]. Treatment was with either prednisolone (60 mg/day for 2 months, then tapered) or the same dose of prednisolone together with azathioprine (2 mg/kg per day). Non-renal clinical features of patients in the two groups were similar. Although symptomatic improvement was noted in both groups, no difference in creatinine clearance or biopsy activity scores was apparent at 6 months. Follow-up of the same patients after 3 years showed a similar incidence of acute disease flares, both renal and non-renal, in the two groups. Thus the addition of azathioprine in this study did not confer any additional benefit over prednisolone alone. Hahn *et al.* also failed to detect a benefit in creatinine clearance, extrarenal manifestations or overall survival in patients treated with azathioprine and prednisolone as compared with prednisolone alone [31].

By contrast, a number of studies showed that the addition of azathioprine to prednisolone conferred a renal protective effect over prednisolone alone [25, 28]. Sztejnbok *et al.* reported significantly higher mortality, hospitalization rates, incidence of end-stage renal disease and reduced creatinine clearance in patients treated with prednisolone alone when compared with those treated with prednisolone and azathioprine [25]. Similarly, Cade *et al.* showed a renal protective effect in lupus patients using a combination of azathioprine plus prednisolone [28].

The question remains, then, as to whether the addition of azathioprine is a useful adjunct to corticosteroids in renal preservation in lupus nephritis. The balance of the evidence is that azathioprine does not confer any major advantage in inducing remission of lupus nephritis. However, azathioprine may play a role in maintaining remission and preventing relapses, since withdrawal of azathioprine was associated with disease exacerbations in a number of studies [25, 43, 44]. This tendency to relapse upon withdrawal of azathioprine was confirmed in a controlled, but not double-blind, trial by Sharon *et al.* in which seven of nine patients who had azathioprine withdrawn had flares of their disease compared with only one of seven patients who continued on azathioprine [44].

Toxicity of azathioprine. Some patients are intolerant of azathioprine and develop nausea, vomiting and diarrhoea with this drug. Azathioprine causes marrow suppression, and this can be severe in individuals who have a deficiency of thiopurine methyltransferase. Other toxicities include an increased risk of infection, abnormal liver function tests and the development of malignancies with prolonged usage.

Oral cyclophosphamide

Cyclophosphamide has emerged as an important therapy in conjunction with corticosteroids for the induction of remission in focal and diffuse proliferative glomerulonephritis [35–40]. Steinberg *et al.* at the National Institutes of Health performed one of the first randomized studies comparing cyclophosphamide plus prednisolone with prednisolone alone in 13 patients with lupus nephritis [26]. At the end of 10 weeks, patients receiving cyclophosphamide plus prednisolone had a greater improvement in anti-DNA antibodies, serum complement, urine sediment, proteinuria, and extrarenal manifestations. No difference was seen in the creatinine clearance between the two groups. In a further study from the same group, 38 patients, of whom 34 had diffuse proliferative glomerulonephritis, were assigned to low-dose prednisolone plus either: azathioprine (up to 4 mg/kg), cyclophosphamide (up to 4 mg/kg) or placebo [30]. Cyclophosphamide- and azathioprine-treated patients had a reduction in extrarenal manifestations of lupus. Although cyclophosphamide was superior to azathioprine and placebo in reducing proteinuria, creatinine clearance was comparable between the three groups at 10 weeks. These initial studies failed to support the notion that cyclophosphamide was superior to prednisolone alone in preserving renal function. The outcome of this group of patients was further examined at 28 months [32]. Of the 11 patients with unfavourable outcomes (eight deaths and three end-stage renal disease – ESRD), two occurred in the cyclophosphamide group, four in the azathioprine group and five in the placebo group. Gradual deterioration of renal function occurred in all three groups, but deterioration of renal function was most frequent in those patients who received prednisolone plus placebo. A final report of outcome at 85 months was reported by Carette *et al.* [35]. Cyclophosphamide plus prednisolone was shown to be only marginally superior to prednisolone for maintaining renal function ($p = 0.03$) and preventing ESRD ($p = 0.07$). From these studies a marginal advantage of cyclophosphamide, but not of azathioprine, was evident for both loss of renal function and ESRD.

In contrast, others failed to see an impact on renal survival with cyclophosphamide [33, 53]. In a study of 50 patients, Donadio *et al.* at the Mayo Clinic evaluated the effectiveness of cyclophosphamide in the treatment of diffuse proliferative glomerulonephritis [33]. Patients were randomized to receive either prednisolone alone or prednisolone and cyclophosphamide for 6 months, followed by maintenance prednisolone. Although there was a higher incidence of nephritis relapse in the prednisolone group, the proportion of patients alive after 4 years with stable or improved renal function was similar in the two treatment groups.

From the early NIH studies, oral cyclophosphamide appeared to be effective at preserving renal function, but this was evident only with prolonged follow-up [35]. The rate of side-effects associated with the use of long-term oral cyclophosphamide, particularly infections, gonadal toxicity and bladder toxicity, was high. This led to clinical trials of pulse intravenous cyclophosphamide, in the hope that intermittent administration might be associated with fewer adverse events.

Intravenous cyclophosphamide
In the continuation of the clinical trial from the NIH, intravenous cyclophosphamide was included as one of the treatment modalities [34, 36, 37]. In 1986 Austin *et al.* reported the clinical outcomes in 107 patients, with a median follow-up time of 7 years [36]. Most patients had diffuse proliferative glomerulonephritis, but a few patients with membranoproliferative, focal proliferative, membranous and mesangial glomerulonephritis were also enrolled. Treatment was with either: high-dose oral prednisolone (1 mg/kg per day for 4–8 weeks, then tapered), oral azathioprine (up to 4 mg/kg per day), oral cyclophosphamide (up to 4 mg/kg per day), combined oral azathioprine and cyclophosphamide (up to 1 mg/kg per day) or intravenous cyclophosphamide (0.5–1 g/m^2 3-monthly). Most patients received a background of maintenance low-dose prednisolone. Unlike other studies in which therapy had been given only for a few months, protocol drugs in this study were given for at least 4 years. This trial showed that a therapeutic regimen using intravenous cyclophosphamide every 3 months plus low-dose daily prednisolone resulted in a significant reduction in the incidence of renal failure as compared with prednisolone alone, and this was most striking in patients followed up for 10 years or more [37]. Marginally but not significantly better preservation of renal function was seen in patients who had prednisolone plus oral cyclophosphamide, or oral cyclophosphamide plus azathioprine, when compared with patients treated with prednisolone alone. Results in the azathioprine group did not differ from those in the prednisolone-only group. In this study the presence of chronic histological changes was found to be a predictor of poor renal outcome. The 72 patients with any combination of glomerular sclerosis, fibrous crescents, tubular atrophy, or interstitial fibrosis were at a significantly greater risk of ESRD as compared with the 29 patients who had none of these histological lesions.

The major NIH randomized studies of treatment in lupus nephritis have demonstrated the benefit of intravenous cyclophosphamide in reducing ESRD after a prolonged follow-up.

Pulse oral cyclophosphamide
Pulse oral cyclophosphamide may be an acceptable alternative to pulse intravenous cyclophosphamide in the treatment of lupus nephritis. In a small, uncontrolled study by Dawisha *et al.*, oral cyclophosphamide administration (0.5–1 g/m^2 for 6 months) plus low-dose prednisolone led to an improvement in disease activity score, and reduction of proteinuria and urinary cellular casts, in the majority of the nine patients with nephritis who completed the study [54].

Pulse oral cyclophosphamide has similar pharmacokinetics to intravenous cyclophosphamide [55] and avoids the need for intravenous cannulation and hospital attendance. However, controlled studies with more patients, comparing the efficacy and long-term toxicity of pulse oral with pulse intravenous cyclophosphamide, as well as comparison with other disease-modifying agents, are needed before pulse oral cyclophosphamide can be advocated.

Toxicity of cyclophosphamide. Intravenous cyclophosphamide often leads to nausea and vomiting, but this can be controlled by serotonin antagonists, such as ondansetron, given together with dexamethasone. The most common toxic effect is depression of normal haematopoiesis [56]. This toxicity is dose-dependent and is reversible on discontinuing therapy. A further major side-effect is an increased risk of infections, and this is worsened by the concomitant use of corticosteroids [36, 57, 58]. In particular, an increased incidence of herpes zoster is seen with cyclophosphamide [36]. Cyclophosphamide is metabolized to phosphoramide mustard and acrolein, which are excreted by the kidneys, and acrolein can lead to a haemorrhagic cystitis [36, 58, 59]. This is particularly common with oral cyclophosphamide. The incidence of haemorrhagic cystitis in the initial NIH studies ranged from 15% to 43% [60, 61]. The use of intravenous cyclophosphamide with vigorous hydration and concomitant administration of 2-mercaptoethane sulphonate sodium (mesna) has essentially eliminated bladder complications. Prolonged oral cyclophosphamide is associated with an increased risk of malignancy and it is likely that intravenous cyclophosphamide also carries this risk [58, 60, 61]. Cyclophosphamide, unlike azathioprine, is a potent teratogen and must not be used in pregnancy [62].

Cyclophosphamide also causes dose- and age-related gonadal toxicity with oligospermia in men and premature ovarian failure in women [36, 58, 63–66]. Few data on gonadal toxicity in men with lupus are available. In one study of six men treated with oral cyclophosphamide at a daily dose of 50–100 mg, germinal aplasia occurred after a cumulative dose of 9–18 g [67]. All studies show that the risk of ovarian toxicity rises substantially with age and is correlated with the duration of treatment and the cumulative dose of cyclophosphamide [36, 64–66]. In patients aged less than 25 the risk of ovarian failure after 6 months of monthly intravenous cyclophosphamide was nil, whilst a further 24 months of quarterly cyclophosphamide increased this risk to 17% [65]. Comparable figures for women aged over 31 years were 25% and 100% respectively [65]. In another study, 19 out of 35 patients (54%) treated with cyclophosphamide developed ovarian failure as compared with one out of 20 patients (5%) treated with azathioprine [68]. Since lupus nephritis chiefly afflicts women of reproductive age, one must balance this risk of premature ovarian failure, which is usually permanent, with the benefits of treatment. While intermittent intravenous pulse therapy is associated with less bladder toxicity, there is still concern over dose accumulation with chronic administration and the potential to develop malignancy and gonadal toxicity.

Pulse methylprednisolone

Pulse methylprednisolone has been used in at least two different ways. In the first, pulse methylprednisolone has been used in three consecutive daily doses of 0.5–1 g at the initiation of treatment of severe proliferative lupus nephritis or for the treatment of renal flares. This approach has been used together with cyclophosphamide and azathioprine, and in conjunction with oral prednisolone [3, 42]. The long-term results of this approach are good, although the regimen has not been examined in a randomized controlled study. The second way that methylprednisolone has been used is as monthly pulses together with continuous low-dose prednisolone. Boumpas *et al.* examined the impact of intravenous methylprednisolone versus intravenous cyclophosphamide in 65 patients with lupus nephritis, of whom 56 had diffuse proliferative glomerulonephritis [38]. Methylprednisolone (1 g/m^2) was given for 3 consecutive days at induction, followed by monthly infusion for 6 months. Intravenous cyclophosphamide (0.5–1 g/m^2) was given monthly for 6 months, and in some patients quarterly administration of cyclophosphamide was continued for 2 years. All patients received in addition low-dose oral prednisolone. Renal insufficiency (doubling of the serum creatinine) was significantly greater in the methylprednisolone group compared with the long-term cyclophosphamide group. There was a significantly greater cumulative probability of exacerbations of lupus nephritis or extrarenal lupus in patients on short-term cyclophosphamide when compared with those receiving long-term treatment.

The question of whether a 6-month course of methylprednisolone was sufficient to have had a therapeutic impact was raised. To address this, Gourley *et al.* compared the effects of: monthly methylprednisolone given for at least 1 year; monthly intravenous cyclophosphamide (0.5–1 g/m^2) given for 6 months, reduced to quarterly for at least two years; and both methylprednisolone and cyclophosphamide, in 82 patients with lupus nephritis. All patients in addition received low-dose prednisolone [40]. Renal remission occurred in seven of 24 patients in the methylprednisolone group (29%), 13 of 21 patients in the cyclophosphamide group (62%), and 17 of 20 patients in the combination therapy group (85%). Thus, the likelihood of remission was significantly greater in the combination therapy group than in the methylprednisolone group.

Sesso *et al.* evaluated the effects of pulse cyclophosphamide alone versus pulse methylprednisolone in a prospective, randomized trial [39]. Twenty-nine patients with lupus nephritis (WHO II, III, and IV) received either: monthly pulse cyclophosphamide (0.5–1 g/m^2) for 4 months, followed by bimonthly doses for 4 months and quarterly doses for 6 months; or pulse methylprednisolone (10–20 mg/kg) for 3 days, and thereafter at the same intervals as the cyclophosphamide regimen. After a mean follow.up of 15 months, two patients in the cyclophosphamide group and three in the methylprednisolone group had died. There was no significant difference in the risk of death, renal failure, or rate of remission between the two groups. This negative result may reflect the small patient numbers and the short follow-up. From these studies it appears that intermittent methylprednisolone and oral prednisolone are not as effective in the treatment of severe lupus nephritis as pulse cyclophosphamide and oral prednisolone.

Meta-analysis of controlled trials of treatment of lupus nephritis

In a review, Donadio and Glassock argued that the addition of immunosuppressive drugs to corticosteroids did not improve the prognosis of lupus [69]. This question has been formally addressed by meta-analysis. Felson and Anderson, in their analysis of published clinical studies of lupus nephritis, showed that patients treated with prednisolone plus cyclophosphamide or azathioprine had fewer unfavourable outcomes than patients treated with prednisolone alone [70]. The rates of renal deterioration, ESRD and nephritis-related death were all significantly lower in the treatment group receiving immunosuppressive agents. Similarly, Bansal and Beto concluded in their meta-analysis that treatment with cyclophosphamide or azathioprine combined with prednisolone reduced mortality and ESRD when compared with prednisolone alone [71].

To address this question of the usefulness of immunosuppressive drugs in the management of lupus nephritis, we pooled data from all published randomized controlled trials to analyse the effectiveness of corticosteroids versus corticosteroids plus cyclophosphamide or azathioprine [25–40]. The trials included satisfied the following criteria: (1) all patients had systemic lupus erythematosus, with clinical or biopsy evidence of lupus nephritis; (2) treatment was assigned either randomly or consecutively; (3) the concurrent control group in each study received prednisolone only; and (4) the experimental group received cyclophosphamide or azathioprine together with prednisolone. These studies are summarized in Table 8.5. The outcome measures were death and renal failure. The addition of azathioprine to prednisolone, compared with prednisolone alone, was associated with a reduction in the risk of renal failure, but because of a wide confidence interval this was not statistically significant. There was no significant difference in mortality rates between patients treated with azathioprine plus prednisolone and prednisolone alone. Treatment with cyclophosphamide plus prednisolone was associated with a significantly reduced risk of renal failure when compared with treatment with prednisolone alone ($p < 0.01$). Like azathioprine, cyclophosphamide therapy failed to have an impact on mortality reduction. The conclusion from these meta-analyses is that the addition of immunosuppressants, in particular cyclophosphamide, to corticosteroids is effective in reducing the risk of developing renal failure in patients with lupus nephritis.

Table 8.5 Summary of the randomized, controlled trials which compared the effects of immunosuppressive drugs with corticosteroids in the treatment of severe lupus nephritis

Reference	No. of patients	Immunosuppressive regimen	Prednisolone regimen	Patients with biopsy	Patients with DPGN	Median follow-up	Results
Sztejnbok *et al.* (1971) [25]	42	AZA 2.5 mg/kg × 12–48 months	Individualized	NA	NA	24 months	More renal deterioration as defined by decreased clearance and increased ESRD in prednisolone group
Donadio *et al.* (1972, 1974) [27, 29]	18	AZA 2 mg/kg × 6 months	60 mg/day × 2 months,then decreased	All	Most	37 months	No difference in survival or renal outcome
Cade *et al.* (1973 [28]	27	AZA 1–2 mg/kg	60–100 mg/day × 6 months, then tapered	All	All	25 months	More renal deterioration in prednisolone group
Hahn *et al.* (1975) [31]	24	AZA 3–4 mg/kg × 24 months	60 mg/day for at least 6 months	Most	NA	17 months	No difference in outcome
NIH studies Steinberg *et al.* (1971) [30] Steinberg and Decker (1974) [30] Decker *et al.* (1975) [32] Dinant *et al.* (1982) [34] Carette *et al.* (1983) [35] Austin *et al.* (1986) [36] Steinberg and Steinberg (1991) [37]	107	AZA <4 mg/kg at least 4 years CYCLO <4 mg/kg at least 4 years CYCLO+AZA <1 mg/kg of each drug at least 4 years	1 mg/kg per day for 4–8 weeks, then tapered	101	60	7 years	Trend towards less renal deterioration in groups who received cytotoxic-drug therapies, but statistically significant only for IV CYCLO plus PRED vs. PRED alone, especially in patients with moderate chronicity scores

DPGN = diffuse proliferative glomerulonephritis; AZA = azathioprine; CYCLO = cyclophosphamide; MPRED = methylprednisolone; PRED = prednisolone; NA = not available; ESRD = end-stage renal disease; IV = intravenous

Table 8.5 (cont)

Reference	No. of patients	Immunosuppressive regimen	Prednisolone regimen	Patients with biopsy	Patients with DPGN	Median follow-up	Results
Donadio *et al.* (1978) [33]	50	CYCLO 2 mg/kg × 6 months	60 mg/day × 1–3 months, then tapered	All	50	4 years	Increased rate of nephritis recurrence at 4 years in PRED group
Boumpas *et al.* (1992) [38]	65	IV CYCLO 0.5–1 g/m^2 monthly for 6 months	IV MPRED 1 g/m^2 × 6 months	64	56	5 years	Long course of CYCLO was better than MPRED in renal preservation
		IV CYCLO 0.5–1 g/m^2 monthly for 6 months, then 3 monthly for 2 years					
Gourley *et al.* (1996) [40]	82	IV CYCLO 0.5–1 g/m^2 monthly for 6 months, then 3 monthly for 2 years	IV MPRED 1 g/m^2 × 12 months	82	62	5 years	CYCLO alone or in combination with MPRED led to significantly more renal remission than MPRED alone
		IV MPRED+IV CYCLO					
Sesso *et al.* (1994) [39]	29	IV CYCLO 0.5–1 g/m^2 monthly for 4 months, 2 monthly for 4 months, then 3 monthly for 6 months	IV MPRED 10–20 mg/kg × 13 months	27	23	15 months	No significant difference in renal function between groups

DPGN = diffuse proliferative glomerulonephritis; AZA = azathioprine; CYCLO = cyclophosphamide; MPRED = methylprednisolone; PRED = prednisolone; NA = not available; ESRD = end-stage renal disease; IV = intravenous

Plasma exchange

Several studies have examined the role of plasmapheresis in the treatment of patients with SLE and lupus nephritis, following the initial report by Verrier Jones *et al.* in 1976 [72]. Although plasmapheresis was well tolerated with few adverse effects, impact on renal function was disappointing. The controlled trials have either shown slight but insignificant benefit [73], or no benefit from plasmapheresis [45–47].

The largest study in severe lupus nephritis was the Lupus Nephritis Collaborative Study, which recruited 86 patients [47]. This was a multicentre, randomized, controlled clinical study of patients with severe lupus nephritis (WHO III, IV and V) designed to evaluate the addition of a 4-week course of plasmapheresis to a treatment regimen using oral prednisolone and cyclophosphamide, with a median follow-up time of 120 weeks. In this study the addition of plasmapheresis to the treatment regimen did not alter outcomes in patients with severe lupus nephritis. However, this study has been criticized as it was questionable whether the ultimate outcome could be attributed to the brief plasmapheresis period.

Synchronization of plasmapheresis with intravenous cyclophosphamide

The lack of a clinical impact of plasmapheresis in lupus nephritis is not entirely unexpected, since removal of autoantibodies leads to a compensatory enhanced production of autoantibodies by pathogenic B-cell clones [74, 75]. Hence, the concept of synchronizing plasmapheresis with subsequent pulse cyclophosphamide, to target proliferating B-cell clones, was introduced. Lombardo *et al.* examined this combination of plasmapheresis with subsequent pulse cyclophosphamide in 37 lupus patients, including 13 with renal disease [76]. In nine of 13 patients, improvement in renal function and immunological tests were seen. The remaining four patients who had renal failure did not improve, but were described as having 'irreversible lesions'. Euler *et al.* also examined the effects of synchronized plasmapheresis and cyclophosphamide in 14 patients with severe lupus, 10 of whom had nephritis [50]. The protocol included a reduction of all immunosuppressive therapy before plasmapheresis to prevent suppression of pathogenic clones, followed by plasmapheresis to eliminate autoantibodies and then cyclophosphamide. Eight of the 14 patients went into sustained remission, despite withdrawal of immunosuppressive therapy. Of concern is that the dose of cyclophosphamide used was high (1.2–1.4 g/m^2). One patient developed an oropharyngeal squamous cell carcinoma at 17 months and four patients developed irreversible amenorrhoea.

Clearly, controlled trials are needed to clarify the usefulness of the synchronized approach and balance the potential therapeutic gain with the treatment-associated adverse effects. The use of such high doses of cyclophosphamide, with its adverse profile, cannot be justified without further validation. This synchronization approach is currently being investigated in a randomized controlled study by the international Lupus Plasmapheresis Study Group [48–50].

Other treatments used for lupus nephritis

Intravenous immunoglobulin

Uncontrolled studies have shown a temporary benefit in SLE patients from the infusion of high doses of intravenous immunoglobulin [77, 78]. Currently, there are limited data on the use of intravenous immunoglobulin in the treatment of lupus nephritis. Prospective, controlled studies are needed to evaluate critically the efficacy of this therapy.

Cyclosporin A

Several studies have examined the effectiveness of cyclosporin A in the treatment of lupus nephritis [79–81]. None of these studies were controlled, and it is difficult to discern whether cyclosporin was of any benefit. The nephrotoxicity of cyclosporin is a major problem and, pending randomized controlled studies comparing this drug with other immunosuppressive agents, we cannot recommend its use in lupus nephritis.

Methotrexate

Methotrexate may be useful as a steroid-sparing agent in lupus with arthritis and serositis, and may have potential benefits in mild nephritis [82, 83] Methotrexate is, however, renally excreted and cannot be used in patients with renal impairment.

Eicosapentaenoic acids

Fish oils, that are rich in eicosapentaenoic acids, suppressed manifestations of lupus in murine models of SLE [84, 85]. Eicosapentaenoic acids and their metabolites can suppress T-cell proliferation and block the production of certain inflammatory cytokines (TNF, IL-1 and IL-2) [86–88]. A clear benefit of eicosapentaenoic acids has not been shown in controlled studies involving patients with lupus nephritis [89] and cannot be recommended at present.

Androgens or anti-oestrogen therapy

The observation that SLE is a disease predominantly affecting young women [90], with a tendency to flare during pregnancy [91] or with oral contraceptive administration [92], suggests that hormonal factors may be determinants of pathogenesis or severity. Female NZB × NZW mice develop lupus-like disease at a much higher frequency than do males, and disease is ameliorated by androgens [93, 94], or tamoxifen, an oestrogen antagonist [95]. Attempts in humans to control SLE by manipulating oestrogen and testosterone levels have had only modest success [96, 97]. Despite *in-vitro* data, there is little evidence to support the use of androgens or anti-oestrogens in lupus nephritis.

Total lymphoid irradiation

This has been used successfully in patients with proliferative lupus nephritis [98, 99] but has not been prospectively compared with other options.

Monoclonal antibodies

Several studies have examined the use of monoclonal antibody therapy in patients with lupus nephritis [100, 101]. CD5 is a molecule on the surface of T cells and a subpopulation of B cells, and the use of anti-CD5 ricin A chain immunoconjugate (CD5 PLUS) led to an improvement in urine and laboratory parameters in five of eight patients with glomerulonephritis [101]. This approach remains to be validated in clinical practice.

Purine analogues

Adenosine-deaminase resistant analogues, with increased specificity for lymphoid cells, are under preliminary testing in autoimmune diseases [102]. These drugs produce, in effect, a mild deaminase deficiency and accelerate apoptosis of lymphoid cells. Their immunosuppressive properties have not been thoroughly investigated, and warrant further testing before any recommendations can be made for their efficacy in lupus nephritis.

Oral tolerance therapy

Oral tolerance therapy may have a role in the treatment of systemic lupus erythematosus, if the offending antigens can be identified. Since lupus is an autoimmune disease, characterized by the production of autoantibodies, candidates such as DNA or ribonucleic acid may be potential antigens for such therapy in the future.

Prognostic factors

Knowledge concerning prognosis assists physicians in their choice of treatment and provides patients with information on the possible outcomes. Patients with proliferative glomerulonephritis (WHO III and IV) tend to have a worse outcome for renal function when compared with patients with milder lesions [12, 15–18]. The combination of severe active and chronic histological changes on renal biopsy is also reported adversely to affect outcome [35, 103]. Patients without chronic histological changes, even in the face of active lupus nephritis, had a lower risk of developing renal failure: 90% or more remaining free of renal failure after 10 years [36]. A number of clinical variables are associated with a greater probability of renal progression in lupus nephritis. These include: black race, low haematocrit, raised serum creatinine, presence of hypertension, high urinary protein excretion, low C3 complement and poor socioeconomic status [15, 103, 104]. Failure to respond to prednisolone and cyclophosphamide is also a predictor of subsequent development of renal failure [105], as are nephritic flares [8].

Dialysis and transplantation

Between 17% and 30% of patients with lupus nephritis develop ESRD by 10 years [4, 6, 8, 104, 106]. Both haemodialysis and continuous ambulatory peritoneal dialysis are well tolerated and there is a tendency for lupus disease activity to diminish after the start of dialysis [107]. If there is no overt disease activity, then we discontinue immunosuppressants in patients on dialysis and continue with a small dose of prednisolone. Overall survival on dialysis is good with 75% survival at 10 years [108] (Table 8.6). Graft survival and function in patients with lupus after transplantation are comparable to those obtained in patients with other diseases [109], and recurrence of lupus nephritis is uncommon after transplantation [110].

Table 8.6 Overall survival in patients with lupus nephritis, after starting dialysis

Reference	1 year	2 years	5 years	10 years
Pollack *et al.* (1987) [111] (age <50 years)	95		83	
Pollack *et al.* (1987) [111] (age >50 years)	69		38	
Cheigh *et al.* (1990) [107]	95	88	81	75

Conclusion

Immunosuppressive therapy and corticosteroids have had an impact on renal preservation in patients with severe lupus nephritis. Despite numerous studies, the most efficacious treatment with the least toxicity remains to be established. No consensus has yet been reached on a number of therapeutic issues, including: the optimal induction drug regimen, the optimal regimen for treating relapse, and optimal maintenance therapy to prevent relapses. Improvements to the therapy of lupus nephritis will follow a clearer understanding of the immunopathogenesis.

TREATMENT OF NEPHRITIS IN CRYOGLOBULINAEMIA

Classification

The phenomenon of cryoprecipitation has been known for more than 50 years [112, 113]. The current classification of cryoglobulins was proposed by Brouet *et al.* in 1974, and recognizes three types of cryoglobulins based on their immunochemical characteristics [114] (Table 8.7). Type I cryoglobulins are composed of a monoclonal immunoglobulin component only, usually IgM, occasionally IgG and rarely IgA. Type I cryoglobulins are found in association

Table 8.7 Immunochemical classification of cryoglobulinaemias and disease associations

Immunoglobulin		Disease associations
Type I	Monoclonal, usually IgM, occasionally IgG, rarely IgA	Lymphoproliferative diseases (myeloma, Waldenström's macroglobulinaemia, non-Hodgkin's lymphoma, chronic lymphocytic leukaemia, monoclonal gammopathy of undetermined significance)
Type II	Mixture of a monoclonal (usually IgM) rheumatoid factor and polyclonal IgG	Lymphoproliferative diseases; malignancy; infections (viral, especially hepatitis C, bacterial, and parasitic infections, subacute bacterial endocarditis); autoimmune disease (e.g. systemic lupus erythematosus); malignancy; chronic liver disease
Type III	Mixture of polyclonal Ig of different isotypes	Malignancy; infections (viral, bacterial and parasitic infections); autoimmune disease (e.g. systemic lupus erythematosus); chronic liver disease

with lymphoproliferative diseases such as myeloma, Waldenström's macroglobulinaemia or non-Hodgkin's lymphoma [115–117]. Types II and III cryoglobulins are referred to as mixed cryoglobulins simply because they consist of a mixture of immunoglobulins of different isotypes. Type II cryoglobulins are composed of a mixture of monoclonal and polyclonal immunoglobulins. Frequently the monoclonal component is an IgM with rheumatoid factor activity and the second component is a polyclonal IgG [118]. Type II cryoglobulins are found in association with lymphoproliferative disorders, infectious diseases and autoimmune diseases [115–117]. Type III cryoglobulins are composed of a mixture of polyclonal immunoglobulins, usually IgM and IgG [114], and are found in a variety of autoimmune disorders and infections [115–117].

Renal involvement in cryoglobulinaemia

The frequency of renal involvement in cryoglobulinaemia varies, from 35% in non-nephrological studies to 100% in nephrological centres [114, 116, 119–125]. Renal presentation ranges from proteinuria and/or haematuria with active urine sediment and hypertension in most patients, to a nephrotic syndrome, acute nephritic syndrome or acute renal failure [116, 120, 125–127]. Renal manifestations are usually a late manifestation of mixed cryoglobulinaemia, occurring some years after the onset of extrarenal symptoms [116, 120].

Monti *et al.* conducted a study in the largest cohort of patients with cryoglobulinaemia, forming the Italian Group for the Study of Cryoglobulinaemia in 1995 [117]. This multicentre study described the clinical course of 913 patients with cryoglobulinaemia. Renal involvement as defined by proteinuria, haematuria and/or a raised creatinine was present at diagnosis in about 20% of patients. The frequency of renal involvement in the different groups was: essential 21.7%, secondary to chronic liver disease 14%, secondary to lymphoproliferative disease 18.5%, and secondary to connective tissue disease 18.3%. Using Brouet's immunological classification [114], renal involvement was more common in type II than in type III cryoglobulinaemia, 35% versus 12%, respectively. Glomerular involvement in monoclonal type I cryoglobulinaemia is unusual, and only a few cases have been reported [128–130].

Excluding cases of systemic lupus erythematosus and post-streptococcal glomerulonephritis, most patients with mixed cryoglobulinaemia have a membranoproliferative (mesangiocapillary) glomerulonephritis [125, 127, 131–133]. Mesangial proliferative glomerulonephritis and membranous nephropathy have also been infrequently described [125, 127, 131, 133, 134]. A vasculitis of small and medium-sized vessels is commonly seen, but glomerular vasculitis is rare [125, 127, 135]. Immunohistochemistry reveals the same classes of immunoglobulin in the glomerular deposits as are found in the cryoglobulins, usually IgM and IgG together with C3 [114, 131, 136]. Electron microscopy typically shows coarse granular electron-dense deposits, almost exclusively in subendothelial sites within glomeruli, and these on higher magnification contain fibrillary structures typical of cryoglobulins [137, 138] (Figure 8.3).

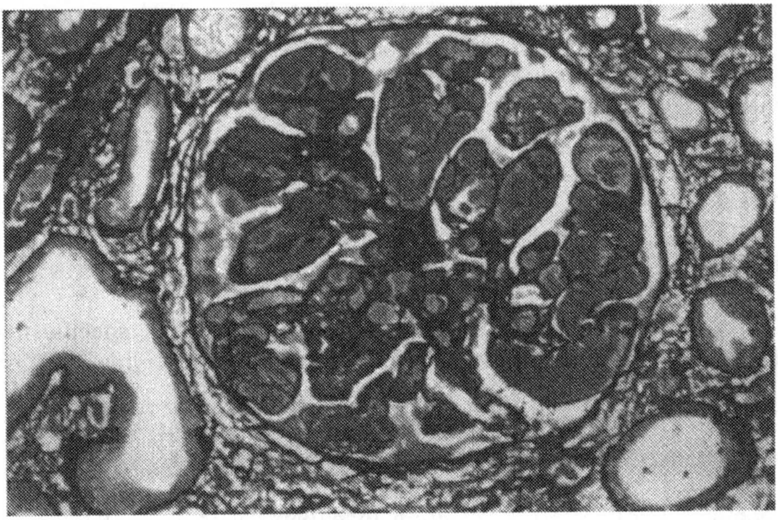

Figure 8.3 Renal biopsy from a patient with mixed cryoglobulinemia showing multiple intraluminal glomerular deposits (PA-silver; original magnification × 100)

Essential mixed cryoglobulinaemia and hepatitis C virus infection

Approximately 30–55 % of the patients with type II and type III cryoglobulinaemia were found to have no obvious associated disease [117, 139, 140]. Because of the high prevalence of coexisting liver dysfunction in these patients with what was termed 'essential' mixed cryoglobulinaemia, it was proposed that hepatototropic viruses may be involved in the pathogenesis of this disease. Initially, hepatitis B infection was implicated as the causative agent in essential mixed cryoglobulinaemia. Although earlier studies did find an association with hepatitis [141–143], subsequent studies did not confirm an association between hepatitis B infection and essential mixed cryoglobulinaemia [144, 145].

Recently, hepatitis C has emerged as the major pathogenetic factor in these patients. Since the initial report of antibodies against hepatitis C virus (HCV) in patients with type II mixed cryoglobulinaemia in 1990 [146], other groups have confirmed the presence of anti-HCV antibodies using ELISA and recombinant immunoblot assay [139, 147–151]. The presence of HCV viral RNA using polymerase chain reaction [139, 147–151] has been demonstrated in over 80% of patients with mixed cryoglobulinaemia. Other supporting evidence for a pathogenetic role of this virus includes the presence of HCV-associated antigens in the skin and liver biopsy specimens of patients with essential mixed cryoglobulinaemia [152], and the finding of HCV RNA that is enriched over serum levels in the cryoprecipitate [139, 153]. Because HCV RNA and antigens have not been detected in the glomerular lesions, the mechanism by which HCV causes glomerulonephritis is unclear. The term 'essential' mixed cryoglobulinaemia should perhaps be obsolete since there is now substantial evidence to suggest that it is almost always HCV-associated. However, HCV has not been consistently detected in cases associated with lymphoproliferative disorders.

Treatment

General

When cryoglobulinaemia develops in association with a specific myeloproliferative disorder, then the treatment is that of the underlying disorder.

Treatment of hepatitis C-associated cryoglobulinaemia

The demonstration of HCV infection in patients with type II mixed cryoglobulinaemia provides the rationale for using antiviral drugs. A number of studies have showed alpha-interferon (α-IFN) to be effective in patients with essential mixed cryoglobulinaemia, with resolution of purpura and neuropathy, reduction of cryoglobulin levels, and normalization of liver enzymes and haemoglobin values [139, 154–157]. The mechanisms of action of α-IFN are not clearly elucidated, but may include a direct antiviral action [158], the inhibition of immunoglobulin synthesis [159], and/or an effect on B-cell proliferation [160].

The effects of α-IFN on renal function are less clear, although a number of studies have examined this question [157, 161, 162]. Misiani *et al.* examined the effects of α-IFN in their randomized controlled study of 53 patients with HCV and type II cryoglobulinaemia [157]. Sixty per cent of the treatment group had no detectable HCV RNA at the end of treatment and these patients had a significant improvement in cutaneous vasculitis, IgM, cryoglobulin levels, rheumatoid factor and serum creatinine, compared with untreated patients. In the study by Johnson *et al.* the effects of α-IFN on renal function were examined in 34 patients with HCV-associated cryoglobulinaemia and nephritis [162]. Fourteen patients received standard α-IFN doses of 3 million units three times per week for at least 6 months. Although treatment was associated with a significant reduction in proteinuria and improved liver function tests, renal function did not improve. Another study compared the effects of α-IFN with methylprednisolone, or a combination of α-IFN plus methylprednisolone, in 65 patients with HCV-associated mixed cryoglobulinaemia [161]. Fifteen patients received α-IFN, 17 patients received α-IFN plus methylprednisolone orally, 18 patients received methylprednisolone alone, and 15 patients were untreated. Complete response was defined as reduction of cryocrit to less than 50% of initial value with one or more of the following: disappearance of purpura, improvement of neuropathy, or improvement of kidney function. This was achieved in 53.3% of patients treated with α-IFN, 52.9% of patients treated with α-IFN plus methylprednisolone, 16.7% of patients treated with methylprednisolone, and 6.7% of control patients after 1 year. Renal involvement, defined as proteinuria, haematuria, and increased creatinine levels, significantly improved in 33% and 40% of patients in the α-IFN and α-IFN plus methylprednisolone groups respectively. No improvement was found in patients who received prednisolone only. Although a greater percentage of patients in the α-IFN plus methylprednisolone group achieved a complete response within 3 months as compared with α-IFN alone (66.7% versus 25%), the addition of methylprednisolone led to increased viraemia. It was concluded that the marginal effects of combined therapy, at the cost of increased viraemia, did not justify the advocation of this combined approach.

Viraemia and renal disease usually relapse after cessation of therapy [149, 157, 161, 162], but some 18–33% of patients with HCV-positive chronic liver disease can eliminate the virus permanently [163, 164]. The reasons behind the different responses to α-IFN are not yet established. It is also unclear at present if a higher dose of α-IFN and/or a more prolonged course of treatment will increase the frequency of response and reduce the relapse rate.

Other therapy for mixed cryoglobulinaemia

Interpretation of studies of treatment are complicated by the lack of controlled studies and also by the fact that many of these studies were performed prior to the recognition of the role of HCV infection in the pathogenesis of mixed cryoglobulinaemia. Corticosteroids are effective in treating the extrarenal symptoms of mixed cryoglobulinaemia, but their effects on renal function are less well substantiated [116, 165, 166]. In one retrospective study, corticosteroids led to a significant fall in proteinuria and creatinine in 15 patients with essential mixed cryoglobulinaemia [165]. A variety of cytotoxic agents, including cyclophosphamide, chlorambucil and azathioprine, have been used together with corticosteroids to treat essential cryoglobulinaemia [116, 134, 167–172] but their role remains unsubstantiated.

Plasma exchange reduces cryoglobulin [173, 174] and immune complex levels, and has been reported to lead to an improvement of renal function [119, 122, 125, 174–176]. However, the effects are usually temporary, since depletion of cryoglobulins leads to rapid rebound immunoglobulin synthesis [177]. This led to the rationale of combined plasma exchange with immunosuppressants in an attempt to curtail rebound immunoglobulin synthesis. L'Abbate *et al.* found that a combined regimen of plasma exchange and cyclophosphamide was effective in suppressing rebound immunoglobulin synthesis [123]. Similarly, Houwert *et al.* showed that a combination of prednisolone, cyclophosphamide and plasma exchange was effective in inducing clinical remission in two patients with type III essential cryoglobulinaemia with glomerulonephritis and neurological involvement [178]. Geltner *et al.* in their prospective study evaluated the effects of steroids, chlorambucil and plasma exchange on five patients with mixed cryoglobulinaemia, with renal or neurological and vasculitic manifestations [119]. This combined regimen led to an improvement of renal function in four patients. However, in the study by Tarantino *et al.* which examined the clinical outcome of 105 patients with a median follow-up of 72 months, therapy with immunosuppressive drugs, corticosteroids and/or plasma exchange had no impact on the final outcome [127]. The traditional therapeutic approach of corticosteroids, immunosuppressives and plasma exchange will probably be modified by the knowledge that HCV represents a pathogenetic factor in essential mixed cryoglobulinaemia. However, this approach may still be appropriate in patients without HCV infection, in whom cryoglobulinaemia represents the activity of a B-cell clone which has yet to become overt as lymphoma or myeloma.

Prognosis of renal disease

Renal involvement is one of the most serious complications in mixed cryoglobulinaemia and heralds a bad overall prognosis [114–116, 121, 125, 127, 133, 175]. In patients with renal disease, survival ranges from a 5-year survival figure of 60% to a 15-year survival rate of 40% [175, 179]. The leading causes of death were primarily related to cardiovascular disease, liver disease or infection [127]. In the study by Tarantino *et al.* in which the clinical outcome of 105 patients with essential mixed cryoglobulinaemia and renal involvement was reported, age older than 50 years, purpura, splenomegaly, cryocrit levels higher than 10%, low C3 levels, and raised creatinine were all independent risk factors for death or dialysis [127].

The course of renal disease is variable. Spontaneous recovery and remission has been described in some patients, whilst others either have an indolent course or have intermittent relapses with slow decline of renal function [120, 179]. Progression to renal failure occurs only in about 10–15% patients [133], but most patients die before end-stage renal disease develops [180]. Recurrence of disease can occur after transplantation [133, 181, 182]. Few data are available on the clinical outcome of patients on renal replacement therapy, but in one study 65% of patients were alive at 5 years after starting dialysis [133].

Conclusion

In patients with cryoglobulinaemia, efforts should be made to look for underlying diseases such as lymphoreticular neoplasia, malignancy, chronic liver disease, and infections. Therapy should then be tailored to the underlying cause. In patients with essential mixed cryoglobulinaemia, HCV infection should be sought and treatment with α-IFN considered. The issue of optimal duration and dosage of α-IFN remains unresolved, and the effects of α-IFN therapy on the long-term outcome of essential mixed cryoglobulinaemia also remain to be established. It is possible that a higher dose of α-IFN taken for a longer period may prevent or delay disease relapses. Although α-IFN has relatively few adverse effects, toxicities associated with long-term usage remain unknown. There are no controlled data at present to show that steroids, cytotoxics, or plasma exhange, either used alone or in combination, offer any long-term benefits in the treatment of nephritis associated with cryoglobulinaemia. The optimal therapy for cryoglobulinaemia-associated nephritis has yet to be defined, and controlled, randomized studies, with a large number of patients, comparing the different forms of therapy, are lacking. In the absence of such studies, treatment will remain empirical and anecdotal.

Acknowledgement

We thank Dr A.J. Howie for provision of photomicrographs.

References

1. Pollak VE, Pirani CL, Schwartz FD. The natural history of the renal manifestations of systemic lupus erythematosus. J Lab Med 1964;63:537–50.
2. Baldwin DS, Lowenstein J, Rothfield NF, Gallo GR, McCluskey RT. The clinical course of the proliferative and membranous forms of lupus nephritis. Ann Intern Med 1970;73:929–42.
3. Ponticelli C, Zucchelli P, Moroni G, Cagnoli L, Banfi G, Pascuali S. Long-term prognosis of diffuse lupus nephritis. Clin Nephrol 1987;28, 263–71.
4. Nossent HC, Henzen-Logmans SC, Vroom TM, Berden JHM, Swaak TJG. Contribution of renal biopsy data in predicting outcome in lupus nephritis. Analysis of 116 patients. Arthritis Rheum 1990;33:970–7.
5. Cameron JS. Lupus nephritis in childhood and adolescence. Pediatr Nephrol 1994;8:230–49.
6. Donadio JV, Hart GM, Bergstralh EJ, Holley KE. Prognostic determinants in lupus nephritis: a long-term clinicopathologic study. Lupus 1995;4:109–15.
7. Neumann K, Wallace DJ, Azen C *et al.* Lupus in the 1980s: III. Influence of clinical variables, biopsy, and treatment on the outcome in 150 patients with lupus nephritis seen at a single center. Semin Arthritis Rheum 1995;25:47–55.
8. Moroni, G Quaglini S, Maccario M, Banfi G, Ponticelli C. 'Nephritic flares' are predictors of bad long-term renal outcome in lupus nephritis. Kidney Int 1996;50:2047–53.
9. Abeles M, Urman JD, Weinstein A, Lowenstein M, Rothfield NF. Systemic lupus erythematosus in the younger patient: survival studies. J Rheum 1980;7:515–22.
10. Ginzler EM, Diamond HS, Weiner M *et al.* A multicenter study of outcome in systemic lupus erythematosus. I. Entry variables as predictors of prognosis. Arthritis Rheum 1982;25: 601–11.
11. Nossent JC, Bronsveld W, Swaak AJG. Systemic lupus erythematosus. III. Observations on clinical renal involvement and follow up of renal function: Dutch experience with 110 patients studied prospectively. Ann Rheum Dis 1989;48:810–16.
12. Gruppo Italiano per lo Studio della Nefrite Lupica (GISNEL). Lupus nephritis: Prognostic factors and probability of maintaining life-supporting renal function 10 years after the diagnosis. Am J Kidney Dis 1992;19: 473–9.
13. Adu D, Cameron JS. Lupus nephritis. Clin Rheum Dis 1982;8:153–82.
14. McCluskey RT. Lupus Nephritis I. In: Sommers SC, editor. Kidney Pathology Decennal 1966–1975. New York: Appleton Century Crofts; 1975: 435–60.
15. Austin HA, Muenz LR, Joyce KM *et al.* Prognostic factors in lupus nephritis: contributions of renal histology. Am J Med 1983;75:382–90.
16. Banfi G, Mazzucco G, Di Belgiojoso GB *et al.* Morphological parameters in lupus nephritis: their relevance for classification and relationship with clinical and histological findings and outcome. Q J Med 1985;55:153–68.
17. Leaker B, Fairley KF, Dowling J, Kincaid-Smith PS. Lupus nephritis: clinical and pathological correlatiosn. Q J Med 1987;62:163–79.
18. McLaughlin J, Gladman DD, Urowitz MB, Bombardier C, Farewell VT, Cole E. Kidney biopsy in systemic lupus erythematosus. II. Survival analysis according to biopsy results. Arthritis Rheum 1991;34:1268–73.
19. Balow JE, Boumpas DT, Austin HA *et al.* Renal disease. In: Schur PH, editor. The Clinical Management of Systemic Lupus Erythematosus. Philadelphia, PA: Lippincott-Raven; 1996; 109–26.
20. Balow JE, Boumpas DT, Fessler BJ, Austin HA. Management of lupus nephritis. Kidney Int 1996;53:S88–92.
21. Donadio VJ. Treatment of membranous nephropathy in systemic lupus erythematosus. Nephrol Dial Transplant 1992;1:97–104
22. Pasquali S, Banfi G, Zucchelli G, Moroni G, Ponticelli C, Zucchelli P. Lupus membranous nephropathy: long-term outcome. Clin Nephrol 1993;39:175–82.

23. Sloan RP, Schwartz MM, Korbet SM, Borok RZ, Lupus Nephritis Collaborative Study Group. Long-term outcome in systemic lupus erythematosus membranous glomerulonephritis. J Am Soc Nephrol 1996;7:299–305.
24. Pollak VE, Pirani CL, Dujovne I *et al.* The clinical course of lupus nephritis: relationship to the renal histologic findings. In: Kincaid-Smith P, Mathew TH, Becker EL, editors. Glomerulonephritis: Morphology, Natural History, and Treatment. New York: Wiley; 1973: 1167–81.
25. Sztejnbok M, Stewart A, Diamond H, Kaplan D. Azathioprine in the treatment of systemic lupus erythematosus. A controlled study. Arthritis Rheum 1971;14:639–45
26. Steinberg AD, Kaltreider HB, Staples PJ, Goetzl EJ, Talal N, Decker JL. Cyclophosphamide in lupus nephritis: a controlled trial. Ann Intern Med 1971;75:165–71.
27. Donadio JV, Holley KE, Wagoner RD, Ferguson RH, McDuffie FC. Treatment of lupus nephritis with prednisolone and combined prednisolone and azathioprine. Ann Intern Med 1972;77:829–35.
28. Cade R, Spooner G, Schlein E *et al.* Comparison of azathioprine, prednisolone, and heparin alone or combined in treating lupus nephritis. Nephron 1973;10:37–56.
29. Donadio JV, Holley KE, Wagoner RD, Ferguson RH, McDuffie FC. Further observations on the treatment of lupus nephritis with prednisolone and combined prednisolone and azathioprine. Arthritis Rheum 1974;17:573–82.
30. Steinberg AD, Decker JL. A double-blind controlled trial comparing cyclophosphamide, azathioprine and placebo in the treatment of lupus nephritis. Arthritis Rheum 1974;6:923–37.
31. Hahn BH, Kantor OS, Osterland CK. Azathioprine plus prednisolone compared with prednisolone alone in the treatment of systemic lupus erythematosus. Ann Intern Med 1975; 83:597–605.
32. Decker JL, Klippel JH, Plotz PH, Steinberg AD. Cyclophosphamide or azathioprine in lupus glomerulonephritis. A controlled trial: results at 28 months. Annal Int Med 1975;83: 606–15.
33. Donadio JV, Holley KE, Ferguson RH, Ilstrup DM. Treatment of diffuse proliferative lupus nephritis with prednisolone and combined prednisolone and cyclophosphamide. N Engl J Med 1978;299:1151–5.
34. Dinant HJ, Decker JL, Klippel JH, Balow JE, Plotz PH, Steinberg AD. Alternative modes of cyclophosphamide and azathioprine therapy in lupus nephritis. Ann Intern Med 1982;96:728–36.
35. Carette, S, Klippel JH, Decker JL *et al.* Controlled studies of oral immunosuppressive drugs in lupus nephritis. A long-term follow-up. Ann Intern Med 1983;99:1–8.
36. Austin HA, Klippel JH, Balow JE *et al.* Therapy of lupus nephritis: Controlled trial of prednisolone and cytotoxic drugs. N Eng J Med 1986;314: 614–19.
37. Steinberg AD, Steinberg SC. Long-term preservation of renal function in patients with lupus nephritis receiving treatment that includes cyclophosphamide versus those treated with prednisolone alone. Arthritis Rheum 1991;34:945–50.
38. Boumpas DT, Austin HA, Vaughn EM *et al.* Controlled trial of pulse methylprednisolone versus two regimes of pulse cyclophosphamide in severe lupus nephritis. Lancet 1992;340: 741–5.
39. Sesso R, Monteiro M, Sato M, Kirsztajn G, Silva L, Ajzen H. A controlled trial of pulse cyclophosphamide versus pulse methylprednisolone in severe lupus nephritis. Lupus 1994;3: 107–12.
40. Gourley MF, Austin HA, Scott D *et al.* Methylprednisolone and cyclophosphamide, alone or in combination, in patients with lupus nephritis. A randomized, controlled trial. Ann Intern Med 1996;125:549–57.
41. Austin HA, Boumpas DT. Treatment of lupus nephritis. Semin Nephrol 1996;16:527–35.
42. Cameron JS. Glomerular and tubular disease. The treatment of severe lupus nephritis. Nephrol 1996;2:S35–41.
43. Levitt JI. Deterioration of renal function after discontinuation of long-term prednisolone–azathioprine therapy in primary renal disease. N Engl J Med 1970;282:1125–7.

44. Sharon E, Kaplan D, Diamond HS. Exacerbation of systemic lupus erythematosus after withdrawal of azathioprine therapy. N Engl J Med 1972;288:122–4.
45. French Cooperative Group. A randomised trial of plasma exchange in severe acute systemic lupus erythematosus: methodology and interim analysis. Plasma Ther Transfus Technol 1985; 6:535–9.
46. Derksen RHWM, Hené RJ, Kallenberg CGM, Valentijn RM, Kater L, on behalf of the Dutch Co-operative Study Group. Prospective multicentre trial on the short-term effects of plasma exchange versus cytotoxic drugs in steroid-resistant lupus nephritis. Neth J Med 1988;33:168–77
47. Lewis EJ, Hunsicker LG, Lan S-P, Rohde RD, Lachin JM, for the Lupus Nephritis Collaborative Study Group. A controlled trial of plasmapheresis therapy in severe lupus nephritis. N Engl J Med 1992;326:1373–9.
48. Clark WF, Dau PC, Euler HH *et al.* Plasmapheresis and subsequent pulse cyclophosphamide versus pulse cyclophosphamide alone in severe lupus: design of the Lupus Plasmapheresis Study Group trial. J Clin Apheresis 1991;6:40–7.
49. Euler HH, Guillevin L. Plasmapheresis and subsequent pulse cyclophosphamide in severe lupus erythematosus. An interim report of the Lupus Plasmapheresis Study Group. Ann Med Interne 1994;145:296–302.
50. Euler HH, Schroeder JO, Harten P, Zeuner RA, Gutschmidt HJ. Treatment-free remission in severe systemic lupus erythematosus following synchronisation of plasmapheresis with subsequent pulse cyclophosphamide. Arthritis Rheum 1994;37:1784–94.
51. Pollak VE, Pirani CL, Kark RM. The effect of large doses of prednisolone on the renal lesions and life span of patients with lupus glomerulonephritis. J Lab Clin Med 1961;57:495–511.
52. Hahn BH, Bagby M, Hamilton T, Osterland CK. Comparison of therapeutic and immunosuppressive effects of azathioprine, prednisolone and combined therapy in NZB/NZW mice. Arthritis Rheum 1973;16:163–70.
53. Ginzler E, Diamond H, Guttadauria M, Kaplan D. Prednisolone and azathioprine compared to prednisolone plus low-dose azathioprine and cyclophosphamide in the treatment of diffuse lupus nephritis. Arthritis Rheum 1976;19:693–9.
54. Dawisha JM, Yarboro CH, Vaughan EM, Austin HA, Balow JE, Klippel KH. Outpatient monthly oral cyclophosphamide therapy in systemic lupus erythematosus. J Rheumatol 1996; 23:273–8.
55. Silverman JA, Pascucci VL, Chatterji DC, Klippel JH. The pharmocokinetics of bolus oral cyclophosphamide in systemic lupus erythematosus. Arthritis Rheum 1984;27:(Suppl.): S64 (abstract).
56. Elion GB, Burgi E, Hitchings GH. Studies on condensed pyrimidine systems. IX. The synthesis of some 6-substituted purines. J Am Chem Soc 1952;74: 411–14.
57. Karnofsky DA. Late effects of immunosuppressive anticancer drugs. Fed Proc 1967;26:925–32.
58. Balow JE, Austin HA, Tsokos GC, Antonovych TT, Steinberg AD, Klippel JH. Lupus nephritis. Ann Intern Med 1987;106:79–94.
59. Plotz PH, Klippel JH, Decker JL *et al.* Bladder complications in patients receiving cyclophosphamide and urinary bladder toxicity. Ann Intern Med 1979;91:221–3.
60. Stillwell TJ, Benson RCJ, DeRemee RA, MacDonald TJ, Weiland LH. Cyclophosphamide-induced bladder toxicity in Wegener's granulomatosis. Arthritis Rheum 1988;31:465–70.
61. Hoffman GS, Kerr Gs, Leavitt RY *et al.* Wegener's granulomatosis. An analysis of 158 patients. Ann Intern Med 1992;116:488–98.
62. Klein NW, Vogler MA, Chatot CL, Pierro LJ. The use of cultured rat embryos to evaluate the teratogenic activity of serum. Cadmium and cyclophosphamide. Teratology 1980;21:199–208.
63. Trompeter RS, Evans PR, Barratt TM. Gonadal function in boys with steroid-responsive nephrotic syndrome treated with cyclophosphamide for short periods. Lancet 1981;i:1177–9.
64. Koyama H, Wada T, Nishizawa T *et al.* Cyclophosphamide-induced ovarian failure and its therapeutic significance in patients with breast cancer. Cancer 1977;39:1403–9.

65. Boumpas DT, Austin HA, Vaughan EM, Yarboro CH, Klippel JH, Balow JE. Risk of sustained amenorrhoea in patients with systemic lupus erythematosus receiving intermittent pulse cyclophosphamide therapy. Ann Intern Med 1993;119:366–9.
66. Wang CL, Wang F, Bosco JJ. Ovarian failure in oral cyclophosphamide treatment for systemic lupus erythematosus. Lupus 1995;4:11–14.
67. Fairley KF, Barrie JU, Johnson W. Sterility and testicular atrophy related to cyclophosphamide therapy. Lancet 1972;i:568–9.
68. McDermott EM, Powell RJ. Incidence of ovarian failure in systemic lupus erythematosus after treatment with pulse cyclophosphamide. Ann Rheum Dis 1996;55:224–9.
69. Donadio JV, Glassock RJ. Immunosuppressive drug therapy in lupus nephritis. Am J Kidney Dis 1993;21:239–50.
70. Felson DT, Anderson J. Evidence for the superiority of immunosuppressive drugs and prednisolone over prednisolone alone in lupus nephritis: results of a pooled analysis. N Engl J Med 1984;311:1528–33.
71. Bansal VK, Beto JA. Treatment of lupus nephritis: a meta-analysis of clinical trials. Am J Kidney Dis 1997;29:193–9.
72. Verrier Jones J, Bucknall RC, Cumming RH *et al.* Plasmapheresis in the management of acute systemic lupus erythematosus. Lancet 1976;ii:709–11.
73. Clark WF, Balfe JW, Cattran DC *et al.* Long-term plasma exchange in patients with systemic lupus erythematosus and diffuse proliferative glomerulonephritis. Plasma Ther Transfus Technol 1984;5:353–60.
74. Nasca T, Muder RR, Thomas DB, Schrecker JC, Ruben FL. Antibody response to pneumococcal polysaccharide vaccine in myasthenia gravis: effect of therapeutic plasmapheresis. J Clin Apheresis 1990;5:133–9.
75. Dau PC. Increased proliferation of blood mononuclear cells after plasmapheresis treatment of patients with demyelinating disease. J Neuroimmunol 1990;30:15–21.
76. Lombardo R, Cepparrone F, Di Pietro G, Franco C, Graziani G, Avanzi G. Plasma exchange in systemic lupus erythematosus. Experience in thirty-seven patients. Int J Artif Org 1993;16: 177–9.
77. Pirner K, Rubbert A, Burmester GR, Kalden JR, Manger B. Intravenous administration of immunoglobulins in systemic lupus erythematosus: review of the literature and initial clinical experience. Infusions Ther Transfusion Med 1993;20:131–5.
78. Francioni C, Galeazzi M, Fioravanti A, Gelli R, Megale F, Marcolongo R. Long term i.v. Ig treatment in systemic lupus erythematosus. Clin Exp Rheumatol 1994;12:163–8.
79. Balletta M, Sabella D, Magri P *et al.* Cyclosporin plus steroids versus steroids alone in the treatment of lupus nephritis. Contrib Nephrol 1992;99:129–30.
80. Miescher PA, Favre H, Lemoine R, Huang YP. Drug combination therapy of systemic lupus erythematosus. Springer Semin Immunopathol 1994;16:295–311.
81. Radhakrishnan J, Kunis CL, D'Agati V, Appel GB. Cyclosporin treatment of lupus membranous nephropathy. Clin Nephrol 1994;42:147–54.
82. Walz LeBlanc BA, Dagenais P, Urowitz MB, Gladman D. Methotrexate in systemic lupus erythematosus. J Rheumatol 1994;21:836–8.
83. Ferraccioli GF, De Vita S, Bartoli E. Methotrexate benefits in patients with lupus with and without nephritis. J Rheumatol 1995;22:1442–7.
84. Prickett JD, Robinson DR, Steinberg AD. Effects of dietary enrichment with eicosapentaenoic acid upon autoimmune nephritis in female NZB × NZW/F_1 mice. Arthritis Rheum 1983; 26:133–9.
85. Robinson DR, Prickett JD, Makoul GT, Steinberg AD, Golvin RB. Dietary fish oil reduces progression of established renal disease in NZB × NZW/F_1 mice and delays renal disease in BXSB and MRL/lpr strains. Arthritis Rheum 1986;29:539–46.
86. Endres S, Ghorbani R, Kelly VE *et al.* The effect of dietary supplementation with n-3 polyunsaturated fatty acids on the synthesis of interleukin-1 and tumor necrosis factor by mononuclear cells. N Engl J Med 1989;320:265–71.

87. Santoli D, Zurier RB. Prostaglandins E precursor fatty acids inhibit human IL-2 production by a PGE-independent mechanism. J Immunol 1989;143:1303–9.
88. Das UN. Beneficial effect of eicosapentaenoic and docosahexaenoic acids in the management of systemic lupus erythematosus and its relationship to the cytokine network. Prostagland Leukotri Essent Fatty Acids 1994;51:207–13.
89. Westberg G, Tarkowski A. Effect of MAXEPA in patients with SLE. Scand J Rheumatol 1990;19:137–43.
90. Lahita RG. Sex, age, and systemic lupus erythematosus. In: Lahita RG, editor. Systemic Lupus Erythematosus. New York: Churchill Livingstone; 1992.
91. Mund, A, Swison J, Rothfield N. Effect of pregnancy on the course of systemic lupus erythematosus. J Am Med Assoc 1963;183:917–25.
92. Jungers, P, Dougados M, Pelissier C *et al.* Influence of oral contraceptive therapy on activity of systemic lupus erythematosus. Arthritis Rheum 1982;25:618–23.
93. Melez, KA, Boegel WA, Steinberg AD. Therapeutic studies in New Zealand mice. VII. Successful androgen treatment of NZB/NZW F_1 females of different ages. Arthritis Rheum 1980;2 41–8.
94. Steinberg AD, Roths JB, Murphy ED. Effects of thymectomy and androgen administration upon the autoimmune disease of MRL/Mo-lpr/lpr mice. J Immunol 1980;125:871–83.
95. Sthoeger ZM, Bentwich ZVI, Zinger H, Mozes E. The beneficial effect of the estrogen antagonist, tamoxifen on experimental systemic lupus erythematosus. J Rheumatol 1994;21: 2231–8.
96. Sturgess AD, Evans DT, Mackay IR, Riglar A. Effects of the estrogen antagonist tamoxifen on disease indices in systemic lupus erythematosus. J Clin Lab Immunol 1984;13:11–14.
97. Lahita, RG, Kunkel HG. Treatment of systemic lupus erythematosus with the androgen 19-nortestosterone. Arthritis Rheum 1984;27:S65 (abstract).
98. Stroeber S, Field E, Hoppe RT *et al.* Treatment of intractable lupus nephritis with total lymphoid irradiation. Ann Intern Med 1985;102:450–8.
99. Strober S, Farinas MC, Field EH *et al.* Lupus nephritis after total lymphoid irradiation. Persistent improvement and reduction in steroid dosage. Ann Intern Med 1987;197:689–91.
100. Wacholtz MC, Lipsky PE. Treatment of lupus nephritis with CD5 PLUS, an immunoconjugate of an anti-CD5 monoclonal antibody and ricin A chain. Arthritis Rheum 1992;35:837–9.
101. Stafford, FJ, Fleisher TA, Brown M *et al.* Clinical and biological effects of anti-CD5 ricin A chain immunoconjugate in systemic lupus erythematosus (SLE). Arthritis Rheum 1993;36: S227.
102. Sipe JC, Romine JS, Koziol JA, McMillan R, Zyroff J, Beutler E. Cladribine in treatment of chronic progressive multiple sclerosis. Lancet 1994;344:9–13.
103. Austin HA, Boumpas DT, Vaughan EM, Balow JE. Predicting renal outcomes in severe lupus nephritis: contributions of clinical and histologic data. Kidney Int 1994;45:544–50.
104. Esdaile JM. Prognosis in systemic lupus erythematosus. Springer Semin Immunopathol 1994; 16:337–55.
105. Levey AS, Lan S-P, Corwin HL *et al.* Lupus Nephritis Collaborative Study. Progression and remission of renal disease in the Lupus Nephritis Collaborative Study. Results of treatment with prednisolone and short-term oral cyclophosphamide. Ann Intern Med 1992;116:114–23.
106. Esdaile JM, Levington C, Federgreen W, Hayslett JP, Kashgarian M. The clinical and renal biopsy predictors of long-term outcome in lupus nephritis: a study of 87 patients and review of the literature. Q J Med 1989;269:779–833.
107. Cheigh JS, Kim R, Stenzel KR *et al.* Systemic lupus erythematosus in patients with end-stage renal disease: long-term follow-up on the prognosis of patients and the evolution of lupus activity. Am J Kidney Dis 1990;16:189–95.
108. Cheigh JS, Stenzel KH. End-stage renal disease in systemic lupus erythematosus. Am J Kidney Dis 1993;21:2–8.
109. Roth D, Milgrom M, Esquenazi V, Strauss J, Zilleruelo G, Miller J. Renal transplantation in systemic lupus erythematosus: one center's experience. Am J Nephrol 1987;7:367–74.

110. Goss JA, Cole BR, Jendrisak MD *et al.* Renal transplantation in systemic lupus erythematosus and recurrent lupus nephritis: a single center experience and a review of the literature. Transplantation 1991;52:805–10.
111. Pollack CA, Ibels LS. Dialysis and transplantation in patients with renal failure due to systemic lupus erythematosus: the Australian and New Zealand experience. Aust NZ J Med 1987;17:321–5.
112. Wintrobe MM, Buell MV. Hyperproteinemia associated with multiple myeloma. Bull Johns Hopkins Hosp 1933;52:156–65.
113. Lerner AB, Watson CJ. Studies of cryoglobulins. I. Unusual purpura associated with the presence of high concentrations of cold precipitate serum globulin. Am J Med Sci 1947;214: 410–15.
114. Brouet JC, Clauvel JP, Danon F *et al.* Biologic and clinical significance of cryoglobulins. A report of 86 cases. Am J Med 1974;57:775–88.
115. Meltzer M, Franklin EC, Elias K, McCluskey RT, Cooper N. Cryoglobulinemia: a clinical and laboratory study. II. Cryoglobulins with rheumatoid factor activity. Am J Med 1966;40: 837–56.
116. Gorevic PD, Kassab HJ, Levo Y *et al.* Mixed cryoglobulinemia: clinical aspects and long term follow-up of 40 patients. Am J Med 1980;69:287–308.
117. Monti G, Galli M, Invernizzi F *et al.* Cryoglobulinaemias: a multi-centre study of the early clinical and laboratory manifestations of primary and secondary disease. Q J Med 1995;88: 115–26.
118. Winfield JB. Cryoglobulinemia. Hum Pathol 1983;14:350–4.
119. Geltner D, Kohn RW, Gorevic P, Franklin EC. The effect of combination therapy (steroids, immunosuppressives and plasmapheresis) on 5 mixed cryoglobulinaemia patients with renal, neurological and vascular involvement. Arthritis Rheum 1981;24:1121–7.
120. Tarantino A, De Vecchi A, Montagnino G *et al.* Renal disease in essential mixed cryoglobulinemia. Long-term follow up of 44 patients. Q J Med 1981;197:1–30.
121. Ben-Bassat M, Boner G, Rosenfeld J *et al.* The clinco-pathologic features of cryoglobulinaemic nephropathy. Am J Clin Pathol 1983;79:147–56.
122. Cassuto-Viguier E, Quaranta JF, Ortonne JP, Cassuto JP, Duplay H, Dujardin P. Effect of plasma exchange on the course of cryoglobulinaemias. In: Nose Y, Malchevsky PS, Smith JW, Krakaw RSJW, Krakaw RS, editors. Plasmapheresis. New York: Raven Press; 1983:299–308.
123. L'Abbate A, Maggiore Q, Caccamo A, Bartolomeo F, Misefari V. Suppression of post-apheresis autoantibody rebound in cryoglobulinaemia and cold agglutinin haemolytic anaemia. Int J Artif Org 1983;6:51–6.
124. Cordonnier DJ, Vialtel P, Dechelette E *et al.* Long-term management of essential mixed cryoglobulinaemia. In: Ponticelli C, Minetti L, D'Amico G, editors. Antiglobulins, Cryoglobulins and Glomerulonephritis. Dordrecht: Martinus Nijhoff; 1986:237–49.
125. Frankel AH, Singer DRJ, Winearls CG, Evans DJ, Rees AJ, Pusey CD. Type II essential mixed cryoglobulinaemia: presentation, treatment and outcome in 13 patients. Q J Med 1992;298: 101–24.
126. Barbiano di Belgioioso G, Montoli A, Tarantino A *et al.* Clinical and histologic correlations in essential mixed cryoglobulinaemia glomerulonephritis. In: Ponticelli C, Minetti L, D'Amico G, editors. Antiglobulins, Cryoglobulins and Glomerulonephritis. Dordrecht: Martinus Nijhoff; 1986:203–10.
127. Tarantino A, Campise M, Banfi G *et al.* Long-term predictors of survival in essential mixed cryoglobulinemic glomerulonephritis. Kidney Int 1995;47:618–23.
128. Ponticelli C, Imbasciati E, Tarantino A, Piertrogrande M. Acute anuric glomerulonephritis in monoclonal cryoglobulinemia. Br Med J 1977;1:948.
129. Lockwood CM. Lymphoma, cryoglobulinemia and renal disease. Kidney Int 1979;16:522–30.
130. Carlos HW, Tavassoli MD. Acute renal failure from precipitation of cryoglobulins in a cool operating room. J Am Med Assoc 1989;244:1472–3.
131. Druet P, Letonturier P, Contet A, Mandet C. Cryoglobulinemia in human renal disease: a study of 76 cases. Clin Exp Immunol 1969;15:483–96.

132. Ferrario F, Colasanti G, Barbiano Di Belgioioso G *et al.* Histological and immunohistological features in essential mixed cryoglobulinemia glomerulonephritis. In: Ponticelli C, Minetti L, D'Amico G, editors. Antiglobulins, Cryoglobulins and Glomerulonephritis. Dordrecht: Martinus Nijhoff; 1986:193–202.
133. Tarantino A, Moroni G, Banfi G, Manzoni C, Segagni S, Ponticelli C. Renal replacement therapy in cryoglobulinaemic nephritis. Nephrol Dial Transplant 1994;9:1426–30.
134. MacIntosh RM, Kaufman DB, Kulvinskas C, Grossman B. Cryoglobulins. I. Studies on the nature, incidence, and clinical significance of serum cryoproteins in glomerulonephritis. J Lab Clin Med 1970;75:566–77.
135. Adam C, Morel-Maroger L, Richet G. Cryoglobulins in glomerulonephritis not related to systemic disease. Kidney Int 1973;3:334–41.
136. Feizi T, Gitlin N. Immune-complex disease of the kidney associated with chronic hepatitis and cryoglobulinemia. Lancet 1969;ii:873–6.
137. Cordonnier DD, Martin H, Groslambert P, Micouin C, Chenais F, Stoebner P. Mixed IgG–IgM cryoglobulinemia with glomerulonephritis. Immunochemical, fluorescent and ultrastructural study of kidney and *in vitro* cryoprecipitate. Am J Med 1975;59:867–72.
138. Feiner H, Gallo G. Ultrastructure in glomerulonephritis associated with cryoglobulinemia. Am J Pathol 1977;88:145–62.
139. Agnello V, Chung RT, Kaplan LM. A role for hepatitis C virus infection in type II cryoglobulinemia. N Engl J Med 1992;327:1490–5.
140. Cacoub P, Musset L, Lunel Fabiani F *et al.* Hepatitis C virus and essential mixed cryoglobulinaemia. Br J Rheumatol 1993;32:689–92.
141. Realdi G, Alberti A, Rigoli A, Tremolada F. Immune-complexes and Australia antigen in cryoglobulinemic sera. Zimmunitatsforsch Exp Klin Immunol 1974;147:114–26.
142. Levo Y, Gorevic PD, Kassab HJ *et al.* Liver involvement in the syndrome of mixed cryoglobulinemia. Ann Intern Med 1977;87:287–92.
143. Galli M, Careddu F, D'Armino A, Monti G, Messina K, Invernizzi F. Hepatitis B virus and essential mixed cryoglobulinemia. Lancet 1980;i:1093.
144. Popp JJ, Dienstag JL, Wands JR, Bloch KJ. Essential mixed cryoglobulinemia without evidence for hepatitis B virus infection. Ann Intern Med 1980;92:379–83.
145. Caporali R, Longhi M, Zorzoli I *et al.* Hepatitis B virus markers in monoclonal (type I and II) and polyclonal (type III) cryoglobulinemias. Haematologica 1988;73:375–8.
146. Pascual M, Perrin L, Giostra E, Schifferli JA. Hepatitic C virus in patients with cryoglobulinaemia type II. J Infect Dis 1990;162:569–70.
147. Ferri C, Greco F, Longombardo G *et al.* Antibodies against hepatitis C virus in mixed cryoglobulinemia patients. Infection 1991;19:417–20.
148. Misiani R, Bellavita P, Fenili D *et al.* Hepatitis C virus infection in patients with essential mixed cryoglobulinemia. Ann Intern Med 1992;117:573–7.
149. Ferri C, Marzo E, Longombardo G *et al.* Interferon-alpha in mixed cryoglobulinemia patients: randomized, crossover controlled trial. Blood 1993;81:1132–6.
150. Mazzaro C, Tulissi P, Moretti M *et al.* Clinical and virological findings in mixed cryoglobulinaemia. J Int Med 19 1995;238:153–60.
151. Sinico RA, Ribero ML, Fornasieri A *et al.* Hepatitis C virus genotype in patients with essential mixed cryoglobulinaemia. Q J Med 1995;88:805–10.
152. Sansonno D, Cornacchiulo V, Iacobelli AR, Stefano RD, Lospalluti M, Dammacco F. Localization of hepatitis C virus antigens in liver and skin tissues of chronic hepatitis C virus-infected patients with mixed cryoglobulinaemia. Hepatology 1995;21:305–12.
153. Lunel F, Musset L, Cacoub P *et al.* Cryoglobulinemia in chronic liver disease: role of hepatitis C virus and liver damage. Gastroenterology 1994;106:1291–300.
154. Bonomo L, Casato M, Afeltra A, Caccavo D. Treatment of idiopathic mixed cryoglobulinemia with alpha interferon. Am J Med 1987;83:726–30.
155. Casuto M, Legana B, Antonelli G, Dianzani F, Bonomo L. Long-term results of therapy with interferon-α for type II essential mixed cryoglobulinaemia. Blood 1991;78:3142–7.

156. Ferri C, Zignego AL, Longombardo G *et al.* Effect of alpha-interferon on hepatitis C virus chronic infection in mixed cryoglobulinemia patients. Infection 1993;2:93–6.
157. Misiani R, Bellavita P, Fenili D *et al.* Interferon alpha-2a therapy in cryoglobulinemia associated with Hepatitis C virus. N Engl J Med 1994;330:751–6.
158. Grossberg SE. An overview of their biological and biochemical properties. In: Pfeffer LM, editor. Mechanisms of Interferon Action. Boca Raton, FL: CRC; 1987:2.
159. Harfast B, Huddlestone JR, Casali P, Merigan TC, Oldstone MBA. Interferon acts directly on B lymphocytes to modulate immunoglobulin synthesis. J Immunol 1991;127:2146–50.
160. Exley R, Nathan P, Walker L, Gordon J, Clemens MJ. Antiproliferative effects of interferons on Daudi Burkitt-lymphoma cells: induction of cell differentiation and loss of response to autocrine growth factors. Int J Cancer 1987;40:53–9.
161. Dammacco F, Sansonno D, Han JH *et al.* Natural interferon-α versus its combination with 6-methyl-prednisolone in the therapy of type II mixed cryoglobulinemia: a long term, randomised, controlled study. Blood 1994;84:3336–43.
162. Johnson RJ, Gretch DR, Couser WG *et al.* Hepatitis C virus-associated glomerulonephritis. Effect of α-interferon therapy. Kidney Int 1994;46:1700–4.
163. Davis GL, Balart LA, Schiff ER *et al.* Treatment of chronic hepatitis C with recombinant interferon alpha. A multicenter randomized controlled trial. N Engl J Med 1989;321:1501–6.
164. Di Bisceglie AM, Martin P, Kassianides C *et al.* Recombinant interferon alpha therapy for hepatitis C. A randomized, double-blind, placebo-controlled trial. N Engl J Med 1989;321: 1506–10.
165. De Vecchi A, Montagnino G, Pozzi C, Locatelli F, Pontivelli C. Intravenous methylprednisolone therapy in essential mixed cryoglobulinemia nephropathy. Clin Nephrol 1983;5:221–7.
166. Vacca A, Dammacco F. Deflazacort versus prednisolone in the treatment of EMC: A between-patient controlled clinical study. Int Arch Allergy Immunol 1992;99:306–10.
167. Hippe E, Jensen KB, Olesen H, Lind K, Thomsen PEB. Chlorambucil treatment of patients with cold agglutinin syndrome. Blood 1970;35:68–72.
168. Mathison DA, Condemi JJ, Leddy JP, Callerame ML, Panner BJ, Vaughan JH. Purpura, arthralgia, and IgM–IgG cryoglobulinemia with rheumatoid factor activity. Response to cyclophosphamide and splenectomy. Ann Intern Med 1971;74:383–90.
169. Grossman J, Abraham GN, Leddy JP. Crystalglobulinaemia. Ann Intern Med 1972;77:395–400.
170. Bengtsson U, Larsson O, Lindstedt G, Svalander C. Monoclonal IgG cryoglobulinemia with secondary development of glomerulonephritis and nephrotic syndrome. Q J Med 1975;175: 491–503.
171. Martelo OJ, Schultz DR, Pardo V, Perez-Stable E. Immunologically-mediated renal disease in Waldenström's macroglobulinemia. Am J Med 1975;58:567–75.
172. Ristow SC, Griner PF, Abraham GN, Shoulson I. Reversal of systemic manifestations of cryoglobulinaemia. Arch Intern Med 1976;136:467–70.
173. Ferri C, Gregmignai G, Bombardieri S *et al.* Plasma-exchange in mixed cryoglobulinemia. Effects on renal, liver and neurologic involvement. Ricerca Clin Lab 1986;16:403–11.
174. Ferri C, Moriconi L, Gregmignai G *et al.* Treatment of the renal involvement in mixed cryoglobulinemia with prolonged plasma exchange. Nephron 1986;43:246–53.
175. Cordonnier D, Vialtel P, Renversez J *et al.* Renal diseases in 18 patients with mixed type II IgM–IgG cryoglobulinaemia: monoclonal lymphoid infiltration (2 cases) and membranoproliferative glomerulonephritis (14 cases). Adv Nephrol 1983;12:177–204.
176. Sinico R, Fornasieri A, Fiorini G *et al.* Plasma exchange in glomerulonephritis associated with systemic lupus erythematosus and essential mixed cryoglobulinaemia. Int J Artif Org 1983;6:21–5.
177. Maggiore Q, L'Abbate A, Bartolomeo F, Martorano C, Cutrupi S. Effects of cryoapheresis on plasma cryoglobulins and renal function in patients with EMC glomerulonephritis. In: Ponticelli C, Minetti L, D'Amico G, editors. Antiglobulins, Cryoglobulins and Glomerulonephritis. Dordrecht: Martinus Nijhoff; 1986:251–64.

178. Houwert DA, Hene RJ, Struyvenberg A, Kater L. Effect of plasmapheresis (PP), corticosteroids and cyclophosphamide in essential mixed cryoglobulinaemia associated glomerulonephritis. Proc EDTA 1980;17:650–4.
179. D'Amico G, Colasanti G, Ferrario F, Sinico RA. Renal involvement in essential mixed cryoglobulinemia. Kidney Int 1989;35:1004–14.
180. Tarantino A, Montagnino G, Baldasarri A *et al.* Prognostic factors in essential mixed cryoglobulins and glomerulonephritis. In: Ponticelli C, Minetti L, D'Amico G, editors. Antiglobulins, Cryoglobulins and Glomerulonephritis. Dordrecht: Martinus Nijhoff; 1986: 219–25.
181. Andrejak M, Bariety J, Bedrossian J *et al.* Cryoglobulinaemia in renal transplant recipients. Transplantation 1978;26:446–7.
182. Hiesse C, Bastuji-Garin S, Santelli G *et al.* Recurrent essential mixed cryoglobulinemia in renal allografts. Am J Nephrol 1989;9:150–4.

9. Recurrence of glomerulonephritis following renal transplantation

M.D. DENTON and M.H. SAYEGH

Introduction

Glomerulonephritis is a major cause of end-stage renal disease (ESRD) and is the primary disease in over a third of patients undergoing renal transplantation. Recurrence of glomerulonephritis in the renal allograft represents a significant problem. Large data registries from the United States and Europe report a 4% to 7% incidence of graft loss secondary to recurrent glomerulonephritis in adults [1, 2]. Recurrence of glomerulonephritis imposes a greater impact on graft survival in paediatric transplant recipients [3]. Moreover, the relative impact of recurrent glomerulonephritis on allograft function and survival is predicted to increase as advances in transplant immunobiology and the development of specific immunosuppressive strategies reduce rejection-mediated graft loss. All forms of glomerulonephritis have been reported to recur *histologically* following renal transplantation, but the incidence and severity of *clinical* recurrence varies greatly according to the type of glomerular disease. This chapter attempts to clarify some of the salient clinical features of recurrent glomerulonephritis from a body of literature full of anecdotal reports and retrospective studies. Development of *de-novo* glomerulonephritis in the transplant will also be discussed. There are several excellent reviews on recurrent glomerulonephritis [4–8] and this chapter aims to complement these by focusing on more recent developments in the field.

Incidence of recurrence and effect on graft survival

Table 9.1 lists glomerular diseases, both primary and secondary to systemic disease, that recur in renal allografts, and gives approximate values for the incidence of histological recurrence and graft loss. There are several issues one must bear in mind when interpreting rates of recurrence. Firstly, due to the small number of cases within any nephrology centre, the literature predominantly consists of anecdotal reports or small retrospective studies. Results from such small studies must be interpreted with extreme caution, particularly when subgroup analysis is performed. Secondly, in order to define recurrent disease, one must have an accurate histological diagnosis both pre- and post-transplant. However, many patients with chronic glomerulonephritis enter ESRD without

C.D. Pusey (ed.), The Treatment of Glomerulonephritis, 177–200.

Table 9.1 Recurrent glomerulonephritis in renal allografts: rate of recurrence and graft loss

Type of glomerulonephritis	Rate of recurrence (%)	Graft loss (%)	Comments
Focal segmental glomerulosclerosis	20–40	15	Well-defined risk factors for recurrence. Variable clinical course confirms heterogeneity of disease.
IgA nephropathy	50	15	Clinical recurrence increases with time. Overall graft survival excellent.
Membranous nephropathy	20	5	Generally minor clinical manifestations. Early NS associated with poor prognosis.
Mesangiocapillary type I	25	25	Difficult to distinguish from transplant glomerulopathy. Complement levels do not predict activity. Association with HCV.
Mesangiocapillary type II	90	10	Often absence of C3 nephritic factor.
Haemolytic uraemic syndrome	10–50	10–50	Recurrence and outcome depend on aetiology of primary HUS. Frequency complicated by *de-novo* HUS.
Henoch-Schonlein purpura	30–80	10	Clinical outcome worse in LRD. Histology identical to IgA nephropathy.
Wegener's granulomatosis	5–20	5–20	Azathioprine is better than CsA in preventing relapse. Cyclophosphamide is an effective treatment in relapses.
Anti-GBM disease	0	0	No recurrence if anti-GBM titres are undetectable prior to Tx. *De-novo* disease may occur in Alport's syndrome.
Lupus nephritis	1	1	Disease activity diminishes in ESRD.

CsA: cyclosporin A; ESRD: end-stage renal disease; HCV: hepatitis C virus; HUS: haemolytic uraemic syndrome; LRD: living related donor; NS: nephrotic syndrome; Tx: transplantation

ever having a renal biopsy; and often renal allograft biopsies are not performed in transplant patients with mild proteinuria or even chronic graft dysfunction, so leading to underdiagnosis and underestimation of the recurrence rate. Thirdly, the lack of specificity in the pathological features of some conditions may lead to errors in diagnosis; examples include the non-specificity of the histological lesion of primary focal segmental glomerulosclerosis (FSGS), the similarity between transplant glomerulopathy and mesangiocapillary glomerulonephritis (MCGN), and the common vascular changes observed in haemolytic uraemic syndrome (HUS), malignant hypertension, and cyclosporin toxicity. Fourthly, recurrence rates can be complicated by the existence of *de-novo* disease (e.g. membranous nephropathy). Common types of *de-novo* glomerulonephritis in renal allografts are outlined in Table 9.2.

Table 9.2 De-novo glomerulonephritis in renal allografts

Disease	Incidence	Pathology	Aetiology
Transplant glomerulopathy	5%	Widening of subendothelial space. Duplication and interposition of GBM. No immune complex deposition.	Graft rejection, ? T cell-mediated graft endothelial cell injury, ? CMV infection.
De-novo membranous nephropathy	2%	GBM thickening and spike formation. Associated changes of rejection.	Associated with graft rejection. *In-situ* immune complex formation with neoantigens formed during graft injury.
De-novo HUS	1–3%	Fibrin thrombi in capillary loops. Reduplication of internal elastic lamina.	Cyclosporin, graft ischaemia, graft rejection, OCP.
De-novo type I MCGN	? 2%	Mesangial hypercellularity. Thickened capillary loops with interpositioning and IC deposition.	Hepatitis C virus. Cryoglobulins, ? deposition of HCV antigen.
Anti-GBM disease in Alport's syndrome	Rare	Necrotizing focal segmental disease with linear deposition of IgG.	IgG production and binding to previously 'unseen' alpha chain of type IV collagen.

CMV: cytomegalovirus; GBM: glomerular basement membrane; HCV: hepatitis C virus; IC: immune complex; OCP: oral contraceptive pill; RF: rheumatoid factor.

Precautions must also be taken when estimating the incidence of graft loss secondary to recurrence. Histological appearances of acute or chronic rejection may coexist with glomerular pathology and it may therefore be difficult to determine the precise cause of graft loss. Particular attention must be paid to the duration of follow-up; risk of recurrent disease increases with time post-transplantation and length of graft survival [9]. Finally, it is important to appreciate that the primary disease may influence graft survival by mechanisms independent of disease recurrence. For example patients with IgA nephropathy have a higher than average graft survival despite frequent recurrence, whereas patients with systemic lupus erythematosus (SLE) have a low cadaveric graft survival despite a negligible recurrence rate. A recent study of recurrent FSGS shows that a large proportion of grafts with recurrence fail due to an increased rate of acute cellular rejection and not to recurrent disease itself [10].

Recurrence of primary glomerulonephritis

Primary focal segmental glomerulosclerosis

Recurrent FSGS is the most worrisome problem in the spectrum of recurrent disease owing to its frequency and the severity of the recurrent lesion. Overall the incidence of recurrence is estimated at between 20% and 40%, and half of these grafts will fail as a direct consequence of recurrent disease [11–13]. The coexistence of certain well-defined risk factors, such as recipient age of less than 6 years, a rapid progression into ESRD, mesangial hypercellularity on the native biopsy and recurrence in a previous transplant, markedly increase the risk of recurrence [12, 14, 15]. Paediatric patients with rapid progression to ESRD and mesangial expansion have an 85–100% chance of recurrence [5]. The high risk predicted in certain subgroups has led to the suggestion that these patients should be placed on intensive prophylactic treatment regimens, including plasmapheresis, prior to transplantation (see below). There is no convincing evidence linking the use of living related donor (LRD) transplants with an increased risk of recurrence; however, some centers advocate not using LRD grafts in high-risk patients simply because of the high failure rate [16]. Black patients have a reduced incidence of recurrence [17]. A variant of FSGS occurs in a familial pattern and is characterized by a high rate of progression to ESRD but a low rate of recurrence in renal allografts [18]. Since the introduction of cyclosporin as an immunosuppressive agent, the incidence of recurrent FSGS has remained unchanged [19]. Ingulli *et al.* reported recurrence in four of 22 (18%) patients on prednisone and azathioprine immunosuppression compared with two of 18 (11%) on cyclosporin-based immunosuppression [20].

The clinical severity of recurrent FSGS is highly variable, reflecting the heterogeneity of this condition. Classically, heavy proteinuria can occur immediately following vascular anastomosis, leading to frank nephrotic syndrome and rapid graft loss. Other patients may develop low-grade proteinuria months after transplantation with a slow deterioration in renal function if any. Often the severity of recurrence mirrors the severity of the primary disease. Recurrence usually occurs within 1 month post-transplantation and rarely later than 1 year post-transplantation. Spontaneous remission has been reported. Kim *et al.* reported an increased rate of acute cellular rejection in patients with recurrence, and speculate that recurrence may result in molecular changes within the graft which stimulate acute rejection [10].

The rapidity of onset of proteinuria in some patients post-transplantation strongly favours the existence of a circulating factor in the recipient, responsible for increasing graft glomerular permeability. Supporting this hypothesis is the finding of a transient nephrotic syndrome in infants born to nephrotic mothers, and the experimental observation that nephrotic syndrome in rats can be induced by injecting serum from nephrotic patients [22]. This line of investigation has been pursued by Savin and colleagues, leading to partial characterization of a factor which increases both rat and human glomerular permeability to albumen *in vitro* [23]. They found that serum from patients with recurrent FSGS, when incubated with isolated glomeruli, increased their permeability to albumen. Interestingly, this factor was not present in patients transplanted without recurrence or in a group of patients with FSGS not transplanted, approximately half of whom were on dialysis. This may be due to low activity of disease in the latter two groups, or may support the concept of a heterogeneic pathophysiology. By measuring the permeability activity of serum prior to transplantation they were able to predict with some accuracy those patients who would go on to develop recurrent disease.

Initial characterization of this factor revealed it to be an immunoglobulin-like protein of low molecular weight which was removed from serum by plasmapheresis, and bound to a protein A column [23]. Interestingly, they found that cyclosporin ameliorated the effect of this factor on glomerular permeability, and this was associated with an increase in glomerular cAMP [24]. Taken together, these interesting insights into the pathophysiology of recurrent FSGS support the potential benefit of a variety of therapeutic options in this disease. Unfortunately, the results of clinical studies evaluating the use of cyclosporin, plasmapheresis, immunoadsorption and other treatment options are disappointing (Table 9.3). Increasing cyclosporin dosage has been reported to reduce proteinuria following recurrence [20]. This is likely to be a functional effect of cyclosporin mediated by changes in glomerular haemodynamics rather than a direct disease modifying effect [25]. Several case reports, however, have claimed permanent remission of recurrent FSGS with high dose cyclosporin [25, 26]. A controlled trial will need to be performed to determine whether high doses of cyclosporin can alter the natural history of this condition. Finally, conversion to FK 506 has not been shown to improve proteinuria or graft function significantly [27].

Several studies have examined the role of plasma exchange [28–31] and immunoadsorption [32] in the treatment of recurrent FSGS. These small

Table 9.3 Studies examining treatment options in recurrent primary FSGS

Treatment	Ref.	Study design	Patient no.	Mean age (years)	Proteinuria (g/dl) Pre-	Proteinuria (g/dl) Post-	Mean follow-up (months)	Graft loss in recurrence	Comments
Plasma exchange	3	Case series Historic control	9 16(C)	30	12	5.1	17+11	11% cf. 50% in control	6/9 patients had sustained remission. Non-responders had worse glomerulosclerosis on Bx. PE reversed foot process fusion.
Plasma exchange	25	Case control	14	29	8.45	5.6	44	27% cf. 40% in control	In 7/9 patients PE decreased proteinuria but effect lasted <4 months.
Prophylactic plasma exchange +ALG	55	Prospective Controlled	8 6(C)	12	NR	6 51(C)	1	NR	37% recurrence in treatment group cf. 66% in control. Milder recurrence in treatment group.
Plasma exchange	62	Case series	2	12	2.6	0.34	32	0	Sustained remission.
Plasma exchange and high-dose CsA ~20 mg/kg per day	77	Case series	11	9.6	24 61*	NR 2.8*	28	16%	7 in complete remission, 3 in partial remission.
Immunoadsorption	26	Case series	8	32	9	1.9	13+3	12%	Transient effect on proteinuria. Remission in 1 patient. More effective than PE in reducing proteinuria.

Table 9.3 (cont).

Treatment	Ref.	Study design	Patient no.	Mean age (years)	Proteinuria (g/dl)		Mean follow-up (months)	Graft loss in recurrence	Comments
					Pre-	Post-			
High-dose CsA 12 mg/kg per day	76	Case report	1	20	15	8	8	100%	Clinical remission on CsA for 8 months.
OKT3	109	Case report	1	NR	NR	NR	24	100%	2 previous Tx failed on CsA. Remission on FK 506.
FK 506	71	Case series	10	NR	7.2	3.9	NR	100%	No deterioration in RF over study period.
Indomethacin	60	Case series	2	21	20	4	84	0%	Effect on glomerular haemodynamics.
Cyclophosphamide	56	Case series	3	Paediatric	NR	<1	55	100%	Maximum 12-week course of 1–2 mg/kg per day.

*Denotes mean spot urine protein/creatinine ratio.

ALG: antilymphocyte globulin; Bx: biopsy; C: control; CsA: cyclosporine A; NR: not recorded; PE: plasma exchange; RF: renal function; Tx: transplant studies lack appropriate controls, and only limited conclusions can be drawn from them. Both plasma exchange and immunoadsorption can reduce proteinuria, often to baseline levels, but the effect is short-lived, with return of nephrotic range proteinuria within weeks to months after discontinuation of treatment. In one study plasma exchange was shown to improve the histological lesion of podocyte effacement [30]. In patients with more extensive glomerulosclerosis on biopsy, proteinuria responded less well to plasma exchange. There is no convincing evidence, however, to suggest that these treatments can alter the natural history of the disease process. Although some case reports claim long-term remission following the early institution of plasma exchange [33, 34], a prospective controlled trial of suitable size is needed to address this question fully. A small prospective study examining the effect of prophylactic plasma exchange pre- and post-transplant, in patients at high risk of recurrence, showed a reduced incidence and severity of recurrence in the treatment group [35]. Other treatment options include OKT3 [36]; cyclophosphamide, which appeared successful in a case series of three patients [37]; and indomethacin, which reduces proteinuria by affecting glomerular haemodynamics and is unlikely to alter the natural course of the disease [38]. Bilateral native nephrectomy prior to transplantation does not reduce the rate of recurrence, contrary to earlier belief [39].

To summarize, despite recent advances in understanding the pathophysiology of recurrent FSGS, there is currently no definitive treatment. Several unproven treatment protocols are employed by centres in North America. Such protocols may include high-dose steroids, a 12-week course of cyclophosphamide (during which azathioprine or mycophenolate immunosuppression is discontinued), and a 1 week course of plasmapheresis. If stable remission is not achieved with the above measures, patients may be converted from standard to high-dose cyclosporin therapy, starting at 10 mg/kg per day and increasing to a maximum of 30 mg/kg per day, with tapering following remission.

IgA nephropathy

Worldwide, IgA nephropathy is the most frequent form of glomerulonephritis leading to ESRD. Recurrence of IgA nephropathy in renal allografts is common. Most studies report approximately a 50% rate of histological recurrence within 6 months post-transplantation. When regular routine biopsies have been performed, mesangial IgA deposition may be seen within weeks post-transplantation. Interestingly, when kidneys from donors with subclinical IgA nephropathy have been inadvertently transplanted into recipients, mesangial IgA deposits are observed initially, but promptly resolve. Analysis of predictive risk factors for histological recurrence provides an interesting insight into the pathophysiology of this condition. High titres of circulating IgA complexes post-transplantation are associated with increased risk of histological recurrence [40]. Recurrence is reported to be more common following LRD transplantation and in HLA identical grafts, suggesting that genetic factors are important [41, 42]. However, a more recent analysis involving 49 transplants found no difference in the recurrence rate of IgA nephropathy between recipients of cadaveric versus living related grafts [43]. Prolonged time on dialysis prior to transplantation is not associated with reduced recurrence, suggesting that 'burn-out' of the disease process does not occur following ESRD.

Whereas there is general agreement on the rate of histological recurrence, there is less consensus on the clinical course of recurrence. Early studies, including the original description by Berger *et al.* in 1975, report that the clinical manifestations of recurrent disease are mild and that graft loss secondary to recurrence is rare [44]. In this series, seven patients with histological recurrence all had minor clinical features and none had renal impairment. It has been argued, however, that the duration of follow-up in these studies was too short, and failed to allow the relatively indolent nature of IgA nephropathy to manifest. More recent reports, involving longer follow-up, have noted significant graft dysfunction and high rates of graft loss. Kessler reported retrospectively on the outcome of 71 patients transplanted following ESRD secondary to biopsy-proven IgA nephropathy [45]. With a mean follow-up period extending over 5 years they found recurrent mesangial IgA deposition in 50%, and mesangial proliferation in 34% of patients biopsied. Nephrotic syndrome and subsequent graft failure developed in 15% of patients, all of whom had mesangial proliferation on the original transplant biopsy. Odem et al reported on the outcome post transplantation of 43 patients with primary IgA nephropathy [46]. In this study recurrent mesangial IgA deposits were observed in 60% of patients and 15% of patients had graft dysfunction secondary to recurrent disease. The major predictor in this series for recurrent disease was the length of time post-transplantation.

Risk factors for the progression of recurrent disease are similar to those for primary IgA nephropathy, namely heavy proteinuria, mesangial proliferation, glomerulosclerosis and hypertension [47]. Crescentic IgA nephropathy with rapid progression to ESRD is more likely to recur following transplantation [48] IgA anti-neutrophil cytoplasmic antibodies (IgA ANCA) have been detected in patients with recurrent crescentic IgA nephropathy, and it has been suggested that these autoantibodies highlight a subgroup of patients with severe disease and a mixed overlap syndrome between IgA nephropathy and microscopic polyarteritis [49]. The introduction of cyclosporin A therapy has not altered the incidence of histological recurrence, but according to one report may reduce the clinical severity of recurrent IgA disease [50]. However, these findings may be a reflection of shorter duration of follow-up in the cyclosporin-treated group. Certainly, studies examining the role of cyclosporin in the treatment of primary IgA nephopathy have shown a limited use for this agent [51]. There are no controlled trials and very few anecdotal data on the treatment of recurrent IgA disease. Due to the indolent nature of the disease most cases should probably be managed conservatively with good blood pressure control. In cases presenting with the nephrotic syndrome or deteriorating renal function in the absence of histological features of rejection then several unproven therapeutic options exist, including alternate-day steroids, cyclophosphamide or fish oil [51].

Despite the risk of recurrent disease, overall graft survival in patients whose primary disease was IgA nephropathy is good. Indeed several studies have shown higher graft survival in this transplant population compared with those transplanted for ERSD due to other forms of renal disease [52]. Closer observation shows that the benefit in graft survival occurs within 3 months of transplantation, perhaps due to less severe acute rejection. It has been proposed that immunological defects in IgA nephropathy favour allograft acceptance. Lim *et al.* found that the presence of high pretransplant serum levels of IgA antibodies to HLA class I molecules correlated with increased graft survival, and hypothesized that anti-HLA antibodies subserve an immunoprotective effect either by blocking anti-HLA IgG immunoglobulin or by somehow altering the cellular immune response [53].

Recurrent and de-novo *membranous glomerulonephritis*

Assessment of the rate of recurrence of membranous nephropathy is difficult, partly owing to the small numbers of reported cases (a consequence of the low prevalence of membranous as a causal nephropathy in ESRD), and partly due to the frequency of the condition arising *de novo* in the graft. Couchoud *et al.* reported on 19 patients with membranous nephropathy who were subsequently transplanted, and noted recurrence in five (26.6%) allografts [54]. Only one graft failed as a direct consequence of recurrence and mean graft survival was no worse than in the group without recurrence. The use of cyclosporin did not influence the recurrence rate and unexpectedly the only risk factor for recurrence identified was a prolonged period on dialysis prior to transplantation. A similar incidence of recurrence was reported in a review of anecdotal literature involving 24 cases [55]. A more recent, albeit smaller, retrospective study reported a higher rate of recurrence of 50% [56] of which two out of three patients developed progressive renal impairment. Recurrence in successive transplants has been reported [57].

There are few reports on the treatment of recurrent membranous nephropathy. Rapid remission of the nephrotic syndrome was reported with intravenous methylprednisolone and alternate-day steroids in a transplant patient with membranous nephropathy who reached ESRD with a diagnosis of chronic glomerulonephritis [58]. It is unclear whether this was a case of recurrent or *de-novo* membranous nephropathy.

De-novo membranous nephropathy in renal allografts is far more common (estimated incidence of 1–2% of all transplants) and is second only to transplant glomerulopathy (a feature of chronic rejection) as the major cause of nephrotic syndrome in the transplant recipient. The glomerular changes are identical to those seen in recurrent membranous nephropathy, and differentiation between the two relies on an accurate pretransplant diagnosis. Clinically, *de-novo* membranous nephropathy is reported to occur later and to have a more severe clinical course than recurrent membranous nephropathy; however, not all studies confirm this. In a large retrospective study of 1000 renal transplant patients, all of whom had a known primary histological diagnosis, *de-novo* membranous nephropathy developed in 19 patients (1.9%) [59]. Onset of proteinuria ranged from 2 to 58 months post-transplant. Nephrotic syndrome was present in six patients (33%). However, renal function was stable in all patients except four who lost grafts from chronic rejection. In another retrospective study of 872 renal transplants, *de-novo* membranous nephropathy was observed in 30 renal allografts (2%) at a mean time post-transplant of 62 months [60]. Nephrotic syndrome occurred in 62% and was not responsive to steroids. In this series, graft loss due to *de-novo* membranous glomerulopathy occurred in one patient and overall graft survival was the same as in controls.

De-novo membranous nephropathy is often associated with histological features of graft rejection and this may account for the high rates of graft loss reported in some series. In a series of 10 cases of *de-novo* membranous nephropathy reported by Troung *et al.*, six out of 10 patients developed the nephrotic syndrome and graft failure occurred in five (50%) of these patients [61]. All graft biopsies showed additional features of either humoral or cellular rejection. It is hypothesized that rejection-mediated graft injury uncovers previously hidden epitopes which leads to *in-situ* immune complex formation [61]. In keeping with this association, Montagnino *et al.* reported that the incidence of *de-novo* membranous nephropathy has decreased in the cyclosporin era [62], although a subsequent study found no difference in the incidence of *de-novo* membranous nephropathy in those patients receiving cyclosporin compared with those on azathioprine-based immunosuppression [60].

Hepatitis B and C infections are often observed in patients with *de-novo* membranous nephropathy. In one study 12 out of 19 patients with *de-novo* membranous nephropathy were positive for either hepatitis B or C, suggesting an important role for these viruses in the aetiology of this condition [59]. Other studies have found that the incidence of HCV infection in patients with *de-novo* membranous nephropathy is no different from that found in the total transplant population [63].

Mesangiocapillary glomerulonephritis

Both type I and type II mesangiocapillary glomerulonephritis (MCGN) can recur in renal allografts. The true incidence of recurrence of either condition is difficult to determine due to the paucity of reports in the literature. A confounding factor in the study of type I MCGN is the histological similarity to transplant glomerulopathy, a rejection-mediated phenomenon that also manifests as heavy proteinuria. Electron microscopy and immunofluorescence techniques help distinguish the former by the presence of subendothelial deposits and capillary wall C3 deposition.

In adults, the incidence of recurrence of type I MCGN has been estimated at 25% [11] and most of these patients underwent a progressive deterioration in graft function. Aggressive disease in the native kidneys is associated with a higher incidence of recurrence following transplantation. An extended interval on dialysis prior to transplantation does not appear to influence the recurrence rate [64]. Recurrence may occur within weeks, and manifests clinically as severe proteinuria and the nephrotic syndrome, and histologically by marked crescentic changes. When recurrence occurs, early graft failure is the rule rather than the exception [65]. Unlike in the native kidney, hypocomplementaemia is a poor marker of disease activity in the renal allograft [64]. Cyclosporin has not significantly altered the rate of recurrence or the severity of the disease in renal allografts [50]. Cahan *et al.* reported successful treatment of a case of recurrent crescentic type I MCGN, with nephrotic syndrome and progressive renal impairment, with intravenous steroids, dipyridamole and cyclophosphamide [66]. Muczynski reported remission of type I MCGN with plasmapheresis but lack of effect of cyclophosphamide in the same patient [67].

Type II MCGN has a much higher rate of histological recurrence, estimated at 88% in one major study [11], but unlike type I MCGN the clinical manifestations are often mild with lower rates of graft loss (approximately 10%). More aggressive disease associated with crescentic activity has been reported [68]. Recurrence in the second graft after loss of the first graft from recurrence has been described, but does not necessarily follow the same course. Neither hypocomplementaemia nor serum C3 nephritic factor is a marker of recurrent disease, casting doubt on the pathogenetic role of these serum factors [64, 69]. There is no proven treatment for recurrent type II MCGN, although plasma exchange has been reported to be successful in severe disease [70].

Recurrence of glomerulonephritis associated with systemic disease

Hepatitis C virus-associated type I MCGN

Hepatitis C virus (HCV) is the aetiological factor in a major proportion of previously described idiopathic type I MCGN [71]. Indeed it has been recently confirmed that hepatitis C infection may result in *de-novo* MCGN in renal allografts [72]. This is of particular concern given the high incidence of HCV infection in the ESRD population. In a cohort of 98 HCV-infected transplant patients, eight patients developed the nephrotic syndrome, of whom five patients (5%) had biopsy-proven MCGN [72]. Time of onset post-transplantation varied from 2 months to 10 years. Complement levels were low in only two patients and cryoglobulins were absent in all patients. Greater quantities of circulating immune complexes containing anti-HCV antibody and HCV antigen were found in patients with glomerular disease compared with a control group of HCV-infected transplant patients without MCGN. Gallay *et al.* reported two cases of *de-novo* MCGN in HCV-infected transplant recipients. Both presented with heavy proteinuria and progressive renal impairment, and disease progressed despite treatment with α-interferon [73]. The authors highlight the similarity of the histological and ultrastructural appearance (subendothelial electron-lucent material and poverty of capillary wall electron-dense deposits) of HCV-associated MCGN with transplant glomerulopathy, and question whether HCV infection is an aetiological agent in transplant glomerulopathy.

Haemolytic uraemic syndrome

Haemolytic uraemic syndrome (HUS) constitutes a triad of acute renal failure, microangiopathic haemolytic anaemia and thrombocytopenia. It represents a common pathophysiological response to a heterogeneous group of aetiological agents that mediate endothelial cell injury in the renal microvasculature. Both recurrent and *de-novo* HUS can occur in the renal allograft. The reported rate of recurrence varies (between 10% and 50%) and is almost certainly related to the aetiology of the original disease [4 74]. Whilst verotoxin-induced HUS in children is unlikely to recur, familial HUS can result in the repeated loss of renal allografts. The type of immunosuppression used may also influence the recurrence rate. However, a recent study showed that a positive family history of HUS was a much greater predictor of recurrence than the type of immunosuppression used [75]. In this series of 13 transplants in 11 patients, two of five grafts (40%) in patients on cyclosporin were lost from recurrence, whereas two of eight grafts were lost with FK 506 therapy (25%) [75]. The prognosis of recurrent HUS is poor with approximately 50% graft loss within 1 year post-transplantation. Several precautions should be taken to reduce the likelihood of recurrence. Firstly, transplantation should be delayed for at least 6 months after the primary disease has completely remitted. The choice of initial immunosuppression is dependent on the predicted likelihood of recurrence. Cyclosporin should not be used if recurrence occurred in the first transplant, and should be withheld initially, or dosage reduced, when a non-heart-beating donor kidney is transplanted. LRD grafts should be avoided owing to the familial pattern of prostacyclin synthesis abnormality and the report of early recurrence with LRD [74]. Finally, oral contraceptives should not be used, and there is sound theoretical basis for the prophylactic use of antiplatelet agents, e.g. aspirin and dipyridamole.

De-novo HUS in renal allografts is often associated with cyclosporin A usage and tends to occur early post-transplantation when cyclosporin levels are high. The mechanism of cyclosporin-induced HUS is complex and only partially resolved. Cyclosporin has been reported to decrease endothelial production of prostacyclin and nitric oxide and increase the production of thromboxane and endothelin, so promoting vasospasm, platelet aggregation and thrombosis [76]. Although FK 506 is often used as an alternative immunosuppressive agent in established transplant HUS, it is important to note that this agent, in addition to ALG and OKT3, has been associated with transplant HUS [77]. Other risk factors for *de-novo* HUS include the use of grafts from non-heart-beating donors, retransplantations, sensitized recipients [78], and combined kidney/pancreas transplantation. It is predicted that these factors amplify endothelial injury via ischaemic and immunological mechanisms. Caution should be taken when two or more risk factors coexist, and for this reason cyclosporin is often withheld in the early post-transplant period of non-heart-beating donor grafts.

The diagnosis of recurrent or *de-novo* HUS in the transplant patient is fraught with difficulties. Firstly, the extrarenal manifestations of HUS, such as thrombocytopenia and microangiopathic haemolytic anaemia, are often very mild and may only be indicated by small changes in serum lactate dehydrogenase and haptoglobin. Secondly, the histopathological features of HUS are shared by a variety of other disorders which may affect the transplant, including acute vascular rejection, malignant hypertension, and cyclosporin nephrotoxicity. Distinguishing cases of HUS from these other conditions is clearly important owing to the distinct treatment options required. Importantly, acute rejection may provoke both recurrent and *de-novo* HUS in the graft, making an accurate histological evaluation for rejection essential in patients with HUS.

Several studies have examined treatment options in transplant HUS [78–90]. All of these are small case series and are subject to the usual limitations. The mainstay of treatment is early institution of dialysis, rigorous blood pressure control and replacement blood transfusions. Platelets should not be transfused as this can further promote microvascular platelet aggregation. Cyclosporin should be discontinued, or dosage reduced, and appropriate alternative immunosuppression instituted. This is particularly important in view of the fact that recurrent HUS can be associated with acute rejection and that the pathological features can be representative of vascular rejection. Conversion to FK 506 has been associated with improved outcome in some reports [27]. To date recurrent or *de-novo* HUS has not been described with the newer immunosuppressive agents, including mycophenolate mofetil and rapamycin. There are no controlled trials assessing the effects of plasma exchange or plasma infusion in transplant HUS, and anecdotal data have given conflicting results [78, 83, 89]. It is interesting that two early studies reported successful treatment with thrombolytic therapy [85, 86].

Systemic lupus erythematosus

Recurrence of lupus nephritis in the renal allograft is extremely rare [91, 92]. Indeed the serological and clinical activity of SLE usually diminishes following the onset of ESRD and rarely returns, despite transplantation [93]. Several mechanisms have been proposed to explain this disease 'burn-out' following ESRD, including the immunosuppressive effects of uraemia, the removal of 'lupus factors' by dialysis or loss of renally produced mediators. None of these suggestions satisfactorily explain the low rate of recurrence of disease following transplantation. A recent review of the literature reports the incidence of recurrent lupus nephritis as 2.7%, and the incidence of positive lupus serology post-transplantation as 11% [94]. Some groups claim that the low rate of recurrence post-transplantation is secondary to immunosuppressive treatment. Indeed some studies [95, 96], but not all [91], have reported that recurrence is lower and graft survival better in patients on cyclosporin-based regimens, than on steroids and azathioprine alone. An increased risk of recurrence is seen in patients whose primary disease led to rapid onset of renal failure, and in these patients the histology of the recurrent disease mirrors that of the primary disease [94]. Recurrence is more likely in living related grafts; however, this does not significantly influence overall allograft survival in this group, which is better than in cadaveric allografts [94]. A recent large single-centre study involving 80 transplants in 69 patients whose primary disease was SLE, reported a mean 1- and 5-year graft survival of 82% and 64% respectively, results which compare favourably to renal transplantation irrespective of the primary disease [97]. Analysis of subgroups, however, showed that graft survival for cadaveric grafts was significantly worse than that for LRD (44% vs. 89%). Lower graft survival in cadaveric grafts was associated with an increased incidence of acute and chronic rejection.

The optimal timing of transplantation following ESRD is also controversial. Whilst it is pertinent to wait 6 months to allow possible return of renal function following a relapse of lupus nephritis, an important issue is whether transplantation should go ahead despite serological markers of active lupus. Several studies, but not all, report poorer outcome if transplantation occurs in patients with positive serological markers of disease [98]. Radhakrisham *et al.* compared the outcome of renal allografts in patients with or without anti-cardiolipin antibodies [99]. Predictably, the number of venous thromboses was greater in the anticardiolipin antibody positive group, supporting the use of prophylactic long-term antioagulation in these patients; however, there was no difference in the rate of graft loss or graft function. Renal transplant vein thrombosis has been reported in patients with anticardiolipin antibodies [99]. Recurrence of lupus nephritis is usually heralded by rising anti-DNA antibody titres and may be associated with extrarenal symptoms. Treatment has involved high-dose steroids and pulse cyclophosphamide, with variable success [100]. There is no longer an indication for plasmapheresis in this condition.

Wegener's granulomatosis and microscopic polyarteritis

Both Wegener's granulomatosis (WG) and microscopic polyarteritis (MP) can relapse in the transplant patient, despite chronic immunosuppressive therapy. Unfortunately, with both conditions, particularly the latter, only anecdotal data are available concerning the incidence of relapse and long-term outcome of these patients following transplantation. Based mainly on case reports and small case series, it is estimated that less than 20% of transplant patients with WG have a clinical relapse, and it appears that lung and upper respiratory tract are more commonly involved than the renal allograft [101]. Recurrence can occur at any time and may be several years post-transplantation [102]. Recurrence of renal limited forms of systemic vasculitis (idiopathic necrotizing crescentic glomerulonephritis) is considered rare [4]. Graft involvement usually manifests as deteriorating renal function with crescent formation, although nephrotic syndrome has been reported [103]. Extrarenal involvement resulting in ureteric stenosis and graft dysfunction has been reported [70].

Several studies show that relapse is more common and occurs earlier on cyclosporin than on azathioprine-based immunosuppression. A review of 15 patients by Clarke *et al.* found the relapse rate of WG to be appreciably lower (20% vs. 71%) in patients receiving azathioprine than in those receiving cyclosporin [104]. No recurrence was observed in 20 patients on triple-therapy immunosuppression combining the two agents [105]. When relapse does occur, cyclophosphamide has been shown to be very effective at inducing remission [101, 106]. Much interest concerns the role of antineutrophil cytoplasmic antibodies (ANCA) in guiding the time of transplantation and predicting future relapses following transplantation. ANCA levels correlate well with disease activity, and it is generally believed that one should wait until the ANCA titres are low before transplantation. However, successful transplantation has been reported by several groups even in the presence of elevated ANCA titres. One study reports successful transplantation of three patients with MP during clinical remission but persistently high antimyeloperoxidase ANCA titres. Following transplantation and initiation of triple-therapy immunosuppression, ANCA titres fell and no relapse occurred over a follow-up period of 38 months [107]. Rostaing *et al.* reported on eight patients with systemic vasculitis, of whom seven had raised ANCA titres before transplantation. Only one patient suffered a relapse over a mean follow-up of 38 months, and this patient was the only patient not receiving azathioprine in the immunosuppressive regimen [108]. Although studies support the value of ANCA in predicting a relapse of WG in native kidneys [109], such longitudinal studies have not been performed in transplant patients. It would be unwise to institute treatment on the basis of a rising ANCA titre alone; rather this should be an indicator of impending clinical relapse. To summarize, the post-transplant patient should receive both azathioprine- and cyclosporin-based immunosuppression, and when clinical and serological markers of relapse occur, azathioprine should be replaced by a 4–8 week course of cyclophosphamide. Cascade filtration apheresis reversed graft dysfunction and nephrotic syndrome in a case of recurrent ANCA positive WG occurring 5 years post-transplantation [103].

Anti-GBM disease

Despite a paucity of recent literature on recurrent anti GBM disease, there is a general consensus that the disease almost never recurs in renal allografts, providing anti-GBM titres are absent prior to transplantation. Cameron reports successful transplantation without recurrence in 20 patients with this condition [7]. Patients should wait for 6–12 months on dialysis, until anti-GBM antibodies are absent, prior to transplantation. If anti-GBM antibodies persist, and transplantation is considered urgent, then some centres advocate lowering titres with prednisolone, cyclophosphamide and plasma exchange prior to transplantation [110]. Native nephrectomy has no influence on anti-GBM antibody titres or recurrence. Even when anti-GBM titres are detectable at the time of transplantation, most patients develop only mild clinical features despite the presence of linear IgG deposition in the capillary walls [4]. Almkuist *et al.* report a case of recurrence in an isograft donated from an identical twin sibling [111]. Clinical renal function was not seriously impaired despite the presence of a crescentic nephritis, and the abnormalities resolved with steroid and azathioprine treatment. Recurrence is usually immediate, rarely accompanied by pulmonary haemorrhage, and should be treated with cyclophosphamide and plasma exchange.

De-novo anti-GBM disease may arise in renal allografts transplanted into patients with Alport's syndrome. Indeed this observation provided important clues to understanding the aetiology of Alport's syndrome. Patients with Alport's syndrome have one of several possible mutations in the genes encoding alpha chains of type IV collagen. The most common mutation is in the alpha 5 chain, but this also results in deficiency of the Goodpasture antigen (an epitope in the alpha 3 chain). When these patients receive a renal transplant, a proportion generate an immune response to the previously 'unseen' antigen within the graft glomerular basement membrane. A small percentage of these patients develop detectable circulating antibodies and crescentic nephritis [1]. Severe disease is seen more frequently in the second transplant due to sensitization. Clinical features usually develop within months post-transplantation of the first graft, and within weeks of a second tranplant. Treatment regimens involve cyclophosphamide and plasma exchange.

Henoch–Schönlein purpura

Although the natural history of Henoch–Schönlein purpura (HSP)-associated glomerulonephritis is usually one of complete resolution, a small subpopulation of patients with crescentic glomerulonephritis progress to ESRD. In areas where HSP is common, these cases make up a significant proportion of transplanted patients; greater than 10% in a Japanese centre [112]. Since the first case report in 1972, it is now well established that HSP can recur in both adult and paediatric transplant recipients. Recurrence often manifests in isolated renal allograft involvement, which is histologically indistinguishable from IgA nephropathy, so forging a link between these two diseases. Extrarenal manifestations of HSP, such as rash, arthralgia and abdominal pain, are not always associated with transplant recurrence. Histological recurrence can range in severity from isolated mesangial IgA deposition with normal glomerular histology, to mesangial and capillary wall IgA deposition associated with a membranoproliferative pattern and crescents. Histological recurrence occurs in both living related and cadaveric grafts; however, there is evidence to suggest that the use of living related grafts is associated with more severe renal involvement and worse outcome. In a Japanese series of living related transplants, nine out of 12 showed histological recurrence, of whom five had proteinuria and haematuria and two developed graft failure. None of the five cadaveric grafts in this series developed histological or clinical recurrence [112]. Meulders *et al.* pooled data from their own centre with those from the Japanese group and estimated the actuarial risk for renal recurrence and resulting graft loss to be 35% and 11% respectively at 5 years [113]. A factor associated with an increased recurrence rate was rapid progression of the original disease. A 1-year delay on dialysis prior to transplantation was not associated with reduced recurrence, nor was triple-therapy immunosuppression.

Conclusion

There are limited data on the treatment of recurrent glomerulonephritis in renal allografts. Even in recurrent primary focal segmental glomerulosclerosis (FSGS), a prominent threat to graft survival in paediatric transplantation, there are no large, prospective, controlled trials assessing treatment options. With the recent establishment of the United States Renal Allograft Recurrent Disease Registry (RARDR) and other registers, it is hoped that management strategies for recurrence, based on multicentre trials, will be developed that ultimately lead to improved outcome and graft survival in these patients. Until this information is available therapeutic decisions must be based on anecdotal data and information extrapolated from studies assessing treatment of glomerulonephritis in native kidneys. The impact that new immunosuppressive agents, including mycophenolate and rapamycin, will have on the development and outcome of recurrent disease is unknown. Finally, the study of recurrent and *de-novo* glomerulonephritis will continue to yield interesting insights into both the pathophysiology of glomerulonephritis and the immunobiology of transplant rejection.

References

1. Hariharan S, George V, Adams M *et al.* Recurrent and *de novo* glomerular disease after renal transplantation: a report from the Renal Allograft Recurrent Disease Registry (RARDR). Abstract: American Society of Transplant Physicians 1997; 309.
2. United Kingdom Transplant Support Services Authority. Renal Transplant Audit 1984–1993. Bristol: UKTSSA, 1995.

3. Broyer M, Selwood N, Brunner F. Recurrence of primary renal disease in kidney grafts: a European paediatric experience. J Am Soc Nephrol 1992;2:S255–7.
4. Matthew T. Recurrence of disease following renal transplantation. Am J Kidney Dis 1988;12: 85–96.
5. Cameron J. Recurrent primary disease and *de novo* nephritis following renal transplantation. Pediatr Nephrol 1991;5:412–21.
6. Michielsen P. Recurrence of the original disease. Does this influence renal graft failure?. [Review]. Kidney Int 1995;48:S79–84.
7. Cameron J. Recurrent disease in grafted kidneys. In: Tilney N, Strom T, Paul L, editors. Transplantation Biology: Cellular and Molecular Aspects. New York: Lippincott Raven; 1995:619–27.
8. Kotanko P, Pusey CD, Levy J. Recurrent glomerulonephritis following renal transplantation. Transplantation 1997;63:1045–52.
9. Hariharan S, Peddi V, First M *et al.* Recurrent and *de novo* renal disease after renal transplantation in the cyclosporine era: report from the Renal Allograft Recurrence Disease Registry. J Am Soc Nephrol. 1996;7:1910.
10. Kim EM, Striegel J, Kim Y, Matas AJ, Najarian JS, Mauer SM. Recurrence of steroid-resistant nephrotic syndrome in kidney transplants is associated with increased acute renal failure and acute rejection. Kidney Int 1994;45:1440–5.
11. Cameron J. Glomerulonephritis in renal transplants. Transplantation 1982;34:237–45.
12. Senguttuvan P, Cameron J, Hartley R. Recurrence of focal semental glomerulosclerosis in transplanted kidneys: analysis of incidence and risk factors in 59 allografts. Pediatr Nephrol 1990;4:21–8.
13. Garcia V, Abbud FM, Keitel E, Neumann J, Goldani JC. Recurrent focal glomerulosclerosis in renal allografts. Transplant Proc 1995;27:1084–5.
14. Tejani A, Stablein D. Recurrence of focal segmental glomerulosclerosis post transplantation: a special report of the North American Pediatric Renal Transplant Cooperative Study. J Am Soc Nephrol 1992;2(Suppl.3):S258–63.
15. Stephanian E, Matas AJ, Mauer SM *et al.* Recurrence of disease in patients retransplanted for focal segmental glomerulosclerosis. Transplantation 1992;53:755–7.
16. First MR. Living-related donor transplants should be performed with caution in patients with focal segmental glomerulosclerosis. [Review]. Pediatr Nephrol 1995;9:S40–2.
17. Ingulli E, Tejani A. Focal segmental glomerulosclerosis in children. [Review]. Curr Opin Pediatr 1995;7:176–81.
18. Conlon PJ, Butterly D, Albers F, Rodby R, Gunnells JC, Howell DN. Clinical and pathologic features of familial focal segmental glomerulosclerosis. Am J Kidney Dis 1995;26:34–40.
19. Banfi G, Colturi C, Montagnino G, Ponticelli C. The recurrence of focal segmental glomerulosclerosis in kidney transplant patients treated with cyclosporine. Transplantation 1990;50:594–6.
20. Ingulli E, Tejani A. Incidence, treatment, and outcome of recurrent focal segmental glomerulosclerosis posttransplantation in 42 allografts in children – a single-center experience. Transplantation 1991;51:401–5.
21. Fydrik J, Waldherr R, Mehls O, Scharer K. Long term follow up of transplanted children with focal segmental glomerulosclerosis. Pediatr Nephrol 1991;5:C49.
22. Zimmerman S. Increased urinary protein excretion in the rat produced by serum from a patient with recurrent focal glomerulosclerosis after renal transplantation. Clin Nephrol 1984; 22:32–8.
23. Savin VJ, Sharma R, Sharma M *et al.* Circulating factor associated with increased glomerular permeability to albumin in recurrent focal segmental glomerulosclerosis. N Eng J Med 1996; 334:878–83.
24. Sharma R, Sharma M, Ge X, McCarthy E, Savin V. Cyclosporine protects glomeruli from FSGS factor via an increase in cAMP. Transplantation 1996;62:1916–20.

25. Morales J, Andres A, Prieto C, Parag M, Guterriez Millet V, Rodicio J. Cyclosporin-induced partial and transient improvement of nephrotic syndrome in recurrent focal segmental glomerulosclerosis. Nephron 1989;53:283–4.
26. Srivastava R, Kalia A, Travis L, Diven S, Gugliuzza K, Rajaraman S. Prompt remission of post-renal transplant nephrotic syndrome with high-dose cyclosporine. Pediatr Nephrol 1994; 8:94.
27. McCauley J, Shapiro M, Jordan V *et al.* FK 506 in the management of nephrotic syndrome after renal transplantation. Transplant Proc. 1993;25:1351–4.
28. Laufer J, Ettenger R, Ho W, Cohen A, Marik J, Fine R. Plasma exchange for recurrent nephrotic syndrome following renal transplantation. Transplantation 1988;46:540–2.
29. Dantal J, Baatard R, Hourmont M, Cantarovich D, Buzelin F, Soullilou J. Recurrent nephrotic syndrome following renal transplantation in patients with focal glomerulosclerosis. Transplantation 1991;52:827–31.
30. Artero ML, Sharma R, Savin VJ, Vincenti F. Plasmapheresis reduces proteinuria and serum capacity to injure glomeruli in patients with recurrent focal glomerulosclerosis. Am J Kidney Dis 1994;23:574–81.
31. Mowry J, Marik J, Cohen A, Hogg R, Sahney S, Ettenger R. Treatment of recurrent focal segmental glomerulosclerosis with high-dose cyclosporine A and plasmapheresis. Transplant Proc 1993;25:1345–6.
32. Dantal J, Bigot E, Bogers W *et al.* Effects of plasma protein adsorption on protein excretion in kidney transplant recipients with recurrent nephrotic syndrome. N Eng Med J 1994;330:7–14.
33. Zimmerman S. Plasmapheresis and dipyridamole for recurrent focal glomerulosclerosis. Nephron 1985;40:241–5.
34. Torretta L, Perotti C, Costamanga L, Tarantino A, Salvaneschi L. Usefulness of plasma exchange in recurrent nephrotic syndrome following renal transplantation. Artif Org 1995;19: 96–8.
35. Kawaguchi H, Hattori M, Ito K, Takahashi K, Ota K. Recurrence of focal glomerulosclerosis of allografts in children: the efficacy of intensive plasma exchange therapy before and after renal transplantation. Transplant Proc 1994;26:7–8.
36. Zamora I, Simon J. OKT3: a therapeutic alternative in recurrence of focal glomerulosclerosis in the transplanted kidney? [letter]. Nephrol Dial Transplant 1993;8:11.
37. Kershaw DB, Sedman AB, Kelsch RC, Bunchman TE. Recurrent focal segmental glomerulosclerosis in pediatric renal transplant recipients: successful treatment with oral cyclophosphamide. Clin Transplant 1994;8:546–9.
38. Kooijmans CM, Tegzess AM, Bruijn JA, Florijn KW, Van Es L, Van der Woude F. Indomethacin treatment of recurrent nephrotic syndrome and focal segmental glomerulosclerosis after renal transplantation. Nephrol Dial Transplant 1993;8:469–73.
39. Odorico JS, Knechtle SJ, Rayhill SC *et al.* The influence of native nephrectomy on the incidence of recurrent disease following renal transplantation for primary glomerulonephritis. Transplantation 1996;61:228–34.
40. Lesavre P, Diegeon M, Bach J. Analysis of circulating IgA and detection of immune complexes in primary IgA nephropathy. Clin Exp Immunol 1982;48: 61–9.
41. Bachman U, Biava C, Amend W *et al.* The clinical course of IgA nephropathy and Henoch-Schönlein purpura following renal transplantation. Transplantation 1986;42:511–15.
42. Brensilver J, Mallat S, Scholes J, McCabe R. Recurrent IgA nephropathy in living related donor transplantation: recurrence or transmission of familial disease. Am J Kidney Dis 1988; 12:147–51.
43. Frohnert P, Velosa J, Donadio J, Sterioff S. Renal transplantation in IgA nephropathy: the effect of HLA matching on recurrence of primary disease. Transplant Proc 1994;26:1892.
44. Berger J, Yaneva H, Nabarra B, Barbanel C. Recurrence of mesangial deposition of IgA after renal transplantation. Kidney Int 1975;7:232–4.
45. Kessler M, Hiesse C, Hestin D, Mayeux D, Boubenider K, Charpentier B. Recurrence of immunoglobulin A nephropathy after renal transplantation in the cyclosporine era. Am J Kidney Dis 1996;28:99–104.

46. Odem J, Peh C, Clarkson A *et al.* Recurrent mesangial IgA nephritis following renal transplantation. Nephrol Dial Tranplant 1994;9:309–12.
47. Kimata N, Tanabe K, Ishikawa N *et al.* Correlation between proteinuria and prognosis of transplant IgA nephropathy. Transplant Proc 1996;28:1537–9.
48. Streather C, Scoble J. Recurrent IgA nephropathy in a renal allograft presenting as crescentic glomerulonephritis. Nephron 1994;66:113–14.
49. Martin S, Audain M, Baranger T *et al.* Recurrence of IgA nephropathy with IgA anti-neutrophil cytoplasmic antibodies following renal transplantation. Am J Kidney Dis 1997; 29:125–31.
50. Tomlanovich S, Vincenti F, Amend W *et al.* Is cyclosporine effective in preventing the recurrence of immune mediated glomerular disease after tranplantation? Transplant Proc 1988;20:285–8.
51. Galla J. IgA nephropathy. Kidney Int 1995;47:377–87.
52. Lim E, Terasaki P. High survival rate of kidney transplants in IgA nephropathy patients. Clin Transplant 1992;6:100.
53. Lim E, Chia D, Gjertson D, Koka P, Terasaki P. *In vitro* studies to explain high renal allograft survival in IgA nephropathy patients. Transplantation 1993;55:996–9.
54. Couchoud C, Pouteil-Noble C, Colon S, Touraine JL. Recurrence of membranous nephropathy after renal transplantation: incidence and risk factors in 1614 patients. Transplantation 1995;59:1275–9.
55. Davison AM, Johnston PA. Allograft membranous nephropathy. [Review]. Nephrol Dial Transplant 1992;1:114–8.
56. Marcen R, Mampaso F, Teruel F, Rivera M, Orofino L. Membranous nephropathy: recurrence after kidney transplantation. Nephrol Dial Transplant 1996;11:1129–33.
57. Innes A, Woodrow G, Boyd SM, Beckingham IJ, Morgan AG. Recurrent membranous nephropathy in successive renal transplants. Nephrol Dial Transplant 1994;9:323–5.
58. Johnston PA, Goode NP, Aparicio SR, Davison AM. Membranous allograft nephropathy: remission of nephrotic syndrome with pulsed methylprednisolone and high-dose alternate-day steroids. Transplantation 1993;55:214–6.
59. Levy M, Charpentier B. *De novo* membranous glomerulonephritis in renal allografts: report of 19 cases in 1550 transplant recipients. Transplant Proc 1983;15:1099–101.
60. Schwarz A, Krause PH, Offermann G, Keller F. Impact of *de novo* membranous glomerulonephritis on the clinical course after kidney transplantation. Transplantation 1994;58:650–4.
61. Troung L, Gelfand J, D'Agati V *et al. De novo* membranous glomerulonephropathy in renal allografts: a report of ten cases and review of the literature. Am J Kidney Dis 1989;14:131–44.
62. Montagnino G, Colturi C, Banfi G, Aroldi A, Tarantino A, Ponticelli C. Membranous nephropathy in cyclosporine-treated renal transplant recipients. Transplantation 1989;47: 725–7.
63. Hammond H, Haem J, Laurent B, Alamartine E, Diab N. Glomerular disease during HCV infection in renal transplantation. Nephrol Dial Transplant 1996;11(Suppl.4):54–5.
64. Curtis J, Wyatt R, Bhathena D. Renal transplantation for patients with type 1 and type 2 membranoproliferative glomerulonephritis. Serial complement and nephritic factor measurements and the problem of recurrent disease. Am J Med 1979;66:216–25.
65. Cheigh J, Mouradien J, Suslin M. Kidney transplant nephrotic syndrome: relationship between allograft histopathology and natural course. Kidney Int 1980;18:358–65.
66. Cahen R, Trolliet P, Dijoud F, Megri K, Francois B. Severe recurrence of type I membranoproliferative glomerulonephritis after transplantation: remission on steroids and cyclophosphamide. Transplant Proc 1995;27:1746–7.
67. Muczynski KA. Plasmapheresis maintained renal function in an allograft with recurrent membranoproliferative glomerulonephritis type I. Am J Nephrol 1995;15:446–9.
68. Eddy A, Sibley R, Mauer S, Kim Y. Renal allograft failure due to recurrent dense intramembranous deposit disease. Clin Nephrol 1984;21:305–13.

69. Fremeaux BV, Weiss L, Brun P, Kazatchkine MD. Selective disappearance of C3NeF IgG autoantibody in the plasma of a patient with membranoproliferative glomerulonephritis following renal transplantation. Nephrol Dial Transplant 1994;9:811–4.
70. Oberkircher O, Enama M, West J, Campbell P, Moran J. Regression of recurrent membranoproliferative glomerulonephritis Type II in a transplanted kidney after plasmapheresis therapy. Transplant Proc 1988;20:418.
71. Johnson R, Gretch D, Yamabe H. Membranoproliferative glomerulonephritis associated with hepatitis C virus infection. N Eng J Med 1993;328:465–70.
72. Roth D, Cirocco R, Zucker K *et al. De novo* membranoproliferative glomerulonephritis in hepatitis C virus-infected renal allograft recipients. Transplantation 1995;59:1676–82.
73. Gallay BJ, Alpers CE, Davis CL, Schultz MF, Johnson RJ. Glomerulonephritis in renal allografts associated with hepatitis C infection: a possible relationship with transplant glomerulopathy in two cases. Am J Kidney Dis 1995;26:662–7.
74. Hebert D, Kim E, Sibley R, Mauer S. Post transplantation outcome of patients with hemolytic uremic syndrome: update. Pediatr Nephrol 1991;5:162–7.
75. Scantlebury VP, Shapiro R, McCauley J *et al.* Renal transplantation under cyclosporine and FK 506 for hemolytic uremic syndrome. Transplant Proc 1995;27:842–3.
76. Agarwal A, Mauer SM, Matas AJ, Nath KA. Recurrent hemolytic uremic syndrome in an adult renal allograft recipient: current concepts and management. [Review]. J Am Soc Nephrol 1995; 6:1160–9.
77. Doutrelepont JM, Abramowicz D, Florquin S, de PL, Goldman M, Kinnaert P, Vereerstraeten P. Early recurrence of hemolytic uremic syndrome in a renal transplant recipient during prophylactic OKT3 therapy. Transplantation 1992;53:1378–9.
78. Candinas D, Keusch G, Schlumpf R, Burger HR, Weder W, Largiader F. Prognostic factors of hemolytic uremic syndrome in renal allografts. Transplant Proc 1993;25:1041–2.
79. Buturovic J, Kandus A, Malvorth M, Bren A, Drinovec J. Cyclosporine associated hemolytic uremic syndrome in four renal allograft recipients: resolution without specific therapy. Transplant Proc 1990;22:1726–7.
80. Epstein M, Landsberg D. Cyclosporine induced thrombotic microangiopathy resulting in renal allograft loss and its successful reuse: a report of two cases. Am J Kidney Dis 1991;17: 346–8.
81. Giroux l, Smeesters C, Corman J. Hemolytic uremic syndrome in renal allografted patients treated with cyclosporine. Can J Physiol Pharmacol 1987;65:1125–31.
82. Grino J, Caralps A, Carreras L. Apparent recurrence of hemolytic uremic syndrome in azathioprine treated allograft recipients. Nephron 1988;49:301–4.
83. Hochstetler L, Flanigan M, Lager D. Transplant associated thrombotic microangiopathy: the role of IgG administration as initial therapy. Am J Kidney Dis 1994;23:444–50.
84. Noel C, Daunier P, Hazzen M. Incidence and clinical profile of microvascular complications in renal allografted patients treated with cyclosporine. Ann Intern Med. 1992;143:33–6.
85. Schlanger R, Henry M, Sommer B, Ferguson R. Identification and treatment of cyclosporine-associated allograft thrombosis. Surgery 1986;100:329–33.
86. Sommer B, Henry M, Ferguson R. Obliterative renal arteriopathy following cyclosporine therapy. Transplant Proc 1986;17:1285–6.
87. Conlon P, Brennan D, Pfaf W *et al.* Renal transplantation in adults with thrombotic thrombocytopenic purpura/haemolytic uraemic syndrome. Nephrol Dial Transplant 1996;11:1810–4.
88. Van Den Berg-Wolf M, Kootte A, Weening J, Paul L. Recurrent hemolytic uremic syndrome in a renal transplant patient and review of the Leiden experience. Transplantation 1988;45: 248–51.
89. Venkat K, Tkach D, Kupin W *et al.* Reversal of cyclosporine associated hemolytic uremic syndrome by plasma exchange with fresh frozen plasma replacements in renal transplant recipients. Transplant Proc 1991;23:1256–7.

90. Young B, Marsh C, Alpers C, Davis C. Cyclosporine-associated thrombotic microangiopathy/hemolytic uremic syndrome following kidney and kidney–pancreas transplantation. Am J Kidney Dis 1996;28:561–71.
91. Bumgardener G, Mauer S, Payne W. Single-center 1–15 year results of renal transplantation in patients with systemic lupus erythematosus. Transplantation 1983;46:703–9.
92. Sumrani N, Miles AM, Delaney V *et al.* Renal transplantation in cyclosporine-treated patients with end-stage lupus nephropathy. Transplant Proc 1992;24:1785–7.
93. Coplon N, Disken C, Peterson J, Swenson R. The long term clinical course of systemic lupus erythematosus in end-stage renal disease. N Eng J Med 1983;308:186–90.
94. Mojcik CF, Klippel JH. End-stage renal disease and systemic lupus erythematosus. [Review]. Am J Med 1996;101:100–7.
95. Zara C, Lipkowitz G, Perri N. Renal transplantation and end-stage lupus nephropathy in the cyclosporine and precyclosporine eras. Transplant Proc 1989;21:2031–2.
96. el Shahawy M, Aswad S, Mendez RG, Bangsil R, Mendez R, Massry SG. Renal transplantation in systemic lupus erythematosus: a single-center experience with sixty-four cases. Am J Nephrol 1995;15:123–8.
97. Lochhead K, Pirsch J, D'Alessandro A. Risk factors for renal allograft loss in patients with systemic lupus erythematosus. Kidney Int 1996;49:512–17.
98. Yakub Y, Freeman R, Pabico R. Renal transplantation in systemic lupus erythematosus. Nephron 1981;27:197–201.
99. Radhakrishnan J, Valeri A, Kunis C, Appel GB. Use of cyclosporin in lupus nephritis. [Review]. Contrib Nephrol 1995;114:59–72.
100. Goss J, Cole B, Jendrisak M. Renal transplantation for systemic lupus erythematosus and recurrent lupus nephritis: a single centre experience and review of the literature. Transplantation 1991;52:512.
101. Rosenstein ED, Ribot S, Ventresca E, Kramer N. Recurrence of Wegener's granulomatosis following renal transplantation. [Review]. Br J Rheumatol 1994;33:869–71.
102. Fogazzi GB, Banfi G, Allegri L, Bignardi L. Late recurrence of systemic vasculitis after kidney transplantation involving the kidney allograft. Adv Exp Med Biol 1993;336:503–6.
103. Branger B, Zabadani B, Vecina F, Mayor M, Dracon M. Late relapse of rapidly progressive glomerulonephritis (RPGN) in a transplant patient: efficacy of apheresis. Transplant Proc 1995;27:1748.
104. Clarke A, Bitton A, Eappen R, Danoff D, Esdaile J. Treatment of Wegener's granulomatosis after renal transplantation: Is cyclosporin the preferred treatment? Transplantation 1990;50: 1047–51.
105. Schmitt WH, Haubitz M, Mistry N, Brunkhorst R, Erbsloh MB, Gross WL. Renal transplantation in Wegener's granulomatosis [letter]. Lancet 1993;342:8875.
106. Grotz W, Wanner C, Rother E, Schollmeyer P. Clinical course of patients with antineutrophil cytoplasm antibody positive vasculitis after kidney transplantation. Nephron 1995;69:234–6.
107. Frasca G, Neri L, Martello M, Sestigiani E, Borgnino L, Bonomini V. Renal transplantation in patients with microscopic polyarteritis and antimyeloperoxidase antibodies: report of three cases. Nephron 1996;72:82–5.
108. Rostaing L, Modesto A, Oksman F, Cisterne J, Mao G, Durand D. Outcome of patients with antineutrophil cytoplasmic autoantibody-associated vasculitis following cadaveric kidney transplantation. Am J Kidney Dis 1997;29:96–102.
109. Cohen Tervaert J, Huitema M, Hene R. Prevention of relapses in Wegener's granulomatosus by treatment based on antineutrophil cytoplasmic antigen titre. Lancet 1990;336:709–11.
110. Couser W, Wallace A, Monaco A, Lewis E. Successful renal transplantation in patients with circulating antibody to glomerular basement: report of two cases. Clin Nephrol 1973;1:381.
111. Almkuist R, Buckalew V, Hirszel P, Maher J. Recurrence of anti-glomerular basement membrane antibody mediated glomerulonephritis in an isograft. Clin Immunol Immunopathol 1981;18:54–60.
112. Hasegawa A, Kawamura T, Ito H, Hasegowa O, Ogawa O. Fate of renal grafts with recurrent Henoch–Schönlein purpura nephritis in children. Transplant Proc 1989;21:2130–3.

113. Meulders Q, Pirson Y, Cosyns JP, Squifflet JP, van Ypersele de Strihou C. Course of Henoch–Schönlein nephritis after renal transplantation. Report on ten patients and review of the literature. [Review]. Transplantation 1994;58:1179–86.

10. Glomerulonephritis in pregnancy

S. ABE and M.D. LINDHEIMER

Introduction

Nephrologists are often asked to advise women with glomerulonephritis, who wish to conceive and to participate in the management of their pregnancies. This requires an awareness both of the influence pregnancy has on the natural history of many kidney disorders, and how specific diseases influence gestational outcome. This chapter will review data pertinent to these issues and suggest guidelines for counselling and managing gravidas with a variety of glomerular diseases. First, however, will be a brief review of the changes in the renal tract which occur during gestation, the knowledge of which is important for the detection and treatment of renal disease in pregnant women.

The influence of pregnancy on the urinary system and haemodynamics

Functional changes

Pregnancy is characterized by marked changes in renal function [1–3]. A significant elevation of glomerular filtration rate (GFR), as estimated by endogenous creatinine clearance (Ccr), is apparent 4 weeks after conception, peaking approximately 50% above the pre-pregnant value 9–11 weeks later, then sustained through gestational week 36, after which a 15–20% decrement may occur. Studies in which GFR was measured by inulin clearance have confirmed the marked increase in renal haemodynamics which occurs in human pregnancy. Renal plasma flow (RPF), measured by para-aminohippurate clearance (C_{PAH}), is also 50–80% higher than the non-pregnant value during the first and second trimesters, and then decreases by approximately 25% near term (Figure 10.1) [1].

The mechanisms responsible for these renal haemodynamic changes during pregnancy are not fully understood. Though cardiac output and plasma volume increase during pregnancy, the time courses of these changes may not parallel those of GFR and RPF increases. Hormones whose circulating levels increase during gestation, including aldosterone, deoxycorticosterone, progesterone, prolactin and chorionic gonadotropin (hCG), may augment renal haemodynamics but none appears to have a sufficient effect to account for all of the changes seen [1, 2].

C.D. Pusey (ed.), The Treatment of Glomerulonephritis, 201–218.

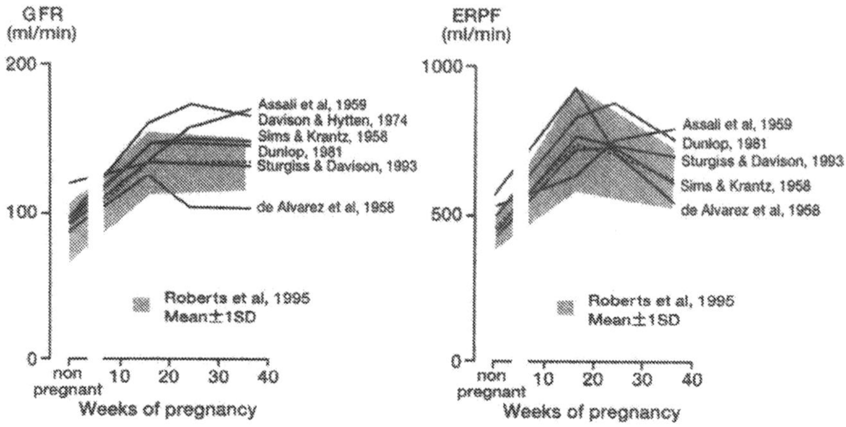

Figure 10.1 Serial changes in glomerular filtration rate (GFR) (left panel) and effective renal plasma flow (ERPF) (right panel) during pregnancy. Changes reported by several workers are superimposed on the mean (dashed line) ±1 standard deviation (shaded area), from a study by Roberts M, Lindheimer MD and Davison JM (Am J Physiol 1996;270:F338–43). (Reproduced from reference 1, with permission)

Micropuncture studies in pregnant animals, and the measurement of glomerular permselectivity to neutral dextrans in gravid humans have shed light into what may occur in individual nephrons during gestation [1, 3]. First, GFR increases during pregnancy in the rat due to a rise in the single nephron plasma flow rate, the renal vasodilatation involving an even reduction of afferent and efferent arteriolar pressures with glomerular capillary pressure remaining constant. Similarly, theoretical analysis of dextran sieving curves measured during human pregnancy also suggests the GFR rise to be due to increased renal plasma flow without an increase in glomerular capillary pressure. Thus, failure of glomerular capillary pressure to rise despite marked increases in renal haemodynamics should allay the fears of some that hyperfiltration in normal pregnancy is potentially harmful to the kidney.

An appreciation of the rise in GFR is essential when evaluating renal disease in normal pregnant women. The average ± SD value of serum creatinine is 0.46 ± 0.13 mg/dl (41 ± 12 μmol/L) and that of serum urea nitrogen (SUN) 8.7 ± 1.5 mg/dl (3.1 ± 0.5 mmol/L). A serum creatinine of 0.8 mg/dl (71 μmol/L) or higher, or a SUN of 14 mg/dl (5.0 mmol/L) or higher, thus suggests decreased renal function. In essence, non-pregnant values may reflect renal dysfunction in pregnant women [1].

GFR varies with position, especially in late pregnancy when GFR may be 20% lower in the supine than in the lateral recumbent position [1]. Patients with mild renal dysfunction also show GFR increments, as indicated in Figure 10.2 [4]. Therefore, results from a single GFR measurement should always be evaluated with caution.

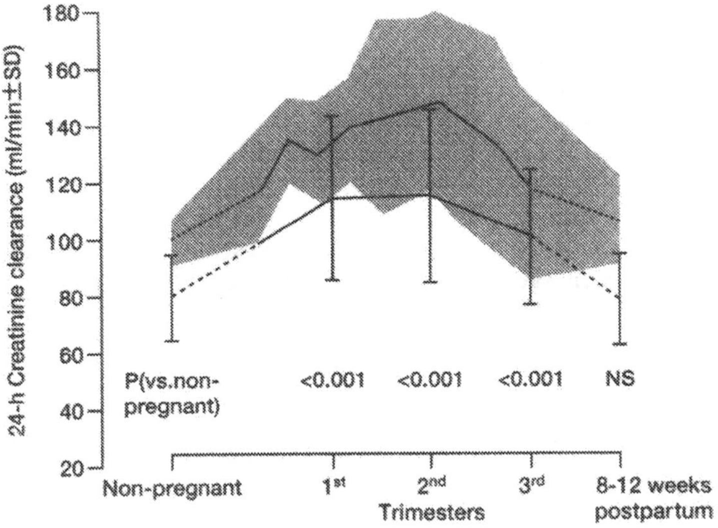

Figure 10.2 Serial 24-h creatinine clearance (mean ± 1 SD) before, during and after pregnancy in 26 women with mild chronic renal disease (solid line). Data from 10 healthy subjects (mean ± 1 SD) shown by hatched area. (From reference 4, with permission)

Tubular function also changes. Glucosuria of pregnancy can occur even with normal blood glucose concentrations and glucose tolerance. The increase in urinary glucose is due to the large filtered load, which in some gravidas may exceed the tubular resorptive capacity for this sugar. However, pregnancy-related change in the glucose threshold and/or features of the glucose titration curve may also contribute to glucosuria [1, 2].

The increased GFR also leads to increased clearance of uric acid (C_{UA} increases from 6–12 ml/min to 12–20 ml/min). This is due to changes in both GFR and the tubular handling of urate, and results in a corresponding decrease in serum uric acid (from 4.0–6.0 mg/dl to 3.0–4.0 mg/dl or from 238–357 μmol/L to 178–238 μmol/L) [1]. Therefore, a uric acid level of more than 5.5 mg/dl (327 μmol/L) is abnormal, and a rise to such levels in the absence of a concomitant increase in creatinine levels may be a sign of superimposed pre-eclampsia. Furthermore, the plasma uric acid increment correlates roughly with the severity of pre-eclampsia.

Haemodynamics

Blood pressure decreases in early pregnancy and in mid-pregnancy diastolic pressures are generally 10–15 mmHg lower than postpartum levels. Blood pressure rises after mid-pregnancy and may reach pre-pregnancy levels at term.

Since cardiac output rises dramatically in the first trimester, and remains elevated until term, the decrease in blood pressure is due to a marked decrement in peripheral vascular resistance. The reasons for these changes are discussed elsewhere [5].

These alterations in blood pressure are clinically relevant. Mild essential hypertension can be masked by a first trimester fall in blood pressure. Similarly, an erroneous diagnosis of pre-eclampsia may be made when blood pressure rises near term. In these respects, diastolic pressures of 75 mmHg and 85 mmHg in the second and third trimester respectively, considered normal in non-pregnant women, should be watched closely when present in gravidas.

Altered anatomy

Anatomical changes occur in the kidney during pregnancy [1, 3]. Renal length increases by nearly 1 cm during gestation, based on data obtained immediately after delivery and at 6 months postpartum. Ultrasound studies indicate that renal parenchymal volume is also increased. The most evident changes are dilatation of the calyces, renal pelvis and ureter, and during gestation it is difficult to differentiate between the 'physiological' dilatation of the urinary tract and obstructive uropathy. The etiology of these changes is poorly understood, but both hormonal factors and obstruction of the ureters by the enlarged uterus have been implicated [1].

Stasis of urine in the collecting system predisposes to urinary tract infections, which may rapidly become virulent, as well as difficulties in obtaining timed urine collections for kidney function tests. One should always hydrate the patient before starting and ending a 24-h collection when measuring clearances and excretion rates in order to minimize errors. There is also an 'overdistension syndrome' characterized by abdominal pain, variable increases in serum creatinine, an exaggeration of the physiological hydronephrosis on ultrasonography or pyelography, and even hypertension. Some patients have been treated successfully by the placement of ureteral stents, with renal function improving and blood pressure normalizing; the stents are removed postpartum without recurrence of the syndrome [1].

Pregnancy in women with glomerulonephritis

An older view that pregnancy was dangerous with pre-existing renal disease has been replaced with cautious optimism. This is based on a growing number of studies, the authors of which have concluded that with close supervision, and when renal function is stable and hypertension absent prior to conception, the gestation succeeds without evidence of progression of the renal disease [1, 3].

Prognosis based on histological diagnosis

Nowadays it is common for women with chronic glomerulonephritis (CGN) to consider seriously pregnancy. However, the clinical diagnosis of CGN includes multiple aetiologies and varies markedly in severity. Since renal biopsy has become a routine clinical examination in nephritic patients, the actual histological diagnosis has replaced the general term 'CGN' in many cases. Several investigators have attempted to analyse the relationship between histological diagnosis and pregnancy outcome [4, 6–11]. Imbasciati *et al.* [12] summarized six studies of pregnancy in women with various forms of underlying glomerulonephritis, reported in the 1980s, as shown in Table 10.1. Percentages of perinatal loss, decreased renal function and increased blood pressure were slightly higher among patients with focal glomerulosclerosis (FGS) and IgA nephropathy than the averages of all patients. The courses of these two diseases during and after gestation have been sources of controversy.

Packham *et al.* [13] reported hypertension in 74% of their pregnant FGS patients, 45% of whom were severely hypertensive, together with renal functional deterioration in 49% and a fetal loss rate of 45%. On the other hand, Surian *et al.* [6] and Jungers *et al.* [9] reported favourable outcomes in FGS patients whose renal function before or in early pregnancy was preserved, and who were normotensive. As the number of patients is limited, it is difficult to compare these data according to the severity of histological involvement. Some patients with FGS apparently progress to end-stage renal failure as part of the natural course of their disease. Thus, evaluation of pregnancy in FGS is difficult. More data are necessary to resolve this issue.

IgA nephropathy is another disorder of which the clinical course during and after pregnancy is disputed. As this is the most common renal disease among women of child-bearing age, it is a clinically significant problem [14]. Kincaid-Smith and Fairley [10] reported substantial declines in renal function, often irreversible, in 22% of their patients. They also described the *de-novo* appearance of hypertension in 63%, the high blood pressure persisting postpartum in 16%. The fetal loss rate in their series was 27%. In contrast, Jungers *et al.* [9] detected no adverse effects of pregnancy on the natural course of IgA nephropathy.

Our results are consistent with those of Jungers *et al.* We performed a prospective study during pregnancy in 36 women with IgA nephropathy, and continued to measure their renal function for an average of 5 years following the index pregnancy [15]. Table 10.2 summarizes the serial measurements of endogenous creatinine clearance in these subjects, as well as in a control group who chose not to conceive. Notably, the index pregnancy had no adverse effects on the remote renal prognosis of these women. There were, however, several patients who progressed to renal failure during the follow-up period. Of interest, they had comparatively severe histological changes not only in the glomeruli but also in the tubules, interstitium and arterioles, prior to conception. In fact, in three of the pregnant and two of the non-pregnant patients,

Table 10.1 Fetal and maternal outcome of pregnancies in women with primary glomerulonephritis

Histology	Pregnancies/ patients	Spontaneous abortion[a]	Perinatal loss[b]	Preterm delivery[bc]	Renal function decrease[c]		Blood pressure increase[c]	
					Reversible	Progressive	Reversible	Permanent
Focal glomerulosclerosis	85/61	2/58 (3%)	19/81 (23%)	25/79 (32%)	11/84 (13%)	4/84 (5%)	27/84 (32%)	8/84 (10%)
Membranous nephropathy	110/70	11/95 (12%)	4/92 (4%)	28/79 (35%)	3/97 (3%)	2/97 (2%)	21/97 (22%)	3/97 (3%)
Membranoproliferative	165/98	23/138 (17%)	11/133 (8%)	25/134 (19%)	9/164 (6%)	5/164 (3%)	31/164 (20%)	20/164 (12%)
IgA nephritis	268/166	12/229 (5%)	36/246 (15%)	43/208 (21%)	28/230 (12%)	5/230 (2%)	58/230 (25%)	27/230 (12%)
Mesangial proliferative[d]	278/163	14/275 (5%)	32/261 (12%)	19/223 (9%)	14/243 (2%)	7/243 (3%)	88/243 (36%)	16/243 (7%)
All types	906/558	62/795 (8%)	102/813 (13%)	140/723 (19%)	65/818 (8%)	23/818 (3%)	225/818 (27%)	74/818 (9%)

Cumulative data from six studies [4, 6–9, 11]. Therapeutic abortions were excluded from calculation of pregnancy outcome.

[a]The series of Surian *et al.* [6] was not considered since it does not include early spontaneous abortion.
[b]Referred to fetuses >20 weeks.
[c]Excluding the series of Abe *et al.* [7] who do not report data on preterm deliveries and on outcomes of renal diseases for each type of nephritis.
[d]Including focal and diffuse proliferative nephritis [4, 7, 11]. (From reference 12, with permission of S. Karger AG, Basel).

Table 10.2 Course of GFR (ml/min) in pregnant and non-pregnant women with IgA nephropathy

	Pregnant (n=36)	Non-pregnant (n=35)
Initial check-up	83±13	87±15
1 year	93±22	87±18
2 years	85±19	80±17
3 years	80±19	78±18
4 years	73±23	73±22
5 years	69±28	69±24
Difference between initial and 5 year GFRs	16±20	19±15

In the above data, all pregnancies occurred within 2 years of the renal check-up with biopsy (mean ± 1 SD) (From reference 15, with permission of Dustri-Verlag Dr Karl Feistle)

maintenance haemodialysis was initiated during follow-up. The number of patients is small but these outcomes appear to reflect the natural course of IgA nephropathy, i.e. approximately 30% of patients gradually progress to end-stage renal failure [16]. Thus, knowledge of histology from a renal biopsy, as well as pre-pregnancy renal function and blood pressure, aid in the pre-conception counselling of women with IgA nephropathy.

Prognosis based on degree of renal dysfunction

Overview

Table 10.3 summarizes a review of the literature on 2813 pregnancies in 1902 women with renal disease published by Davison and Baylis [3]. The authors reported the short- and long-term maternal prognosis as well as fetal outcome, breaking the data down in terms of mild (serum creatinine ⩽1.4 mg/dl or ⩽125 μmol/L), moderate (1.4–2.8 mg/dl or 125–250 μmol/L) and severe (>2.8 mg/dl or >250 μmol/L) renal impairment. Not surprisingly, those with severe renal impairment had significantly more problems during pregnancy, a higher fetal loss rate and more long-term problems. In contrast, women with normal or mildly decreased renal function usually had a successful obstetric outcome, and pregnancy did not adversely affect the course of their renal disease. This latter point has been further supported by a case–control study by Jungers and colleagues, based on their 25-year experience with 360 women with CGN who did (n = 171) or did not (n = 189) conceive (Figure 10.3) [17]. These data underscore the importance of stable, and at most a modest, decrement in renal function prior to conception as a predictor of uneventful pregnancy.

Table 10.3 Pregnancy implications for women with chronic renal disease

Renal status	Serum creatinine mg/dl (μmol/L)	Problems in pregnancy (%)	Successful obstetric outcome (%)	Problems over the long term (%)
Mild	<1.4 (<125)	26	96 (85)	<3 (9)
Moderate	1.4–2.8 (125–250)	47	89 (59)	25 (71)
Severe	>2.8 (>250)	86	46 (8)	53 (92)

Estimates based on 1902 women per 2813 pregnancies (1973–93) having attained at least 28 weeks of gestation. Figures in parentheses by the last two columns refer to outcome when complications developed before 28 weeks of gestation. Collagen diseases are not included. (Modified from reference 3, with permission of Mosby-Year Book, Inc.)

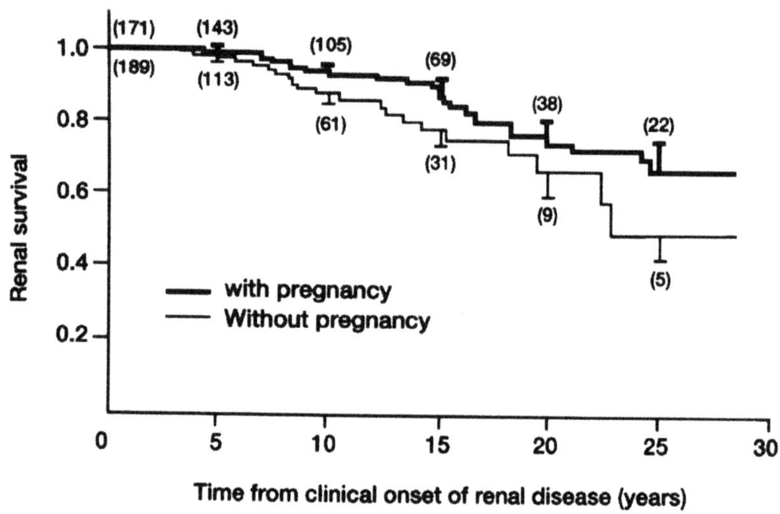

Figure 10.3 Renal survival in women with preexisting renal disease who were pregnant at least once (heavy line) compared with those who never conceived. The long-term renal prognosis was similar in the two groups. (From reference 17, with permission)

The presence of moderately or severely decreased renal function

Some investigators have noted that when serum creatinine exceeds 1.4 mg/dl (125 μmol/L) there is a decrease in fertility. However, these women can and do become pregnant. Through early 1996 there were few reports, all of limited size, concerning pregnancy in patients with moderate or severe renal impairment [1, 18–21]. More recently, Jones and Hayslett assessed maternal and fetal outcomes in 62 women who had 82 pregnancies [22]. All had serum creatinine levels exceeding 1.4 mg/dl (125 μmol/L). The levels rose significantly between the first and third trimester, while the incidence of hypertension increased from 28% at baseline to 48% by the third trimester, and that of high-grade proteinuria (urinary protein excretion above 3000 mg/L), from 23% to 41%. Forty-three percent of the pregnancies were associated with a deterioration in renal function, at times rapid and substantial, and in 10% of these instances the deterioration did not reverse postpartum. Although the infant survival rate was high (93%), rates of premature delivery (59%) and growth retardation (37%) underscored the high potential for obstetric complications in these patients.

The results of Jones and Hayslett confirm the previous reports, of limited size, in which one-third to one-half of gravidas with moderate to severe renal insufficiency experienced functional loss more rapid than would have been expected from the natural course of their renal disease [18, 19, 21, 22]; also, good blood pressure control did not guarantee the preservation of maternal renal function. Finally, there are no reliable criteria, except from Jungers' data, allowing prediction of which women will experience this rapid loss of renal function, and terminating the pregnancy does not necessarily reverse the decline.

A more recent view by Jungers *et al.* [23] is more optimistic. They note that, with recent progress in obstetric and neonatal care, more women with impaired renal function will contemplate pregnancy and can anticipate a good obstetric outcome. They suggest that this view holds as long as serum creatinine is <2.3 mg/dl (200 μmol/L). They further note, however, that once creatinine levels exceed 2.8 mg/dl (250 μmol/L) there is a substantial risk of both an unsuccessful fetal outcome and accelerated loss of maternal renal function. We find these values too high, and recommend the guidelines suggested in Table 10.3, which are closer to the experience of Jones and Hayslett [22].

The need for prospective data

Although our overview suggests that the majority of women with renal disorders, especially those with mild dysfunction, do well, we must inject some caution; most of these views reflect a literature that is primarily retrospective, and to a certain degree selective. In essence, confirmation of our guidelines requires large multicentre prospective trials of an observational nature.

Pregnancy in women with secondary glomerulonephritis

Pregnancy and the kidney in systemic disorders

Systemic lupus erythematosus (SLE)

This disease occurs most often in women of child-bearing age, and its prognosis in pregnancy is more complex than that of women with primary glomerular disorders [1, 24–26]. The outcome is poorest when the disease is active at conception, or has flared in the 6 months preceding pregnancy. Even those who conceive after 6 months of disease quiescence have a 30% chance of experiencing a 'flare', which may only reflect the natural history of SLE in non-pregnant subjects [1, 25, 26]. Women with SLE have an increased incidence of spontaneous abortion, associated at times with placental vasculopathy, and their prognosis is also poorer if the lupus anticoagulant and/or anti-phospholipid antibody is present. Women with these circulating factors are at risk for thrombotic episodes, and rarely a rapidly progressive form of renal failure [1]. The fetus is at risk of developing congenital heart block, and the newborn at risk for a 'neonatal lupus syndrome' as described elsewhere [25, 26]. Still, when renal function is preserved and hypertension absent or well controlled, 85–90% of the fetuses survive (excluding first trimester losses), and there is little evidence that gestation adversely affects the long-term prognosis of the disease.

Lupus 'flares' are treated in a manner similar to the approach used in non-pregnant patients, and pulse steroids should not be withheld in gestation. However, azathioprine, rather than cyclophosphamide, is the chemo-therapeutic drug of choice during pregnancy. If the latter drug must be used in the initial trimester some recommend therapeutic abortion, while use of cyclophosphamide later in gestation may be associated with bone marrow suppression and raises concerns about childhood malignancies [27].

Other connective tissue disorders

Experience with other forms of vasculitis, including scleroderma, polyarteritis nodosa and Wegener's granulomatosis, is sparse and the literature appears to be quite selective and anecdotal [1, 26]. The older literature concerning women with renal involvement due to scleroderma and polyarteritis nodosa was quite dismal. There were instances of maternal death secondary to malignant hypertension, and fetal survival was poor. More recently there have been reports of scleroderma successfully managed with angiotensin-converting enzyme inhibitors, but since these drugs are essentially contraindicated in gestation (as they cause fetopathy and neonatal renal failure), we counsel against conception in this disorder and suggest termination when it is present in the first trimester. Patients with primary systemic vasculitis can be main-tained in remission on prednisolone and azathioprine, and successful preg-nancy on these agents is possible.

Diabetic nephropathy

Diabetic nephropathy is the most common chronic renal disorder encountered in pregnant women [1]. Maternal hyperglycaemia, and the resulting fetal hyperinsulinaemia, have been suggested to contribute significantly to the development of fetal complications [28]. According to the literature [29–31], however, patients with well-preserved renal function usually experience live births (up to 95%) and maternal long-term renal prognosis does not appear to be adversely influenced by pregnancy, despite nephrotic range proteinuria and hypertension complicating 71% and 61% of these pregnancies respectively [29].

The increases in proteinuria and blood pressure often occur in the third trimester and may be difficult to distinguish from superimposed pre-eclampsia [1]. This often leads to early delivery and thus a high incidence of prematurity. Neonatal complications include respiratory distress syndrome (RDS) (19%), hyperbilirubinaemia (26%) and congenital malformations (10%) [29]. The rate of RDS is particularly high, around 50%, in diabetic women with impaired renal function [31]. Hou described nine of 14 pregnancies in women with diabetic nephropathy, whose serum creatinine was 1.4 mg/dl or more, as being associated with an acceleration in the rate of renal functional loss [27].

Reflux nephropathy

While reflux nephropathy is often considered a disorder primarily associated with urinary infections and pathological changes within the interstitium, it frequently leads to focal glomerular sclerosis followed by progressive renal failure. The disorder begins in childhood and thus affects substantial numbers of women of reproductive age. One should always consider a diagnosis of reflux nephropathy in gravidas manifesting relapsing and resistant urinary tract infections, especially if accompanied by unexplained hypertension. Some researchers stress that pregnancy adversely influences the course of the disease, but careful review of their data reveals that such pessimism is primarily restricted to patients with reflux nephropathy who already have hypertension and moderate or severe renal dysfunction prior to conception [1]. The largest series, 335 patients, is that of Jungers and colleagues [32], who noted successful pregnancies in 92% of the women presenting with preserved or only modestly compromised renal function. Finally, because of the nature of this disorder, such patients should be screened frequently throughout gestation for urinary tract infection which, when detected, should be treated aggressively.

Detection and management of renal disease in pregnancy

Renal biopsy

This procedure was once considered contraindicated during pregnancy, perhaps because it was widely practised on women with hypertensive complications, many of whom manifested coagulation abnormalities, and thus serious bleeding episodes were recorded. We now know that in the hands of experienced practitioners, using sonography to locate the kidney, the complication rate is similar to that in non-pregnant subjects [33–35].

Though some authors [34] stress liberal use of the renal biopsy procedure in the investigation of renal disease in pregnancy, including asymptomatic haematuria and proteinuria, we find few indications for its use, as most disorders can be managed by surveying renal function and blood pressure.

Thus, we recommend the following guidelines. Biopsy should be considered in face of a sudden deterioration of function with no apparent cause. This is because certain forms of rapidly progressive glomerulonephritis may respond to aggressive treatment with high-dose steroids and chemotherapy when diagnosed early. There are rarely 'surprises' such as the discovery of renal sarcoidosis, another disorder where progressive renal failure may be reversed by steroids [1]. Second, biopsy is helpful in face of symptomatic nephrotic syndrome (or when the biochemical abnormalities such as hypoalbuminaemia and hypercholesterolaemia are extreme), if the nephrosis is present prior to gestational week 32. Although some might undertake a 'blind' therapeutic trial of steroids in such patients, we prefer to determine if a treatable lesion is present, and thus avoid the complications associated with corticosteroid treatment during pregnancy, including hyperglycaemia, propensity to infection, poor wound healing, and the possibility, albeit small, of fetal anomalies. Nephrotic range proteinuria, alone, in an otherwise asymptomatic patient, is not an indication for biopsy, and the procedure can be deferred until after pregnancy. Similarly, biopsies are postponed to the postpartum period in gravidas manifesting asymptomatic haematuria (though such patients should be examined with ultrasonographic techniques for evidence of stones or tumour). Finally, renal biopsies should not be performed after gestational week 31, since at this late stage of pregnancy the decision to deliver the baby is usually made independent of the biopsy results, and fetal survival is excellent, making even the very minimal risks of an invasive procedure unnecessary.

Dialysis

Conception is exceedingly rare in dialysis patients; and while a rate of only 0.5%/year has been noted, the actual incidence is probably higher [36, 37]. This is especially true with the increasing use of erythropoietin [1]. Hou [38] has suggested that pregnancy is 2–3 times more frequent in women receiving haemodialysis than in those receiving continuous ambulatory peritoneal dialysis (CAPD). In any event, women of child-bearing age receiving renal replacement therapy need contraceptive counselling, a fact often overlooked by the treating nephrologist.

There is a paucity of data regarding both the maternal physiological adaptation to pregnancy and the risks of these patients. In this respect a registry directed by Dr Hou [37, 39] contains information from more than 330 pregnancies. In women undergoing renal replacement therapy the trend is towards improving pregnancy outcomes, but the risk of problems is high, including uncontrollable hypertension, abdominal haemorrhage in peritoneal dialysis patients, and maternal death, as well as early pregnancy loss, fetal growth retardation, and extreme prematurity [37]. On the other hand, the number of live births has increased substantially in the 1990s. Hopefully, as registries such as that of Dr Hou accrue data, new and more optimistic clinical management guidelines will follow.

Some experts advocate use of CAPD over haemodialysis for patients with end-stage renal disease as it is more 'gentle' and fluid changes are less abrupt. This should theoretically provide a more stable environment for the fetus [40]. As yet, this has not become apparent from data in the registry compiled by Hou and colleagues [37, 41]. Whichever form of replacement therapy is employed, increases of approximately 50% in the dialysis prescription are recommended. Near term, however, due to discomfort from abdominal fullness, modifications of the peritoneal dialysis regimen should be considered, such as decreasing the exchange volume and increasing the exchange frequency [36, 37].

Tentative guidelines for dialysis patients during pregnancy are as follows: (1) maintain serum urea nitrogen below 50 mg/dl (20 mmol/L) which may require daily haemodialysis; (2) avoid hypotension which might damage the fetus; (3) strictly control hypertension; (4) avoid rapid intravascular volume fluctuations, limiting intradialysis weight gain to approximately 1 kg, while maintaining progressive weight gain as anticipated for normal gestation. This usually precludes use of 'high flux' technology; (5) calcium levels should be checked frequently, as vitamin D produced by the placenta may require alteration of the calcitriol dosage. Similarly, the changing coagulation milieu of gestation requires close attention to anticoagulation needs; (6) monitor closely for signs of preterm labour. Some recommend electronic fetal monitoring coordinated with each dialysis as early as gestational week 26, so as to aggressively tocolyse should dialysis provoke contractions.

Anaemia is invariably aggravated by pregnancy. Blood transfusion may be necessary, especially near term, but exacerbation of hypertension and circulatory overload are possible even with extra dialysis. Erythropoietin, possibly at doses 1.5–3 times higher than those used in the non-pregnant state, appear to be helpful and no particular adverse effects have as yet been reported in this group [36, 42]. There have been instances in which a lack of responsiveness to erythropoietin was the first clue suggesting pregnancy in an oligomenorrhoeic patient.

Renal transplantation

Transplantation reverses the many reproductive problems associated with severe renal failure [1, 3, 37, 43]. Approximately 2% of women of child-bearing age, with a functioning transplant, will become pregnant. Nearly one-third of the pregnancies do not go beyond the first trimester, i.e. they are spontaneously or therapeutically aborted. Of the pregnancies that continue past the first trimester, however, more than 90% result in live birth [43]. Most clinicians recommend waiting 18–24 months after renal transplantation before attempting to conceive, which allows full recovery from surgery, stabilization of graft function and maintenance level immunosuppression. Furthermore, well-maintained function at 2 years indicates a high probability of allograft survival at 5 years. Suggested guidelines are summarized in Table 10.4 [43], though the criteria are relative, pending further research in this area.

Table 10.4 Pre-pregnancy guidelines for counselling renal transplant recipients

1.	Good general health for about 2 years after transplantation
2.	Stature compatible with good obstetric outcome
3.	No or minimal proteinuria
4.	Normal blood pressure or easily managed hypertension
5.	No evidence of graft rejection
6.	No pelvicalyceal distension on a recent intravenous urogram or ultrasonography
7.	Stable renal function with serum creatinine less than 2.0 mg/dl (180 μmol/L), preferably less than 1.4 mg/dl (125 μmol/L)
8.	Maintenance level immunotherapy (prednisone: 15 mg per day or less; azathioprine: 2 mg/kg body weight per day or less; cyclosporin A: safe doses not yet clearly established but less than 5 mg/kg per day)

(Modified from reference 43)

Clinically, the key points in managing these women [43, 44] are: (1) renal function often increases in early pregnancy, but less than in normal gravidas – this is a good prognostic sign; (2) transient deterioration in late pregnancy (with or without proteinuria) occurs in some patients and in 10–15% of pregnancies the impairment is irreversible – however, this may just represent the natural history of the graft; (3) there is a complication rate of 46%, mostly of mild or moderate degree, and the probability of a live-born infant is high; (4) complications (e.g. hypertension, renal deterioration and/or rejection) occurring before 28 weeks reduce the probability of a successful obstetric outcome from 93% to approximately 70%; (5) the risk of developing hypertension, pre-eclampsia or both approaches 30%; (6) 45–60% of deliveries are preterm and intrauterine growth retardation affects 20–40% of pregnancies. The transplanted kidney, despite its location, does not usually cause dystocia and is rarely injured during vaginal delivery. Caesarean section is indicated only for obstetric reasons.

Transplant patients are monitored as high-risk obstetric cases. Renal function, blood pressure and signs of rejection and/or infection must be monitored closely and treated promptly. Serial fetal surveillance is also essential. Neonatal complications include respiratory distress syndrome, leukopenia, thrombocytopenia, adrenocortical insufficiency and various infections. Though more data are necessary regarding the intrauterine and postnatal effects of immunosuppression, maintenance levels appear to be harmless [43, 44].

The current consensus is that pregnancy does not adversely effect long-term renal prognosis [43–45]. Furthermore, repeated pregnancies apparently do not have a deleterious effect on either graft function or fetal development, so long as renal function is relatively well preserved before conception [46]. Regular, long-term gynaecological follow-up is essential as these women, like all immunosuppressed patients, have a higher risk of malignancy than the general population [43]. The risk of developing a malignancy is reportedly 14% in the initial 10 years after transplantation and 40% at 20 years, as compared to a 6% cumulative 20-year risk in age-matched subjects [47].

Guidelines for counselling and management

There are few, if any, published guidelines for counselling and managing patients with renal disease who want to be or already are pregnant at their initial clinic visit. However, in most cases we routinely begin by investigating the underlying renal disease in terms of renal function, blood pressure and clinical course (stable vs. unstable). We also attempt to ascertain whether the renal disease is primary or secondary (systemic lupus erythematosus, diabetes mellitus, etc.) in origin. Next, we explain the results of examinations and also the possible renal and obstetric complications associated with continuing pregnancy. We must consider a patient's determination to have a child, and whether she thoroughly understands the risks and difficulties entailed. Some patients, of course, reject medical advice. In such cases we must be prepared for a difficult gestation, which may include serious complications.

As discussed above, the data, mainly retrospective, indicate that primary glomerulonephritic patients with normal or mildly decreased renal function (serum creatinine ⩽1.4 mg/dl or ⩽125 μmol/L) and normal blood pressure prior to conception usually have a successful obstetric outcome, and pregnancy does not adversely affect the clinical course of the underlying renal disease [1, 3, 35]. However, we often caution against attempting pregnancy when serum creatinine exceeds 1.4 mg/dl (125 μmol/L) or poorly controlled hypertension is recognized prior to conception, even though others accept creatinine values of 1.8–2.3 mg/dl (160–200 μmol/L) [23]. Of course, there are exceptions. If a nulliparous nephritic patient with decreased renal function (with or without hypertension) presents, having already conceived, and her desire to continue the pregnancy is strong (desire for motherhood or religious objections to termination), nephrologists must be prepared to participate in managing the pregnancy. One must first ascertain that the patient understands the risks, and that her pregnancy will be managed by an obstetrician who specializes in 'high risk' obstetrics (e.g. a subspecialist in maternal–fetal medicine), and that both renal care and delivery will take place at a tertiary-care centre, preferably one with facilities for the care of very premature infants.

Patients who elect to continue pregnancy should be evaluated every 2 weeks until 32 gestational weeks and then once a week until delivery. The initial investigations should include creatinine, urea nitrogen, uric acid, electrolytes, liver enzymes, cholesterol and albumin. The complete blood count should include a platelet count, and a 24-h urine is obtained for measurement of protein and creatinine excretion. This forms a database for monitoring renal function, as well as for detecting superimposed pre-eclampsia later in gestation [5]. Renal parameters (creatinine, or its clearance, urine sediment, and protein excretion) are determined every 4–6 weeks, or more frequently if indicated.

Hypertension, including superimposed pre-eclampsia, may complicate over 20% of these high-risk gestations. The management of high blood pressure in pregnant women is beyond the scope of this contribution, and is discussed in contemporaneous obstetric texts, a chapter by us [5], and a recent review article [48].

Pregnancy in women with renal insufficiency and end-stage renal disease, although rare, is not impossible. Contraception (e.g. low-dose oestrogen-containing oral contraceptives) should be prescribed for patients who do not want to become pregnant. Though the rate of successful pregnancy in dialysis patients has improved, intensive dialysis is required and some serious risks are involved [36]. In contrast, renal transplant recipients who want a child should not be discouraged, though careful management following the aforementioned guidelines is essential, as 93% of pregnancies which continue beyond the first trimester have a successful outcome [43]. Every patient has unique circumstances, both medical and personal, and must be considered on an individual basis.

References

1. Lindheimer MD, Katz AI. The normal and diseased kidney in pregnancy. In: Schrier RG, Gottshalk CW, editors. Diseases of the Kidney, 6th edn. Boston, MA: Little, Brown; 1997:2063–97.
2. Sturgiss SN, Dunlop W, Davison JM. Renal haemodynamics and tubular function in human pregnancy. Bailliere's Clin Obstet Gynaecol 1994;8:209–34.
3. Davison JM, Baylis C. Pregnancy in patients with chronic renal disease or renal transplant. In: Jacobson HR, Striker GE, Klahr S, editors. The Principles and Practice of Nephrology, 2nd edn. St Louis, MO: Mosby; 1995:459–73.
4. Katz AI, Davison JM, Hayslett JP, Singson E, Lindheimer MD. Pregnancy in women with kidney disease. Kidney Int 1980;18:192–206.
5. Akbari A, Lindheimer MD. Management of high blood pressure during pregnancy. In: Epstein M, editor. Calcium Antagonists and the Kidney, 2nd edn. Philadelphia, PA: Hanley and Belfus Inc; 1998:321–44.
6. Surian M, Imbasciati E, Cosci P *et al.* Glomerular disease and pregnancy. A study of 123 pregnancies in patients with primary and secondary glomerular diseases. Nephron 1984;36: 101–5.
7. Abe S, Amagasaki Y, Konishi K, Kato E, Sakaguchi H, Iyori S. The influence of antecedent renal disease on pregnancy. Am J Obstet Gynecol 1985;153:508–14.
8. Barcelo P, Lopez-Lillo J, Cabero L, Del Rio G. Successful pregnancy in primary glomerular disease. Kidney Int 1986;30: 914–19.
9. Jungers P, Forget D, Henry-Amar M *et al.* Chronic kidney disease and pregnancy. Adv Nephrol 1986;15:103–41.
10. Kincaid-Smith P, Fairley KF. Renal disease in pregnancy. Three controversial areas: mesangial IgA nephropathy, focal glomerular sclerosis (focal and segmental hyalinosis and sclerosis), and reflux nephropathy. Am J Kidney Dis 1987;9:328–33.
11. Packham DK, North RA, Fairley KF, Kloss M, Whitworth JA, Kincaid-Smith P. Primary glomerulonephritis and pregnancy. Q J Med 1989;71:537–53.
12. Imbasciati E, Ponticelli C. Pregnancy and renal disease: predictors for fetal and maternal outcome. Am J Nephrol 1991;11:353–62.

13. Packham DK, North RA, Fairley KF, Ihle BU, Whitworth JA, Kincaid-Smith P. Pregnancy in women with primary focal and segmental hyalinosis and sclerosis. Clin Nephrol 1988;29:185–92.
14. Abe S. Pregnancy in IgA nephropathy. Kidney Int 1991;40:1098–102.
15. Abe S. The influence of pregnancy on the long-term renal prognosis of IgA nephropathy. Clin Nephrol 1994;41:61–4.
16. Chauveau D, Droz D. Follow-up evaluation of the first patients with IgA nephropathy described at Necker Hospital. In: Bene MC, Faure GC, Kessler M, editors. Contributions to Nephrology Vol. 104. IgA Nephropathy: The 25th Year. Basel: Karger; 1993:1–5.
17. Jungers P, Houillier P, Forget D *et al.* Influence of pregnancy on the course of primary chronic glomerulonephritis. Lancet 1995;346:1122–4.
18. Hou SH, Grossman SD, Madias NE. Pregnancy in women with renal disease and moderate renal insufficiency. Am J Med 1985;78:185–94.
19. Imbasciati E, Pardi G, Capetta P *et al.* Pregnancy in women with chronic renal failure. Am J Nephrol 1986;6:193–8.
20. Cunningham FG, Cox SM, Harstad TW, Mason RA, Prichard JA. Chronic renal disease and pregnancy outcome. Am J Obstet Gynecol 1990;163:453–9.
21. Abe S. Pregnancy in glomerulonephritic patients with decreased renal function. Hypertens Preg 1996;15:305–12.
22. Jones DC, Hayslett JP. Outcome of pregnancy in women with moderate or severe renal insufficiency. N Engl J Med 1996;335:226–32.
23. Jungers P, Chauveau D, Choukroun G *et al.* Pregnancy in women with impaired renal function. Clin Nephrol 1997;47:281–8.
24. Hayslett JP. Maternal and fetal complications in pregnant women with systemic lupus erythematosus. Am J Kidney Dis 1991;17:123–6.
25. Hayslett JP. The effect of systemic lupus erythematosus on pregnancy and pregnancy outcome. Am J Reprod Immunol 1992;28:199–204.
26. Lockshin MD, Druzin ML. Rheumatic disease. In: Barron WM, Lindheimer MD, editors. Medical Disorders During Pregnancy, 2nd edn. St Louis, MO: Mosby; 1995:307–37.
27. Hou S. The kidney in pregnancy. In: Greenberg A, editor. Primer on Kidney Diseases. San Diego, CA: Academic Press; 1994:237–42.
28. Hayslett JP, Reece EA. Managing diabetic patients with nephropathy and other vascular complications. Bailliere's Clin Obstet Gynaecol 1994;8:405–24.
29. Reece EA, Coustan DR, Hayslett JP *et al.* Diabetic nephropathy: Pregnancy performance and fetomaternal outcome. Am J Obstet Gynecol 1988;159:56–66.
30. Grenfell A, Brudenell JM, Doddridge MC, Watkins PJ. Pregnancy in diabetic women who have proteinuria. Q J Med 1986;59:379–86.
31. Kimmerle R, Zass RP, Cupisti S *et al.* Pregnancies in women with diabetic nephropathy: long-term outcome for mother and child. Diabetologia 1995;38:227–35.
32. Jungers P, Houillier P, Chauveau D *et al.* Pregnancy in women with reflux nephropathy. Kidney Int 1996;50:593–9.
33. Lindheimer MD, Davison JM. Renal biopsy during pregnancy: 'To b . . . or not to b . . .?' Br J Obstet Gynaecol 1987;94:932–4.
34. Packham D, Fairley KF. Renal biopsy: indications and complications in pregnancy. Br J Obstet Gynaecol 1987;94:935–9.
35. Lindheimer MD, Katz AI. Gestation in women with kidney disease: prognosis and management. Bailliere's Clin Obstet Gynaecol 1994;8:387–404.
36. Hou SH. Pregnancy in women on haemodialysis and peritoneal dialysis. Bailliere's Clin Obstet Gynaecol 1994;8:481–500.
37. Hou S. Fertility and pregnancy in end stage disease. In: Brady HR, Wilcox CS, editors. Therapy in Nephrology and Hypertension: A Companion to Brenner and Rector's The Kidney. Philadelphia, PA;WB Saunders; 1998:358–62.
38. Hou SH. Pregnancy in women treated with peritoneal dialysis: viewpoint. Peritoneal Dial Int 1996;16:442–3.

39. Hou SH. Frequency and outcome of pregnancy in women on dialysis. Am J Kidney Dis 1994; 23:60–3.
40. Redrow M, Cherem L, Elliott J *et al.* Dialysis in the management of pregnant patients with renal insufficiency. Medicine 1988;67:199–208.
41. Hou S. Pregnancy in women treated with dialysis. Saudi J Kidney Dis Transplant 1997;8:3–7.
42. McGregor E, Stewart G, Junor BJR, Rodger RSC. Successful use of recombinant human erythropoietin in pregnancy. Nephrol Dial Transplant 1991;6:292–3.
43. Davison JD. Pregnancy in renal allograft recipients: problems, prognosis and practicalities. Bailliere's Clin Obstet Gynaecol 1994;8:501–25.
44. Davison JM. Towards long-term graft survival in renal transplantation: pregnancy. Nephrol Dial Transplant 1995;10(Suppl.1):85–9.
45. Sturgiss SN, Davison JM. Effect of pregnancy on the long-term function of renal allografts: an update. Am J Kidney Dis 1995;26:54–6.
46. Ehrich JHH, Loirat C, Davison JM *et al.* Repeated successful pregnancies after kidney transplantation in 102 women (Report by the EDTA registry). Nephrol Dial Transplant 1996; 111:314–17.
47. London NJ, Farmery SM, Will EJ, Davison AM, Lodge JPA. Risk of neoplasia in renal transplant patients. Lancet 1995;346:403–6.
48. Sibai BM. Drug therapy: treatment of hypertension in pregnant women. N Engl J Med 1996; 335:257–65.

Index

Note: Since the main subject of this book is glomerulonephritis, entries have been kept to a minimum under this keyword and readers are advised to seek more specific entries.

C.D. Pusey (ed.), The Treatment of Glomerulonephritis, 219–227.

Developments in Nephrology

1. J.S. Cheigh, K.H. Stenzel and A.L. Rubin (eds.): *Manual of Clinical Nephrology of the Rogosin Kidney Center.* 1981 ISBN 90-247-2397-3
2. K.D. Nolph (ed.): *Peritoneal Dialysis.* 1981 ed.: out of print
   3rd revised and enlarged ed. 1988 (not in this series) ISBN 0-89838-406-0
3. A.B. Gruskin and M.E. Norman (eds.): *Pediatric Nephrology.* 1981 ISBN 90-247-2514-3
4. O. Schück: *Examination of the Kidney Function.* 1981 ISBN 0-89838-565-2
5. J. Strauss (ed.): *Hypertension, Fluid-electrolytes and Tubulopathies in Pediatric Nephrology.* 1982 ISBN 90-247-2633-6
6. J. Strauss (ed.): *Neonatal Kidney and Fluid-electrolytes.* 1983 ISBN 0-89838-575-X
7. J. Strauss (ed.): *Acute Renal Disorders and Renal Emergencies.* 1984 ISBN 0-89838-663-2
8. L.J.A. Didio and P.M. Motta (eds.): *Basic, Clinical, and Surgical Nephrology.* 1985 ISBN 0-89838-698-5
9. E.A. Friedman and C.M. Peterson (eds.): *Diabetic Nephropathy.* Strategy for Therapy. 1985 ISBN 0-89838-735-3
10. R. Dzúrik, B. Lichardus and W. Guder: *Kidney Metabolism and Function.* 1985 ISBN 0-89838-749-3
11. J. Strauss (ed.): *Homeostasis, Nephrotoxicy, and Renal Anomalies in the Newborn.* 1986 ISBN 0-89838-766-3
12. D.G. Oreopoulos (ed.): *Geriatric Nephrology.* 1986 ISBN 0-89838-781-7
13. E.P. Paganini (ed.): *Acute Continuous Renal Replacement Therapy.* 1986 ISBN 0-89838-793-0
14. J.S. Cheigh, K.H. Stenzel and A.L. Rubin (eds.): *Hypertension in Kidney Disease.* 1986 ISBN 0-89838-797-3
15. N. Deane, R.J. Wineman and G.A. Benis (eds.): *Guide to Reprocessing of Hemodialyzers.* 1986 ISBN 0-89838-798-1
16. C. Ponticelli, L. Minetti and G. D'Amico (eds.): *Antiglobulins, Cryoglobulins and Glomerulonephritis.* 1986 ISBN 0-89838-810-4
17. J. Strauss (ed.) with the assistence of L. Strauss: *Persistent Renalgenitourinary Disorders.* 1987 ISBN 0-89838-845-7
18. V.E. Andreucci and A. Dal Canton (eds.): *Diuretics.* Basic, Pharmacological, and Clinical Aspects. 1987 ISBN 0-89838-885-6
19. P.H. Bach and E.H. Lock (eds.): *Nephrotoxicity in the Experimental and Clinical Situation,* Part 1. 1987 ISBN 0-89838-997-1
20. P.H. Bach and E.H. Lock (eds.): *Nephrotoxicity in the Experimental and Clinical Situation,* Part 2. 1987 ISBN 0-89838-980-2
21. S.M. Gore and B.A. Bradley (eds.): *Renal Transplantation.* Sense and Sensitization. 1988 ISBN 0-89838-370-6
22. L. Minetti, G. D'Amico and C. Ponticelli: *The Kidney in Plasma Cell Dyscrasias.* 1988 ISBN 0-89838-385-4
23. A.S. Lindblad, J.W. Novak and K.D. Nolph (eds.): *Continuous Ambulatory Peritoneal Dialysis in the USA.* Final Report of the National CAPD Registry 1981–1988. 1989 ISBN 0-7923-0179-X

Developments in Nephrology

24. V.E. Andreucci and A. Dal Canton (eds.): *Current Therapy in Nephrology.* 1989 ISBN 0-7923-0206-0
25. L. Kovács and B. Lichardus: *Vasopressin.* Disturbed Secretion and its Effects. 1989 ISBN 0-7923-0249-4
26. M.E. de Broe and J.W. Coburn (eds.): *Aluminum and Renal Failure.* 1990 ISBN 0-7923-0347-4
27. K.D. Gardner Jr. and J. Bernstein (eds.): *The Cystic Kidney.* 1990 ISBN 0-7923-0392-X
28. M.E. de Broe and G.A. Verpooten (eds.): *Prevention in Nephrology.* 1991 ISBN 0-7923-0951-0
29. T.A. Depner (ed.): *Prescribing Hemodialysis.* A Guide to Urea Modeling. 1991 ISBN 0-7923-0833-6
30. V.E. Andreucci and A. Dal Canton (eds.): *New Therapeutic Strategies in Nephrology.* Proceedings of the 3rd International Meeting on Current Therapy in Nephropology (Sorrento, Italy, 1990). 1991 ISBN 0-7923-1199-X
31. A. Amerio, P. Coratelli and S.G. Massry (eds.): *Turbulo-Interstitial Nephropathies.* Proceedings of the 4th Bari Seminar in Nephrology (April 1990). 1991 ISBN 0-7923-1200-7
32. M.G. McGeown (ed.): *Clinical Management of Renal Transplantation.* 1992 ISBN 0-7923-1604-5
33. C.M. Kjellstrand and J.B. Dossetor (eds.): *Ethical Problems in Dialysis and Transplantation.* 1992 ISBN 0-7923-1625-8
34. D.G. Oreopoulos, M.F. Michelis and S. Herschorn (eds.): *Nephrology and Urology in the Aged Patient.* 1993 ISBN 0-7923-2019-0
35. E.A. Friedman (ed.): *Death on Hemodialysis: Preventable or Inevitable?* 1994 ISBN 0-7923-2652-0
36. L.W. Henderson and R.S. Thuma (eds.): *Quality Assurance in Dialysis.* 1994 ISBN 0-7923-2723-3
37. J.G. Abuelo (ed.): *Renal Failure: Diagnosis and Treatment.* 1995 ISBN 0-7923-3438-8
38. J. Talati, R.A.L. Sutton, F. Moazom and M. Ahmed (eds.): *The Management of Lithiasis.* The Rational Deployment of Technology. 1997 ISBN 0-7923-4198-8
39. L.W. Henderson and R. S. Thuma (eds): *Quality Assurance in Dialysis, 2nd edition.* 1998 ISBN 0-7923-5281-5
40. C.D. Pusey (ed.): *The Treatment of Glomerulonephritis.* 1998 ISBN 0-7923-5332-3

Kluwer Academic Publishers – Dordrecht / Boston / London

GPSR Compliance
The European Union's (EU) General Product Safety Regulation (GPSR) is a set of rules that requires consumer products to be safe and our obligations to ensure this.

If you have any concerns about our products, you can contact us on

ProductSafety@springernature.com

In case Publisher is established outside the EU, the EU authorized representative is:

Springer Nature Customer Service Center GmbH
Europaplatz 3
69115 Heidelberg, Germany

www.ingramcontent.com/pod-product-compliance
Lightning Source LLC
Chambersburg PA
CBHW060745150926
51501CB00003B/100
9780792353324